Lecture Notes in Computer Science 8423

Commenced Publication in 1973
Founding and Former Series Editors:
Gerhard Goos, Juris Hartmanis, and Jan van Leeuwen

Yanchun Zhang   Guiqing Yao
Jing He   Lei Wang   Neil R. Smalheiser
Xiaoxia Yin (Eds.)

Health Information Science

Third International Conference, HIS 2014
Shenzhen, China, April 22-23, 2014
Proceedings

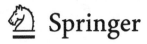 Springer

Volume Editors

Yanchun Zhang
Jing He
Xiaoxia Yin
Victoria University
Melbourne, VIC, Australia
E-mail: {yanchun.zhang, jing.he, xiaoxia.yin}@vu.edu.au

Guiqing Yao
Southampton University, UK
E-mail: g.yao@soton.ac.uk

Lei Wang
Shenzhen Institute of Advanced Technology
Shenzhen, China
E-mail: wang.lei@siat.ac.cn

Neil R. Smalheiser
University of Illinois at Chicago, USA
E-mail: nsmalheiser@psych.uic.edu

ISSN 0302-9743   e-ISSN 1611-3349
ISBN 978-3-319-06268-6   e-ISBN 978-3-319-06269-3
DOI 10.1007/978-3-319-06269-3
Springer Cham Heidelberg New York Dordrecht London

Library of Congress Control Number: Applied for

LNCS Sublibrary: SL 3 – Information Systems and Application,
incl. Internet/Web and HCI

Typesetting: Camera-ready by author, data conversion by Scientific Publishing Services, Chennai, India

Printed on acid-free paper

Springer is part of Springer Science+Business Media (www.springer.com)

Preface

The International Conference Series on Health Information Science (HIS) provides a forum for disseminating and exchanging multidisciplinary research results in computer science/information technology and health science and services. It covers all aspects of health information sciences and systems that support health information management and health service delivery.

The Third International Conference on Health Information Science (HIS 2014) was held in Shenzhen, China, during April 22-23, 2014. Founded in April 2012 as the International Conference on Health Information Science and their Applications, the conference continues to grow to include an ever broader scope of activities. The main goal of these events is to provide an international scientific forum for the exchange of new ideas in a number of fields that intersect with discussions between peers from around the world. The scope of the conference includes: (1) medical/health/biomedicine information resources, such as patient medical records, devices and equipment, software and tools to capture, store, retrieve, process, analyze, and optimize the use of information in the health domain; (2) data management, data mining, and knowledge discovery, all of which play a key role in decision making, management of public health, examination of standards, privacy, and security issues; (3) computer visualization and artificial intelligence for computer-aided diagnosis; and (4) development of new architectures and applications for health information systems.

The conference solicited and gathered technical research submissions related to all aspects of the conference scope. All the papers in the proceeding were peer reviewed by reviewers drawn from the Program Committee. After the rigorous peer-review process, the submitted papers were selected on the basis of originality, significance, and clarity for the purpose of the conference. A total of 29 full-paper submissions were accepted for presentation at the conference. The authors were from six countries, and some will be invited to submit extended versions of their papers to a special issue of the *Health Information Science and System* journal, published by BioMed Central (Springer) and the *World Wide Web* journal.

The high quality of the program—guaranteed by the presence of an unparalleled number of internationally recognized top experts—can be assessed when reading the contents of the program. The conference was therefore a unique event, where attendees were able to appreciate the latest results in their field of expertise, and to acquire additional knowledge in other fields. The program was structured to favor interactions among attendees coming from many diverse areas, scientifically, geographically, from academia, and from industry.

The conference program is further highlighted by four keynote talks. We would like to sincerely thank our keynote speakers: Nobel Laureate Professor Robert Grubbs, California Institute of Technology, USA; Professor Lei Xing,

Stanford University School of Medicine, USA Professor Kendall Ho, The University of British Columbia, Canada, and Professor Yanchun Zhang, Victoria University, Australia.

Our special thanks go to the host organizations: Shenzhen Institutes of Advanced Technology, Chinese Academy of Science; Shenzhen Key Laboratory for Low-cost Healthcare; the University of Chinese Academy of Science (China); the UCAS-VU Joint Lab for Social Computing and E-Health Research; and Victoria University (Australia).

Finally, we acknowledge all those who contributed to the success of HIS 2014 but whose names cannot be listed here.

April 2014

Yanchun Zhang
Guiqing Yao
Jing He
Lei Wang
Neil R. Smalheiser
Xiaoxia Yin

Organization

General Co-chairs

Hairong Zheng   Shenzhen Institutes of Advanced Technology,
     Chinese Academy of Sciences, China
Leonard Goldschmidt   Stanford University, USA
Yanchun Zhang   Victoria University, Australia and University of
     Chinese Academy of Science, China

Program Co-chairs

Jing He   Victoria University, Australia
Neil R. Smalheiser   University of Illinois at Chicago, USA
Lei Wang   Shenzhen Institutes of Advanced Technology,
     Chinese Academy of Sciences, China
Lily Yao   Brunel University, UK

Industry Program Chair

Michael Steyn   Royal Brisbane and Women's Hospital,
     Australia

Workshop Co-chairs

Fengfeng Zhou   Shenzhen Institutes of Advanced Technology,
     Chinese Academy of Sciences, China
Jie Zhao   Hebei University, China

Panel Chair

Xiaohui Liu   Brunel University, UK

Publication Chair

Xiaoxia Yin   Victoria University, Australia

Local Arrangements Chair

Ye Li   Shenzhen Institutes of Advanced Technology,
                                     Chinese Academy of Sciences, China

Publicity Co-chairs

Yunpeng Cai   Shenzhen Institutes of Advanced Technology,
                                     Chinese Academy of Sciences, China
Xiaohui Tao   University of Southern Queensland, Australia
Lodewijk Bos   International Council on Medical and
                                     Care Compunetics (ICMCC),
                                     The Netherlands

Program Committee

Brian W-H. Ng   The University of Adelaide, Australia
Bo Shen   Donghua University, China
Carlo Combi   Università degli Studi di Verona, Italy
Deqin Yan   Liaoning Normal University, Dalian, China
Du Huynh   The University of Western Australia, Australia
Gang Luo   University of Utah, USA
Yi-Ke Guo   University of Utah, USA
Hongli Dong   University of Duisburg-Essen, Germany
Ilvio Bruder   University of Rostock, Germany
Jan Chu   Flinders University, Australia
Jeffrey Kai Chi Chan   University of Melbourne, Australia
Jiming Liu   Hong Kong Baptist University, Hong Kong
Jinhai Cai   University of South Australia, Australia
Juanying Xie   Shaanxi Normal University, China
Kelvin Wong   The University of Western Australia, Australia
Klemens Bhm   Karlsruhe Institute of Technology, Germany
Lei Wang   Shenzhen Institutes of Advanced Technology,
                                     China
Matjaz Gams   Jozef Stefan Institute, Slovenia
Mathias Baumert   The University of Adelaide, Australia
Nigel Martin   University of London, UK
Qixin Wang   The Hong Kong Polytechnic University,
                                     Hong Kong
Ren Ran   Dalian Medical University, China
Sally McClean   Ulster University, UK
Shengxiang Yang   De Montfort University, UK
Sillas Hadjiloucas   University of Reading, UK
Song Chen   University of Maryland, Baltimore County,
                                     USA

Weiqing Sun	University of Toledo, USA
Uyen T.V. Nguyen	The University of Melbourne, Australia
Xi Liang	IBM Research
Xiao He	Tsinghua University, China
Xiuzhen (Jenny) Zhang	Royal Melbourne Institute of Technology (RMIT), Australia
Zhisheng Huang	Vrije University of Amsterdam, The Netherlands
Zhiyuan Luo	University of London, UK
Zidong Wang	Brunel University, UK
Zili Zhang	Deakin University, Australia
Wenjing Jia	University of Technology, Sydney, Australia
Xuan-Hong Dang	The University of California at Santa Barbara, USA

Sponsoring Institutions

Shenzhen Institutes of Advanced Technology, Chinese Academy of Science
Shenzhen Key Laboratory for Low-cost Healthcare
The University of Chinese Academy of Science, China
UCAS-VU Joint Lab for Social Computing and E-Health Research
Victoria University, Australia

Table of Contents

"Machine Beauty" – Should It Inspire eHealth Designers?

Marjo Rissanen

Aalto University School of Science, Finland
mkrissan@gmail.com

Abstract. Features embedded in the scheme of "machine beauty" are worth consideration in the eHealth area. Ideas of minimalism and elegance of design are some key elements of this scheme. One purpose of minimalist design is to increase the understandability of products, which is particularly applicable in the eHealth area. Striving for minimalism in the eHealth area means reasonable choices in production policy and understanding the meaning of quick impressions. Minimalism and aesthetic values in design are considered in this study in relation to different qualities. When the meaning of intended minimalist operations are assessed in the way how they interrelate with quality requirements, the meaning of intended minimalist operations can be better assessed. This article considers this theme from the viewpoints of eHealth design and quality with design science approach.

Keywords: eHealth, machine beauty, minimalism.

1   Introduction

The theme and idea of "machine beauty" [1] have gained some attention in information technology (IT) design [e.g., 2] and in the eHealth area. Machine beauty refers to aspects of "elegance and simplicity in interfaces" [3]. This theme is essential "as our environment becomes rapidly shaped by digital, networked, multifunctional artefacts" [4]. However, aesthetics are also a neglected dimension of research in the area of IT [5], and could be more emphasized in the eHealth area. Minimalism is one key concept in clarifying the essence and ideas of machine beauty. Machine beauty successfully embodied and actualized in designed products may enhance user acceptance, ICT adoption, and dissemination of applications. The main user groups in the eHealth area are health professionals and service consumers, and the appearance and elegance of products are meaningful for both user groups.

In eHealth, it is important that every screen or item in a product has such clarity that one is able to gather, analyze, and evaluate information with flexibility or receive appropriate process support without much extra concentration and time. In this design challenge, understanding the meaning of minimalism can give added value. Aspects of minimalism and elegance of design can be approached from the different viewpoints of a design process or issues in user interface design (e.g., visual, communication, interaction, content design, and from ideological views). This article focuses in particular on the meaning of minimalism in aesthetic design as one of the key tenets

Y. Zhang et al. (Eds.): HIS 2014, LNCS 8423, pp. 1–11, 2014.
© Springer International Publishing Switzerland 2014

of machine beauty. It also focuses on ideas of minimalism, their relation to quality issues, and integration questions in a design process in the eHealth area. This article addresses the following research questions.

- What is meant by machine beauty and what key issues in this theme could be useful in the eHealth area?
- How does this theme interrelate with different views of quality in eHealth?
- How key ideas of machine beauty, such as minimalism, could be utilized in eHealth design area, and what kinds of practical suggestions can be given at a general level?

This study is structured around a literature review and explorative analysis, and connects to design science and the creative foundations that regulate artifact design. Requirements of aesthetic design are considered also from the view of quality facets. Conclusions are connected to findings from the literature and from experiences gathered in a connected case study. Through these sources, gathered experience and materials have produced a set of practical ideas about how to approach the issue of minimalism in the eHealth design area.

2   Minimalism as a Core Area in the Machine Beauty Theme

The concept of machine beauty was created by David Gelernter [1] and is often expressed as "the union of power and simplicity in innovation." With this theme, Gelernter means "the essence of style in information systems design" or a combination "between simplicity and power that drives innovations." According to Nielsen [6], less is more, which means that "every single element in a user interface places some additional burden on the user in terms of having to consider whether to use that element" and that "having fewer will often mean better usability." Therefore, "aesthetic and minimalist design dialogues should not contain information which is irrelevant or rarely needed; every extra unit in information in a dialogue competes with the relevant units of information and diminishes their relative visibility" [7]. Simplicity, minimalist design, and aesthetics are commonly associated with good design [8] and address "users' real goals, helping get on with their work, allowing them to use products productively and effectively as quickly as possible" [9]. Aesthetic design covers many aspects. However, when wielding minimalism in design, one can find some of the key features of aesthetic design, which means striving for the essence in design target and trying to help the system user attain also this essence more easily.

The system designer must be aware of the product's mission and strive to provide a product appearance that makes this mission for users as transparent and obvious as quickly as possible. Aspiration for minimalism in design means concentrating on the essence in design and eliminating unnecessary and disturbing "noise." According to Norman [10], "if a tool must do and be everything, it will become impossible to design, maintain or understand" and thus "it is easier to learn to use two simple tools than a single complex one." Reeves et al [11] refer to Grice about the aspects of clear communication: quality (trustworthiness), quantity (optimal information intensity), relevance (issues relevant to the topic), and clarity. "Style and beauty means harmony" and elegance in design is actually a "courtesy" to its users [11]. According to Santayana [12], beauty is a theory of values. Actually, all design starts from values, and minimalism and elegance are inspired from a certain value frame of design. Elegance in design means better customer attraction, but it may also affect several quality aspects; therefore, it is essential to consider it in new areas such as eHealth.

3   Integrating Ideas of Minimalism into eHealth Design

3.1   Why Does Minimalism Matter in eHealth?

One purpose of minimalism is to enhance clarity in IT applications. Clarity means more user-friendliness and hence it is of great importance. How to find "the essence of style and power that could drive innovations [1]" in eHealth area? It is necessary to find a balance between reasonable simplicity but not to threaten quality issues. Compactness and straightforwardness are worthy aspirations of design targets in complex eHealth design area. However, issues of minimalism are especially useful in complex design areas. Aesthetic and minimalist design is seen in many eHealth criteria lists as a requirement for high-quality design. Applications planned to support patients' self-management in health issues may be too time-consuming to be adopted for daily life [13], as well as applications targeted to serve health professionals [14]. Thus, aspiration for minimalism requires attention when the goal is to produce more adaptive solutions. Some newer technologies in particular require clarity and simplicity at a certain degree. Mobile solution users in eHealth place high emphasis on the simplicity of an application [15]. However, minimalism can be associated with less practical outcomes: very plain applications may be straightforward, visually pleasant, and easy to manage being however not "fitness for use" in professional sense. However, straightforwardness should not be a threat to quality issues (e.g., content design). eHealth represents an area of high knowledge and information intensity. When information filtering is necessary, it should occur with input from professionals in each specialty to secure adequate process support and high-quality customer service.

In a bona fide design, minimalism should increase the degree of professionalism and quality of the product. Carefully and thoughtfully designed minimalism does not threaten information quality or quantity—nor does it diminish a product's power to support its intended function. Minimalism and clarity in design are never all that is needed for a good, elegant design. There are many attributes that reflect aesthetic design, and they are as important and necessary as other factors. However, design that does not take demands of minimalism seriously may also discourage potential users. Minimalism can be implemented in eHealth e.g., in visual, structural, functional, and ideological levels. In eHealth design, it is useful to understand minimalism's meaning not only for aesthetic reasons but also as a concept that may enhance the quality of planned products when successfully integrated. Hence, every project should define what is an appropriate way to integrate such ideas for production policy and which minimalist operations are useful for quality.

3.2   Interrelations of Aesthetic and Minimalist Design and eHealth Quality

Well-designed minimalism can make the product's *mission* more obvious by helping consumers realize the essence and core of applications more easily. Minimalism and aesthetic values, when designed and implemented thoroughly, can give added value that affects several quality aspects. Aesthetically inspiring products with minimalist touches generally means better customer attraction and clarity and hence more *customer quality*. It provides users with the feel of a more manageable and fluent product. According to previous work, aesthetic systems yielded higher satisfaction [16] and perceived goodness of the system [17]. However, the effect on *product quality* is just as central; aesthetics do not always mean more usable [18]. However, more aesthetic systems were perceived to be more usable than were less aesthetic systems [19], and correlations between the interface aesthetics and usability are found [20, 21]. Aesthetics affect users' willingness to buy or adopt the system [5]. Attractive and inviting design may have an impact on *image quality* of products or service providers (e.g., first impressions and features such as navigability and content in a company's web site have an influence of a company's image [22]).

Aesthetics and ethics are often discussed in tandem [23]. Design that takes aesthetic aspects into account may reduce the users' threshold to using offered applications. Minimalist design can often help elder users understand products and applications by giving the impression of a less demanding product, and so achieving better accessibility and equity in utilization. In the health sector, there is evidence that "elder people with little experience with modern technology may find it difficult to identify and report anything other than a general impression such as: I think this is complicated" [24]. In this example, it is understandable that aesthetic values affect *ethical quality* of offered products and services.

Minimalism may also mean a reduction in training costs [25]. Qui and Yu [26] noticed that content structure, functionality, aesthetics, and usability could serve as recommendations for designing an effective online help system for nurses. Minimalism in design when integrated successfully means more clarity. Clarity reduces reaction time; therefore, aesthetic values are also important when trying to meet quality criteria that refer to cost/value determinants and economy improving a product's *efficiency quality*. Minimalism in design can also produce better *process quality* because the product with more embedded clarity may serve more efficiently and fluently than products without these features.

3.3   Ideas to Cultivate Minimalism in eHealth

The task to cultivate minimalism in eHealth is not necessarily as straightforward. Requirements of precision and trust may produce products with many aspects, content, and character. Many IT products try to offer a comprehensive idea of the task in question or support processes in an efficient way, and this may increase the overall complexity of the product. Many systems in the eHealth area are massive, and ideas of minimalism are hard to understand in an entity where system complexity prevails. However, the idea to produce sophisticated and attractive products should not be out of the question. As known, in minimalism the question is not about "brevity", less information or process support; the question is to offer information or process support in a way that is more understandable and pleasant when it comes to the layout and appearance of user interfaces, systems, and applications and their general functioning.

Aesthetic impressions of web pages are formed quickly [27]. In mHealth application design, of the goal is product clarity so that people can get a quick overview of their health status [e.g., 28]. It is useful to strive in eHealth for quick impressions that are positive in an aesthetic sense, but also in an informative sense. A positive *quick impression* in this context means that the user quickly gets an idea of the meaning of each screen, linking information, and the entire application and its functions and features. Giving a rapid impression means that even an informative message is quickly readable and understandable. The idea of quick impressions may therefore mean more clarity, time-savings, and hence better customer quality. When a product looks too laborious and demanding, users tend to struggle to accept it for daily use. Considered minimalism in design, however, may lighten this burden even in cases when the product must have multiple necessary aspects and details. When successfully integrated also in such cases the outcome seems understandable and straightforward. Therefore, in considered minimalism, the question is no doubt about creative design. *Avoidable aspects are so-called "indifferences"*; "indifference attributes" represent features that are rarely needed by users and do not typically result in either customer satisfaction or customer dissatisfaction [29]. A large amount of indifferences may decrease customers' willingness to use and test a novel product because it seems too demanding. *Considered minimalism should always bring more quality. Therefore, planned minimalist operations must be assessed in the context of their added quality value and with understanding the versatile requirements of quality.* The following list presents selected aspects of how to cultivate the idea of minimalism in eHealth at a general level.

- *Avoid projects that are too ambitious in the quick stage.* In the eHealth area, there are many examples of overly ambitious projects and project plans. Novel solutions often mean higher ambitions; however, too much ambition at an early stage of design may frustrate users as well as tire out designers. In the health area, projects typically last a long time. If projects start with plans that are too exhaustive, there is a danger that team members will turn over during development, which means more costs and perhaps even a risk for intended, original plans.
- *Estimate the complexity of products targeted for health consumers; avoid massive, exhaustive, or too time-consuming applications.* Massive products with multiple features are often needed when trying to reach an appropriate level of professionalism in content or in process support in health practice. However, when applications are planned for health service users, exhaustive products with too many aspects may also be discouraging. Products targeting patients' self-management may be too time-consuming for daily life [13] e.g., due to unnecessary steps or options. Because there are different functional environments, an idea is to offer not only a prime version, but also a "light" version for users who do not need all options. Evaluate whether all functions are really necessary or actually add value for the intended target group.

- *Evaluate if modularization could bring better manageability.* Patients go through different phases in their health status; therefore, products for self-health management may contain modules for prevention, curative, and recovery phases. Consider modular product entities if the manageability of a product seems laborious; many eHealth solutions are designed as modular systems for better application management. Share the modules that are easy to use independently but also easy to gather as an entity when necessary by developing product families that can be shared to make big entities smaller and more manageable when it seems reasonable.
- *Evaluate all functions properly; are they all necessary or only causing "noise?"* Carroll [30] states that all learning tasks should be meaningful. Avoid unnecessary features of "indifference" at least in the primary product phase. Indifferences with new products may disturb users' abilities to understand the message of the product. Streamline product plans as much as possible and evaluate if all intended features are really meaningful. Avoid products with diverse functions but without clear justification or a presentation style that is visually or otherwise unnecessarily complex.
- *Remember quick impressions.* Cultivate the idea of the quick impression in every display screen and in every sub-branch of the product. Allowing quick impressions provides added value for users by giving an impression of easy manageability. A positive quick impression of a product may help users understand the product's mission more easily. Quick impressions actualized in the product mean also fewer educational efforts in the implementation phase. In health care this means time savings, which is important for health professionals as well as health consumers. Rosson and Carroll [31] reiterate the importance of "allowing learners to get started quickly." Providing a positive quick impression is one step in this direction.
- *Plan operations that may guarantee maximal self-guidance and self-orientation.* Tutoring and training increase total costs, and the threshold for product adoption may increase when the product requires obvious and too intense training phases. Turner et al [32] states that tools should be usable in training situations with little or no previous instruction. The same idea applies to many products in health care.
- *Use versatile professional help in information filtering.* Most consumers are not able to filter e.g., health-related www-information [33, 34]. In the medical field, it is important to find the relevant levels of knowledge intensity: How deep and thorough of an understanding is needed for appropriate process support? Information content and its depth are critical aspects in applications targeted for eHealth.
- *Gather versatile user feedback for product maturation.* Try to test the product with users who have different skill and knowledge levels of the task in question; it is assumed there are no normal users. In the health area, this is even more important. A versatile user sample in testing or piloting gives more accurate user feedback. Carefully evaluate user feedback: What kinds of desires and ideas are sustainable, reasonable, and meaningful enough for several users and thus essential to integrate into development iterations?
- *Considered minimalism should bring more quality.* Think about added quality value and the ideas of minimalism at the same time. Evaluate planned minimalist operations in the context of their added quality value and use a quality frame versatile enough. Quality views known in quality thinking such as customer, product, process, and production views form essential evaluation areas at a macro level of

eHealth design. It should be determined if the intended operations could improve user-friendliness and user attraction, enhance functionality of products, advance intended process quality, and meet the quality requirements of production. Quality views referring to aspects of ethics, image, and efficiency are as well recognized as meaningful areas in design or in adoption policies in the eHealth area. Innovations must be in balance with ethical values as well as with the mission and values of target organizations. Such minimalist operations are out of the question if they are in contradiction with values of a multifaceted quality frame. Therefore, questions that evaluate planned minimalist operations in relation to settled evaluative questions in each quality facet help to assess the meaning and value of planned minimalist interventions (see the areas of assessment in Table 1). Self-evaluative questions help designers assess the meaning of intended minimalist operations in regard to their quality effects in different areas of quality.

4 An Example: Ideas of Minimalism in an Application Design

In the following example, ideas of minimalism are presented in an application design that concentrates on prevention of neck-and-shoulder disorders in the occupational health area [35]. The aim of the product is to intensify training, which is related to the occupational health area by supporting blended learning intervention with the aid of the application. The common purpose of the product therefore is to improve well-being at work by cultivating self-discipline techniques and strategies that help to maintain good work conditions in areas where neck-and shoulder troubles diminish these abilities.

Table 1 shows how the integrated ideas of minimalism in a product design and facets of quality interrelate. The connected quality frame in the design ideology reiterates versatile quality thinking; however, views that connect the product, customer, and efficiency quality categories are emphasized. Serviceability, flexibility, and user-friendliness underscore design targets. Minimalism in a product design is emphasized by paying special attention to clarity and straightforwardness of interface and structure design and ease in product management.

Design approach emphasizes ideas of minimalism, and these interventions are assessed through a given question pattern (Table 1). The product gives an idea of its content in its main page and hence clarifies its purpose and mission by quick impression (*mission clarity*). Because the occupational health area requires more options for instant health training, the *mission fitness*, alignment with organizational values prevails. The design ideology cultivates ideas of quick impressions. This gives better customer quality by informing the user on every page screen and helps the user understand very quickly what's going on now and next. The purpose of such minimalism is to provide an impression of clarity, understandability, and flexibility. Gained minimalism of the product is attained partially because of the selected tutoring/training ideology that is part of the product idea. Blended training interventions give flexibility because more specific information and knowledge can be handled without loading the product itself with too many details and examples. Flexible and reasonable compactness in training options are one way to enhance image issues in health training. If in this way, more accessibility, equity, and customer autonomy can be acquired this means compatibility with prevailing ethical considerations.

Table 1. Evaluation of minimalist operations in a product

Quality facet; evaluation criteria	Key ideas embodying minimalism in an application	Category emphasis
Mission: clarity & fitness	Observable mission clarity, Example of mission fitness; just-in-time training	Ideological, visual
Customer: user-friendliness, user attraction	*Quick impression* ideology underlined, Clarity with "noise" elimination, Special terminology controlled	Visual, ideological, structural
Product: functionality	Self-guidance operations, content compactness however with professional content intensity	Functional, structural ideological
Process: process support	An intense learner activation with an easy method & logic	Functional, structural, ideological
Efficiency: process efficiency	Tools for control behaviour patterns without heavy interventions	Functional, structural ideological
Production: production process	Quality assessments in minimalism integration	Ideological
Image: image promotion	Image effect with a flexible training idea	Ideological
Ethics: ethical justifications	Alignment with accessibility, equity, customer autonomy	Ideological

5   Conclusions

Aesthetic design can be a value in and of itself. However, it is important that designers understand the connection between aesthetic design and overall quality of products in the eHealth area. The theme of "machine beauty" has much to do with quality issues of design; hence, this concept cannot be associated only with a task that increases a product's aesthetic values. When designers are trying to achieve overall quality with the aid of this element, the outcomes may be more ingenious; in this way, the search for minimalism and beauty may produce even more of an advantage.

"Values have always implicitly driven the decisions of the organization" [36]; hence, all design starts from values. Minimalism and elegance are inspired by a certain value frame of design as well as an understanding about quality that arises from adopted value frames. Continuous evaluation of these frame values forms hence the essence. Also, minimalist operations in the eHealth sector should be assessed against their quality implications. This helps to estimate which kinds of operations are useful and acceptable. In eHealth, aspects of minimalist design are not necessarily straightforward tasks as design targets in this area are demanding.

Minimalism and elegance of design are some issues that describe the concept of machine beauty. It is important to realize that minimalism does not mean brevity or necessarily less information or an approach which is suitable only for simple domains [37]. There may be questions in some cases about reasonable information filtering in this area, but actual minimalist design should provide information in a more understandable and pleasant way or provide support with more ease. Therefore, a product that embodies in eHealth "minimalism and beauty" in a thoughtful way could be even more professional and sophisticated than another product without this emphasis. Such design and implementation may require more creative insights and design efforts; "more skilled developers and greater development efforts [37]". However, only well-implemented and correctly interpreted machine beauty can be a power that makes learning targets more reachable or process support more effective in eHealth. Without understanding the meaning and essence and the design requirements of connected aspects of this theme, results are not necessarily positive in eHealth. Design that takes aesthetic values into account and balances them with quality requirements translates into products that can encompass more power and innovation quality for eHealth.

References

1. Gelernter, D.: Machine Beauty: Elegance and the Heart of Technology. Basic Books, New York (1998)
2. Hevner, A., March, S., Park, J., Ram, S.: Design Science in Information Systems Research. MIS Q. 28, 75–105 (2004)
3. Auerbach, D.: Machine Beauty is in the Eye of the Beholder (1998),
   http://www.yaleherald.com/archive/xxv/2.27.98/ae/machine.html
4. Gajendar, U.: Attention, Attraction, and the Aesthetic Value: Understanding Beauty as a Problem of User Experience. Environment 2 (2003)
5. Tractinsky, N.: Toward the Study of Aesthetics in Information Technology. In: 25th International Conference on Information Systems, pp. 771–780 (2004)
6. Nielsen, J.: Usability Engineering. Elsevier (1994)
7. Nielsen, J., Mack, R.L. (eds.): Usability Inspection Methods. Wiley & Sons, New York (1994)
8. Obendorf, H.: Minimalism (Human-Computer Interaction Series). Springer, London (2009)
9. Hackos, J.: When is Minimalism the Best Course? CIDM Inform. Manage. News. Norman (April 2008)
10. Norman, D.: The Invisible Computer. The MIT Press (1998)
11. Reeves, B., Nass, C.: The Media Equation: How People Treat Computers, Television, and New Media Like Real People and Places. CSLI Publications and Cambridge University Press, Stanford (1996)
12. Santayana, G.: The Sense of Beauty: Being the Outline of Aesthetic Theory. Dover, Mineola (1955)

13. van Gemert-Pijnen, J., Nijland, N., van Limburg, M., et al.: A Holistic Framework to Improve the Uptake of eHealth Technologies. J. Med. Internet Res. 13, e111 (2011)
14. Yapne, J.: Computers and Doctor-Patient Communication. Rev. Port. Med. Geral Fam. 29, 148–149 (2013)
15. Kukec, M., Ljubic, S., Glavinic, V.: Need for Usability and Wish for Mobility: Case Study of Client End Applications for Primary Health Care Providers in Croatia. In: Glavinic, V. (ed.) Information Quality in eHealth, 7th Conference of the Workgroup Human (2011)
16. Lindgaard, G., Dudek, C.: What Is This Evasive Beast We Call User Satisfaction? Interact. Comput. 15, 429–452 (2003)
17. Hassenzahl, M.: The Interplay of Beauty, Goodness, and Usability in Interactive Products. Human-Comput. Interact. 19, 319–349 (2004)
18. Norman, D.: The Psychology of Everyday Things. Basic Books, New York (1988)
19. Tractinsky, N., Shoval-Katz, A., Ikar, D.: What Is Beautiful Is Usable. Interact. Comput. 13, 127–145 (2000)
20. Tractinsky, N.: Aesthetics and Apparent Usability: Empirically Assessing Cultural and Methodological Issues. In: Proceedings of the ACM SIGCHI Conference on Human Factors in Computing Systems, pp. 115–122. ACM (1997)
21. Kurosu, M., Kashimura, K.: Apparent Usability vs. Inherent Usability. In: CHI 1995 Conference Companion, pp. 292–293 (1995)
22. Kuzic, J., Giannatos, G., Vignjevic, T.: Web Design and Company Image. Issues Inform. Sci. Inform. Technol. 7 (2010)
23. Eaton, M.M.: Aesthetics the Mother of Ethics? J. Aesthet. Art Crit. 55, 355–364 (1997)
24. Stojmenova, E., Imperl, B., Zohar, T., Dinevski, D.: User-Centred E-Health: Engaging Users into the e-Health Design Process. In: Proceedings 25th Bled eConference eDependability: Reliable and Trustworthy eStructures, eProcesses, eOperations and eServices. Paper 38, pp. 462–473 (2012)
25. Lazonder, A., Van der Meij, H.: The Minimal Manual: Is Less Really More? Int. J. Man Mach. Studies 39, 729–752 (1993)
26. Qui, Y.: Yu. P.: Study of Characteristics of Effective Online Help Systems to Facilitate Nurses Interacting with Nursing Information Systems. In: Grain, H., Wise, M. (eds.) Health Informatics Conference, pp. 26–32. 2. Health Informatics Society of Australia, Victoria (2005)
27. Tractinsky, N., Cokhavi, A., Kirschenbaum, M., Sharfi, T.: Evaluating the Consistency of Immediate Aesthetic Perceptions of Web Pages. Int. J. Human-Comput. Studies 64, 1071–1083 (2006)
28. Lorenz, A., Oppermann, R.: Mobile Health Monitoring for the Elderly: Designing for Diversity. Pervasive Mobile Comput. 5(5), 478–495 (2009)
29. Kano, N., Seraku, N., Takahashi, F., Tsuji, S.: Attractive Quality and Must-be Quality. J. Jap. Soc. Qual. Control. 14, 39–48 (1984)
30. Carroll, J.M.: The Nurnberg Funnel. MIT Press, Cambridge (1990)
31. Rosson, M., Carroll, J.: Minimalist Design for Informal Learning in Community Computing. In: Communities and Technologies 2005, pp. 75–94. Springer, Netherlands (2005)
32. Turner, S.A., Pérez-Quiñones, M.A., Edwards, S.H.: MinimUML: A Minimalist Approach to UML Diagramming for Early Computer Science Education. J. Educ. Res. Comput. 5(4), 1 (2005)
33. Taylor, H.A., Sullivan, D., Mullen, C., Johnson, C.M.: Implementation of a User-Centered Framework in the Development of a Web-Based Health Information Database and Call Center. J. Biomed. Inform. 44, 897–908 (2011)

34. Bessell, T., McDonald, S., Silagy, C.A., Anderson, J., Hiller, J., Sansom, L.: Do Internet Interventions for Consumers Cause More Harm Than Good? A Systematic Review. Health Expect 5, 28–37 (2002)
35. Rissanen, M.: User-Centred ICT-Design for Occupational Health: A Case Description. In: Huang, G., Liu, X., He, J., Klawonn, F., Yao, G. (eds.) HIS 2013. LNCS, vol. 7798, pp. 273–276. Springer, Heidelberg (2013)
36. Sapienza, A.: Creating Technology Strategies. How to Build Competitive Biomedical R&D. Wiley-Liss, New York (1997)
37. Carroll, J., van der Meij, H.: Ten Misconceptions About Minimalism. IEEE Trans. Prof. Commun. 39, 72–86 (1996)

Mean Shift Based Feature Points Selection Algorithm of DSA Images

Fan Zhang[1,2,*], Congcong Li[2], Shan Kong[2], Shuyue Liu[2], and Yanbin Cui[2]

[1] School of Computer and Information Engineering, Henan University, Kaifeng 475001, China
[2] Institute of Image Processing and Pattern Recognition,
Henan University, Kaifeng 475001, China
zhangfan@henu.edu.cn

Abstract. In Digital Subtraction Angiography (DSA) image registration algorithm, the precision of the control points as well as their number and the distribution in image determine the accuracy of geometric correction and registration. Control points usually adopt the grid points; however, a more effective method is to extract control points adaptively according to the image feature. In this paper, a control point's selection algorithm of DSA images is proposed based on adaptive multi-Scale vascular enhancement, error diffusion and means shift algorithms. Experimental results show that the proposed algorithm can adaptively put the control points to blood vessels and other key image characteristics, and can optimize the number of control points according to practical needs, which will ensure the accuracy of DSA image registration.

Keywords: Digital subtraction angiography, Error diffusion, Mean shift.

1 Introduction

Digital Subtraction Angiography (DSA) is an X-ray imaging. DSA is the technology combined conventional angiography with computer image processing technology. In traditional angiography images are acquired by exposing an area of interest with time-controlled x-rays while injecting contrast medium into the blood vessels. The image obtained would also include all overlying structure besides the blood vessels in this area. This is useful for determining anatomical position and variations but unhelpful for visualizing blood vessels accurately.

In order to remove these distracting structures to see the vessels better, first a mask image is acquired. The mask image is simply an image of the same area before the contrast is administered. Smaller structures require less contrast to fill the vessel than others. Images produced appear with a very pale grey background, which produces a high contrast to the blood vessels, which appear a very dark grey. Tissues and blood vessels on the first image are digitally subtracted from the second image, leaving a clear picture of the artery which can then be studied independently and in isolation from the rest of the body [1,2]. However, DSA image may exist in a variety of

---

* Corresponding author.

Y. Zhang et al. (Eds.): HIS 2014, LNCS 8423, pp. 12–19, 2014.

artifacts which will affect the image quality. The motion artifact is the most common form of artifacts. Recent studies in the elimination of motion artifacts are mainly based on image registration methods. Image registration is the process of transforming different sets of data into one coordinate system. Data may be multiple photographs, data from different sensors, times, depths, or viewpoints [3,4]. Since multiple images that reflect the same or partly same characteristics, so a part of the image pixels should be represented the same point on the corresponding points in the other image.

2   Control Point Selection Based on the Error Diffusion

In DSA images, we can use the image edge, corners and other information to complete the control point extraction. Firstly, detecting image edge, and then picking out specific points according to a threshold value. This gradient threshold approach procedure is as follows:

(1) Edge detection processing for the mask image.

(2) Calculate the gradient magnitude by $\dfrac{\partial f}{\partial x} = f(x+1, y) - f(x, y)$ and

$\dfrac{\partial f}{\partial y} = f(x, y+1) - f(x, y)$, and then compared with a threshold value.

(3) Set the minimum and maximum distances between points to avoid too little or too many points.

To take advantage of image intrinsic characteristics selecting control points adaptively, the proposed feature selection algorithm introduced the error diffusion method. Error diffusion is an important half-tone image algorithm. Because of its efficient and good quality and special expression, error diffusion has been used widely in the image printing, display, as well as non-realistic rendering graphics, and other areas of computer graphics. In the image color conversion process, due to the different color range, the conversion process may introduce some error. Error diffusion algorithm can pass error to surrounding pixels and mitigate their visual error. Error diffusion algorithm is based on human visual characteristics and colorimetric properties of images. We can achieve the optimal binary image reproduction by this algorithm. Digital half-tone technology includes: Dot Diffusion, Error Diffusion, Ordered Dither and so on.

Error diffusion algorithm was proposed firstly by Floyed and Steinberg [5]. This algorithm requires neighborhood processing. Its produces rich tones image, while the distribution of pixel anisotropy. The basic idea is to scan and quantitate image pixel according to certain path with a threshold, then the quantization error is spread to adjacent unprocessed pixels in a certain way. From another angle, error diffusion algorithm can achieve optimal image reproduction because the dots in the image space are proportional to the density and the local image gray [6].

The proposed error diffusion based algorithm of feature point selection can select control point adaptively according to image intrinsic characteristics. The algorithm is designed to distribute control points in image and make the control point's space density is proportional to the local image gray. This paper placed grid points according to Floyd-Steinberg algorithm in the DSA vessel image, so we can as much as possible make the grid points distributing on the vessel, and use these grid points on blood vessels as control points.

For the input image $f(x, y)$, DSA feature point selection algorithm based on the error diffusion is described below:

(1) Beginning with the first point (i_0, j_0), processing pixels according to raster scan order.

(2) $f(i, j)$ represents the value at point (i, j) of input image. For each point (i, j), $f(i, j)$ is compared with the threshold value q to obtain the indicator function $b(i, j)$, and then to obtain the position of the control point, as shown in the Eq.1.

$$b(i, j) \triangleq \begin{cases} 1, & \text{if } f(i, j) \geq q \\ 0, & \text{otherwise.} \end{cases}, \tag{1}$$

where q is a experienced threshold value . $b(i, j) = 1$ means that there is a control point in the point (i, j).

Then at point (i, j), the quantization error $e(i, j)$ is calculated, as shown in the Eq.2.

$$e(i, j) = f(i, j) - (2q) b(i, j), \tag{2}$$

At four direct adjacent to the points of point (i, j), $(i, j + 1)$, $(i + 1, j-1)$, $(i + 1, j)$, $(i + 1, j + 1)$, we   diffuse error $e(i, j)$. The values of these adjacent points are modified. The modified method as Eq.3:

$$\begin{aligned} f(i, j+1) &\Leftarrow f(i, j+1) + w_1 e(i, j), \\ f(i+1, j-1) &\Leftarrow f(i+1, j-1) + w_2 e(i, j), \\ f(i+1, j) &\Leftarrow f(i+1, j) + w_3 e(i, j), \\ f(i+1, j+1) &\Leftarrow f(i+1, j+1) + w_4 e(i, j), \end{aligned} \tag{3}$$

Where $\Leftarrow$ represents that the value of right side in equation is assigned to the left.

(4) Repeat step 2 and 3 until all pixels in the image traversal.

(5) Extracting control point from the points which gray value is 1 in the result binary image.

In the diffusion process, in order to avoid possible omission of error diffusion occurs in the image boundary, the error diffusion pattern should be adjusted in the image border. For example, for a point on the right boundary, the weight w_1 and w_4 should be set to 0; however, the remainder weight should be adjusted so as to their sum is equal to a fixed value. Of course, if no significant features in image boundary, this adjustment can simply be ignored. For the classic Floyd-Steinberg error diffusion algorithm, to produce vivid digital halftone image, weight w_i, $i=1,\cdots,4$ are assigned respectively to 7/16, 3/16, 5/16, 1/16. For the control point setting, a more reasonable approach should adjust the value of weights w_i based on the geometric distance of adjacent points.

In the conventional raster scan order, the pixel will be processed in scan order from left to right. As an alternative, in a so-called zigzag raster scan order, the odd-numbered lines are processed in order from left to right, and the even-numbered rows from right to left. This approach is intended to enable error diffusion from left to right and right to left in the direction with a more balanced spread. Experimental results show that the zigzag raster scan order can generate slightly more accurate results.

In the proposed algorithm, the error diffusion threshold determines the number of control points. This is very important because it allows the error diffusion algorithm predetermined number of grid points, their corresponding number as follows:

$$K \approx \frac{1}{2q} \sum_{i=1}^{M} \sum_{j=1}^{N} f(i, j), \tag{4}$$

Where M, N is ranks number of image $f(i, j)$, q is a threshold.

3   Control Points Simplify Based on Mean Shift

Due to the large number of control points based on above error diffusion method, it cannot adapt to the subsequent image registration. So the proposed algorithm simplifies these control points further using mean shift algorithm.

Mean shift clustering algorithm is a technique of nonparametric kernel density estimation based on Parzen window, which is a process to find local maximum point of density function (also called pattern dot). Starting from any sample point in the data set as the initial point, mean shift procedure converges to the same pattern where pixels can be considered as belonging to the same cluster, and determine the number of clusters automatically, and then describe the clusters boundaries. This algorithm originally developed by Fukunaga et al [7], and later Yizong Cheng applied it to clustering algorithm [8]. Dorin Comaniciu *et al* proposed an adaptive mean shift algorithm based on estimated bandwidth [9], and applied it to image segmentation and clustering [10].

Given n points $X_i \in R^d$, $i=1,\cdots,n$, in d-dimensional space, multivariate kernel density estimation function in point X can be expressed as [9]:

$$\hat{f}_K(\mathbf{x}) = \frac{1}{n} \sum_{i=1}^{n} \frac{1}{h_i^d} k \left(\left\| \frac{\mathbf{x} - \mathbf{X}_i}{h_i} \right\|^2 \right) \tag{5}$$

Where the function $k(x)$ is the profile function of kernel function $K(x)$. Kernel function $K(x)$ is a defined function. It is usually a class of radial symmetry function with special kernel, as follows:

$$K(\mathbf{x}) = c_{k,d} k\left(\|\mathbf{x}\|^2\right) > 0 \quad \|\mathbf{x}\| \le 1 \tag{6}$$

Where $c_{k,d}$ is a normalization constant, to guarantee $K(x)$ integral is 1. In the Eq.5, h_i is called the bandwidth or the window size of kernel function, which determines the kernel scope of X_i. In the proposed algorithm, the clustering algorithm uses Epanechnikov kernel function, which is defined as follows:

$$K(\mathbf{x}) = \begin{cases} \frac{1}{2} c_d^{-1}(d+2)(1-\mathbf{x}^T\mathbf{x}) & \text{if } \mathbf{x}^T\mathbf{x}<1 \\ 0 & \text{otherwise} \end{cases} \tag{7}$$

Epanechnikov kernel function enables the integral mean square error minimized, while the standard deviation is probability density function and kernel density estimation based on the potential integration of data.

The gradient of multivariate kernel density estimation function in Eq.5 is expressed as:

$$
\begin{aligned}
\hat{\nabla} f_K(\mathbf{x}) \equiv \nabla \hat{f}_K(\mathbf{x}) &= \frac{2}{n} \sum_{i=1}^{n} \frac{\mathbf{x}-\mathbf{x}_i}{h_i^d} k'\left(\left\|\frac{\mathbf{x}-\mathbf{x}_i}{h_i}\right\|^2\right) \\
&= \frac{2}{n} \sum_{i=1}^{n} \frac{\mathbf{x}_i-\mathbf{x}}{h_i^{d+2}} g\left(\left\|\frac{\mathbf{x}-\mathbf{x}_i}{h_i}\right\|^2\right) \\
&= \frac{2}{n} \left[\sum_{i=1}^{n} \frac{1}{h_i^{d+2}} \left(\left\|\frac{\mathbf{x}-\mathbf{x}_i}{h_i}\right\|^2\right) \right] \times \left[\frac{\sum_{i=1}^{n} \frac{\mathbf{x}_i}{h_i^{d+2}} g\left(\left\|\frac{\mathbf{x}-\mathbf{x}_i}{h_i}\right\|^2\right)}{\sum_{i=1}^{n} \frac{1}{h_i^{d+2}} g\left(\left\|\frac{\mathbf{x}-\mathbf{x}_i}{h_i}\right\|^2\right)} - \mathbf{x} \right]
\end{aligned}
\tag{8}
$$

Where $g(x) = -k'(x)$. The last section of Eq.8 contains the mean shift vector:

$$M(\mathbf{x}) = \left[\frac{\sum_{i=1}^{n} \frac{\mathbf{x}_i}{h_i^{d+2}} g\left(\left\|\frac{\mathbf{x}-\mathbf{x}_i}{h_i}\right\|^2\right)}{\sum_{i=1}^{n} \frac{1}{h_i^{d+2}} g\left(\left\|\frac{\mathbf{x}-\mathbf{x}_i}{h_i}\right\|^2\right)} - \mathbf{x} \right] \tag{9}$$

Assumed $G(\mathbf{x}) = c_{g,d}\, g\!\left(\|\mathbf{x}\|^2\right)$, Eq.8 can be expressed as [9]:

$$M(\mathbf{x}) = C\,\frac{\hat{\nabla} f_K(\mathbf{x})}{\hat{f}_G(\mathbf{x})}, \tag{10}$$

The Eq.10 shows that mean shift vector is proportional to gradient estimation of density function based on kernel function K. So mean shift vector pointing in the direction of increasing the maximum density. This is basis of mean shift clustering algorithm.

4   Experimental Results

The image used in this experiment is a set of brain DSA images. DSA device model is GE LCV plus. DSA images are stored in multi-DICOM files, totally 25 frames. Experiments using computer with hardware configuration as Intel Xeon dual-core CPU, 3.4GHz, 8.0G RAM, 1TB hard drive and 1G graph card. Software environment is Matlab 2012a.

In the control points simplification based on mean shift, our experiment using an error diffusion threshold value of 20 for the input image point set, as shown in Figure 1. This algorithm simplified result using the control points set is shown in Figure 2, where the initial bandwidth $h_0 = 230$. The number of input control points sets is 2221, and the number of simplified control points set is 25. Observing at Figure 2 we can found that the number of control points set greatly simplified, and the points are located simplify in the vessel at the turning, dramatic changed and bifurcation positions.

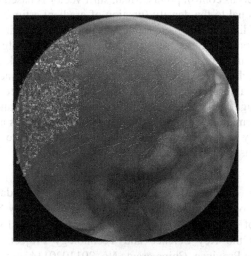

Fig. 1. Control point set of error diffusion image with threshold value 20

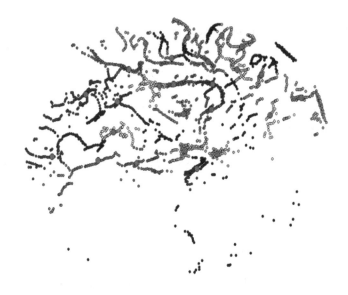

Fig. 2. Simplified control point set by mean shift

5   Conclusions

This paper proposes a DSA feature point selection algorithm based on error diffusion and mean shift. The error diffusion algorithm is introduced in order to take advantage of image intrinsic characteristics and select control point adaptively. The proposed algorithm using Floyd-Steinberg algorithm to place grid points in DSA images, so we can make as many as possible grid points distributed on the vessel, and use these grid points in blood vessels as control points. Mean shift vector is based on kernel function K, which is proportional to the density function of gradient estimation. So mean shift vector pointing the direction of increase of the maximum density. In the proposed algorithm, firstly, control points are grouped by mean-shift algorithm. Secondly, searching the nearest neighbor of each group pattern point, and taking them as simplify control point in each group. Experimental results show that the adaptive multi-scale vessel enhancement algorithm of DSA has good blood enhanced performance, can effectively filter image background and non-vascular structure, and to avoid the increase of blood deformation. This algorithm can set control points adaptively at blood vessels and other key image characteristics, and can optimize the number of control points if needed to ensure the accuracy of DSA image registration.

Acknowledgements. This research was supported by the Foundation of Education Bureau of Henan Province, China grants No. 2010B520003, Key Science and Technology Program of Henan Province, China grants No. 132102210133 and 132102210034, and the Key Science and Technology Projects of Public Health Department of Henan Province, China grants No. 2011020114.

References

1. Schuldhaus, D., Spiegel, M., Redel, T., Polyanskaya, M., Struffert, T., Hornegger, J., Doerfler, A.: Classification-based summation of cerebral digital subtraction angiography series for image post-processing algorithms. Physics in Medicine and Biology 56(1), 1791–1802 (2011)
2. Sang, N., Li, H., Peng, W., Zhang, T.: Knowledge-based adaptive threshold segmentation of digital subtraction angiography images. Image and Vision Computing 25(8), 1263–1270 (2007)
3. Cebral, R., Castro, A., Appanaboyina, S., Putman, M., Millan, D., Frangi, F.: Efficient Pipeline for Image-Based Patient-Specific Analysis of Cerebral Aneurysm Hemodynamics: Technique and Sensitivity. IEEE Transactions on Medical Image 24(4), 457–467 (2005)
4. Zwiggelaar, R., Astley, M., Boggis, R., Taylor, J.: Linear Structures in Mammographic Images: Detection and Classification. IEEE Transactions on Medical Image 23(9), 1077–1086 (2004)
5. Floyd, R., Steinberg, L.: An adaptive algorithm for spatial gray-scale. Proceeding Society Information Display 17(2), 75–78 (1976)
6. Goldschneider, J., Riskin, E., Wong, P.: Embedded multilevel error diffusion. IEEE Transactions on Image Processing 6(7), 956–964 (1997)
7. Fukunaga, K., Hostetler, L.: The estimation of the gradient of a density function, with applications in pattern recognition. IEEE Trans. Information Theory 21(1), 32–40 (1975)
8. Cheng, Y.: Mean Shift, Mode Seeking, and Clustering. IEEE Trans. Pattern Analysis and Machine Intelligence 17(8), 790–799 (1995)
9. Comaniciu, D., Ramesh, V., Meer, P.: The variable bandwidth mean shift and data-driven scale selection. In: IEEE Int. Conf. Computer Vision, vol. 1, pp. 438–445 (2001)
10. Jimenez-Alaniz, J., Pohl-Alfaro, M., Medina-Banuelos, V., Yanez-Suarez, O.: Segmenting brain MRI using adaptive mean shift. In: 28th International IEEE EMBS Annual Conference, pp. 3114–3117 (2006)

Numerical Evaluation of the Effectiveness of the Air Chamber of Shoes Pad for Diabetes with FE-SPH Method

Xin Ye, Linan Zhang, Zaobing Xu, Zengtao Hou, Xueling Bai, and Peng Shang[*]

Centre for Translational Medicine Research and Development,
Shenzhen Institutes of Advanced Technology Chinese Academy of Sciences,
Shenzhen 518055, China
{xin.ye,ln.zhang,zb.xu,zt.hou,xl.bai,peng.shang}@siat.ac.cn

Abstract. The object of this study is to utilize FE-SPH method to simulate the dynamic behavior of the air chamber of shoes pad for diabetes during footing process. The shoes pad' numerical models are discrete as FE mesh, and the air inside is modeled as SPH particles. The fluid structure interaction analysis between air and the shoes pad is carried out with contact algorithms. This explicit dynamic analysis is run on ANSYS software. Results show that: when the shoes pad is loaded, the velocity field concentrated on the central region of air chamber, and the particles in the fringe maintain a zero speed, which means the air flow out in the central region instead of the fringe. Thus, the shoes pad is effective in supplying air for the foot of diabetes.

Keywords: Shoes pad for diabetes, Fluid structure interaction (FSI) analysis, Finite element (FE) analysis, Smoothed particle hydrodynamics (SPH).

1   Introduction

The foot of diabetes is very fragile because of ulceration, thus, it need special care. In our previous work, we designed a shoes pad, which has an air chamber inside. Our goal is that when footing on the shoes pad, the air will be released from the central region to the bottom of foot, thus reducing foot odor. The object of this study is to evaluate the effectiveness of the air chamber of shoes pad.

In this study, a new FSI numerical method is introduced to assess the design of air chamber of shoes pad, and this method is smoothed particle hydrodynamics (SPH), which is a branch of mesh-less methods, and unlike Eulerian method does not use a fixed grid to represent the computation domain [1]. That is the method does not require connectivity data as needed by the finite volume and finite element methods. This gives the method a very useful feature when dealing with complex flows, exhibiting large deformations. In this work, the air will show large deformation, so it needs SPH method to model the air.

---

[*] Corresponding author.

Y. Zhang et al. (Eds.): HIS 2014, LNCS 8423, pp. 20–28, 2014.

2   Method

2.1   Basic Theory of SPH and Model of Air

SPH is a meshless, Lagrangian particle method developed by Lucy and Gingold and Monahan. And then, it has been successfully used for modeling fluid dynamic simulation. As a particle method, SPH uses a set of particles to present fluid flow. All the physical and mathematical properties of the fluid are assigned to the SPH particles. So, instead of using grids in FEM, SPH uses particle interpolation to approximate the field variables at any particle in a support domain which is shown in Fig. 1. Therefore, the interpolated value of a function $f(x)$ at particle i can be written as:

$$f(x_i) = \sum_{j=1}^{N} \frac{m_j}{\rho_j} f(x_j) \cdot W\left(\left|x_i - x_j\right|, h\right) \tag{1}$$

Where, m_j and ρ_j are the mass and density of the particle j and the sum is over all particles N within a radius $2h$ of the support domain Ω_y. Here $W(x_i-x_{j,h})$ is a B-spline based smoothing function with radius $2h$ that resembles a Gaussian function while having a narrower compact support.[2]

In this study, the air is considered as ideal gas, whose mechanical parameters can be determined by the Null material model and the polynomial equation of state. The ANSYS LS-DYNA software provides a *MAT_NULL material model, whose parameters ρ =1.18 kg/m^3 and μ=1.746e-5 Pa/s are selected in this study, to describe the model which has the properties of the fluid. It can describe the deviatoric stress by changing the constitutive model of the material model.

$$\sigma_{ij}^{v} = \sigma'_{ij} = \mu * \xi'_{ij} \tag{2}$$

Then the equation of state can be used to provide the stress components of the pressure behavior, thus they together provide the stress tensor of the material.

$$\sigma_{ij} = \sigma'_{ij} + \frac{1}{3}\sigma_{kk}\delta_{ij} = \mu * \xi'_{ij} + P\delta_{ij} \tag{3}$$

This polynomial equation of state, linear in the internal energy per initial volume, E, is given by.

$$p = C_0 + C_1\mu + C_2\mu^2 + C_3\mu^3 + \left(C_4 + C_5\mu + C_6\mu^2\right)E \tag{4}$$

Here, C_0, C_1, C_2, C_3, C_4, C_5, and C_6 are user defined constants and $\mu = \dfrac{1}{V} - 1$, where V is the relative volume. For this study, C_4 and C_5 are taken as 0.4, C_0, C_1, C_2, C_3, and C_6 are taken as 0 [3,4].

2.2   Mathematical Modeling of Shoes Pad

We construct shoes pad three-dimensional model (Fig. 1) under unloaded state using the SOLIDWORKS software. The inner part of shoes pad is an air chamber, just as showed in Fig. 2. The shoes pad is simplified as linear elastic model whose elastic modulus and Poisson's Ratio are 5.4 MPa, 0.3 MPa, respectively, and its density is 1080 kg/m³.

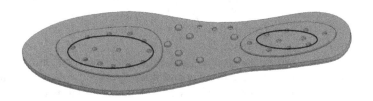

Fig. 1. Three-dimensional model of shoes pad (The areas inside two black oval holes in this figure are central region where foot and shoes pad have a contact, the left oval holes represents the front central region, and the right one represents the back central region)

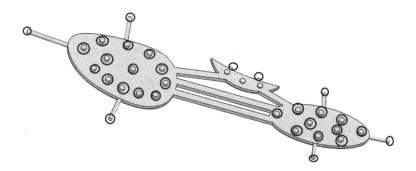

Fig. 2. Air chamber of shoes pad (The black oval holes in this figure are gas holes where the air can flow in and out)

2.3   Load

In order to have a accurate loading, we use the Pressure Distribution Test System to record the pressure distribution of a volunteer's (with a weight of 60kg) foot when he walk with a velocity of 0.5m/s. we take a average of the pressure in these two region (Fig.3) respectively. Then we load these two regions as Fig.4 in ANSYS.

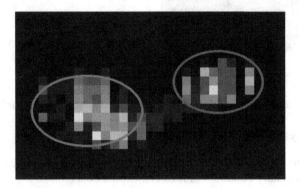

Fig. 3. Pressure distribution in foot of the volunteer when he is walking (the part inside the red circle is the back region in Fig.1, and the part inside blue one is the front central region)

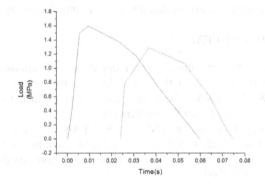

Fig. 4. Load curve for the central regions(the red line is for the front central region, and the black line is for the back region)

2.4   Mesh

The shoes pad is discrete as linear tetrahedral elements (in Fig. 5), 345865 solid elements are generated in ANSYS. The air domain is represented by SPH particle, its total of particles is 35253.

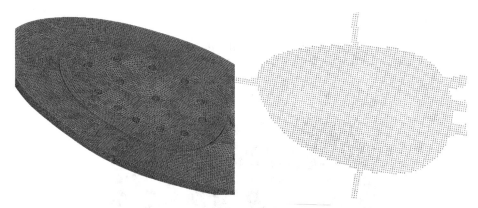

Fig. 5. Mesh of shoes pad and air (left: shoes pad mesh, right: air particles)

2.5   Boundary and Initial Conditions

The bottom of the shoes pad is attached to the ground, thus we fixed the bottom of the shoes pad, the boundary condition of it can be expressed as follows.

$$\{\delta\} = \{\, u\,,v\,,w\,,Qx\,,Qy\,,Qz\,\}^{T} = \{0\,,0\,,0\,,0\,,0\,,0\,\}^{T} \tag{5}$$

The air is modeled as compressible fluid in LS DYNA, and it is represented by SPH particles. These particles are assumed to have an initial velocity of 0 mm/s.

2.6   Coupled SPH with FEM

The coupled FEM and SPH method is implemented by using contact algorithms. The particles impact on the surfaces of the finite elements by contact type of "nodes to surface" in ANSYS LS-DYNA, where the slave part is defined with SPH particles and the master part is defined with finite elements.

This dynamic analysis is run on ANSYS LS DYAN. Considering the numerical stability, the actual load is only part of the theoretical load in Fig. 4. In order to reduce computing time, a time scaling is applied. This calculation procedure runs for 34 hours on Dell Precision T7500.

3   Results and Discussion

An ideal shoes pad should be the one whose air flows out mainly from the central region, which provides more fresh air for the foot of diabetes to ease the ulceration. In order to evaluate the effectiveness of the air chamber of shoes pad, The shoes pad' stress distribution and air chamber' velocity are visualized in a sequence of 'snapshots' in time over the footing phase as showed in Fig. 7. In the air chamber model, when the back central region is loading (from 0.005s to 0.025s in Fig. 7), the SPH particles exhibit a smooth behavior, leading to a contour like round shape. The development of resultant velocity contour is just as a circle whose diameter gradually becomes larger, which indicates the velocity spread from the core of central part to the fringe. The development of the Von –Mises stress presented in Fig. 7 also exhibit a same trend.

From 0.035s to 0.075s, the front central part is loading. The development of resultant velocity contour is just as an ellipse whose value of major axis and minor axis is becoming larger, and the Von –Mises stress on the shoes pad is more like a circle. In fact, shoes pad will transfer it stress value and pattern to the air because of using contact algorithms, thus the contour of the resultant velocity of air chamber resembles the Von –Mises stress development showed in the shoes pad. From above results, we find that the trend of the contour of the resultant velocity on air chamber differs from the Von –Mises stress development, this may be caused by the shape of air chamber. After 0.045s, when the load on the back front region is fading, the trend of the contour of the resultant velocity of air chamber is like a fading circle, which can be aware on the Von –Mises stress development.

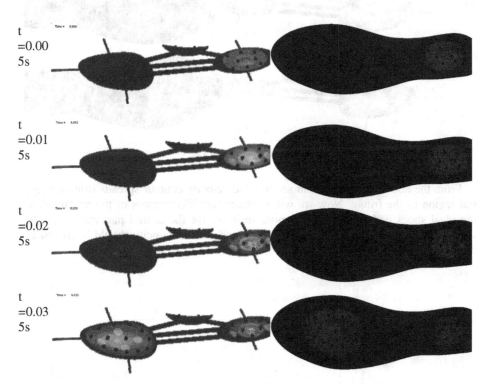

Fig. 6. Contours of resultant velocity of the air chamber of shoes pad (left) and stress development over shoes pad (right)

t =0.04 5s

t =0.05 5s

t =0.06 5s

t =0.07 5s

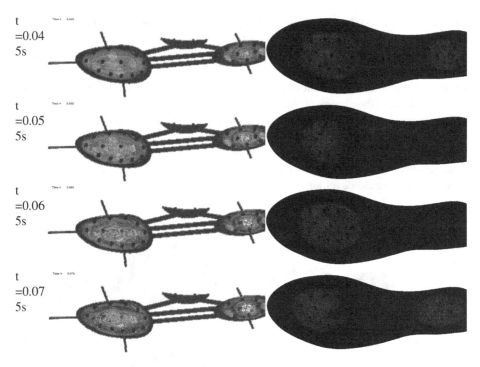

Fig. 6. (*Continued.*)

From the above results, we can see that the velocity contour spreads from the central region to the fringe. Now we will evaluate the effectiveness of the air chamber, the ideal shoes pad should supply more fresh air for the central part instead of the fringe, that is to say, on the fringe, the magnitude of the velocity should be as low as possible.

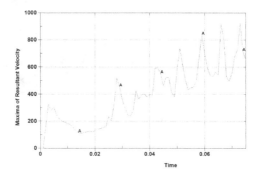

Fig. 7. Development of the peak resultant velocity on air chamber

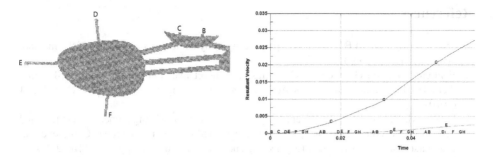

Fig. 8. Development of the resultant velocity on the fringe of air chamber (left: 8 outlets on the fringe, right: velocity development curve for the 8 outlets on the fringe)

From Fig.7, we find that the contour of velocity mainly concentrates on the central region, but the velocity spreads from the central region to the fringe of air chamber. Once the velocity of the particle on the fringe reaches to a large value, this shoes pad will be less effective in providing air for the patient. In order to see whether the velocity of the fringe is large, we depict the peak resultant velocity on air chamber (presented in Fig. 7) and the resultant velocity on the fringe of air chamber (showed in Fig. 8), and we compare these two velocities to assure who domains the process. From Fig. 7, it can be clearly seen that the peak velocity is almost over a value of 200mm/s, and the outlets A, B, D, F, G, H on fringe almost remain a velocity of zero. Only the outlets C, E have developing velocity, which keeps under a magnitude of 0.035 mm/s. The velocity of the fringe is mush small as compared to the whole region, in other words, the impact of the velocity on fringe may be ignored, and the effect of central region domains the shoes pad. To a certain extent, this shoes pad is effective in providing fresh air for the diabetes

This study have some limitations, including the linear elastic material models, the ideal gas model, the simplified loading, the limitation of numerical algorithms, and so on. The numerical analysis must be combined with verification test, which is our next work. This paper only presents a preliminary study to give a qualitative analysis of the effectiveness of the air chamber of shoes pad for diabetes.

4   Conclusion

FE-SPH method is utilized in this study to simulate the dynamic behavior of the air chamber of shoes pad for diabetes during footing process. Results show that to a certain extent, this shoes pad is effective in providing fresh air for the diabetes. This paper only presents a qualitative analysis of the effectiveness of the air chamber of shoes pad for diabetes. Further work is still needed to verify this numerical analysis.

References

1. Liu, G.G.R., Liu, M.B.: Smoothed particle hydrodynamics: a meshfree particle method. World Scientific (2003)
2. Jianming, W., Na, G., Wenjun, G.: Abrasive waterjet machining simulation by SPH method. The International Journal of Advanced Manufacturing Technology 50(1-4), 227–234 (2010)
3. Lavoie, M.A., Gakwaya, A., Ensan, M.N., et al.: Review of existing numerical methods and validation procedure available for bird strike modelling. In: International Conference on Computational & Experimental Engineering and Sciences, vol. 2(4), pp. 111–118 (2007)
4. Varas, D., Zaera, R., López-Puente, J.: Numerical modelling of the hydrodynamic ram phenomenon. International Journal of Impact Engineering 36(3), 363–374 (2009)

Effect of Suture Density on the Dynamic Behavior of the Bioprosthetic Heart Valve: A Numerical Simulation Study

Xin Ye, Linan Zhang, Zaobing Xu, Zengtao Hou, Xueling Bai, and Peng Shang[*]

Centre for Translational Medicine Research and Development,
Shenzhen Institutes of Advanced Technology Chinese Academy of Sciences,
Shenzhen 518055, China
{xin.ye,ln.zhang,zb.xu,zt.hou,xl.bai,peng.shang}@siat.ac.cn

Abstract. This paper constructs the bioprosthetic valve leaflets' parametric model using computer aided design. A series of accurate parameters of the bioproshtetic heart valve, such as radius of the sutural ring, height of the supporting stent and inclination of the supporting stent are determined. Numerical simulation is used to determine the effect of different shape designs and suture density on the mechanical performance of the bioprosthetic valve leaflet. The dynamic behavior of the valve during diastolic phase is analyzed. The finite element analysis results show that the stress distribution of the ellipsoidal leaflet valve is good. The ellipsoidal leaflet valve has the following advantages over the cylindrical leaflet valve: lower peak von Mises-stress, smaller stress concentration area and relatively uniform stress distribution. The suture density also has a significant effect on the dynamic behavior of the valve as it can act to reduce the pressure and improve the stress distribution. It was found that the influence of suture density in the stress of the leaflet differs on the basis of different geometries considered in the model. The degree of influence of the suture density in the bioprosthetic heart valve may also be dependent on the geometries of the valves. This indicates the need to account for the attachment edge, when manufacturing such bioproshetic heart valves for long term durability. Further research is required to assess the effect of suture density on the bioprosthetic heart valve models.

Keywords: Dynamic analysis, Bioprosthetic heart valve, Suture density, Finite element analysis, Computer aided design, Valve behavior.

1 Introduction

The use of bioprosthetic heart valves (BHV) in replacing diseased natural valves has become a routine procedure in the last 50 years. These tissue-derived valves have the advantage of low rates of thromboembolic complications without chronic anticoagulation therapy. However, their long-term durability remains limited due to structural

---

[*] Corresponding author.

Y. Zhang et al. (Eds.): HIS 2014, LNCS 8423, pp. 29–39, 2014.

degradation and failure [1], causes of the structural degradation of BHV tissue include mineralization and associated leaflet damage, and mechanical damage independent of calcification [2]. There is a general consensus that stresses developed in the leaflets during valve operation play a significant role in both calcific and noncalcific related damage. In particular, flexural stresses during valve opening and closing have been thought to play a considerable role in limiting the long-term BHV durability [3].

Thus, the stress state in BHV has been studied by many researchers using experimental or computational analysis. In recent years, Finite element analysis (FEA) has been extensively used for the structural analysis and functional simulation of BHV because of the advantage of a computational model is that material and geometric parameters can be easily changed to determine an optimum design and it enables analysis that may be impractical experimentally. Material models employed in previous studies for simulation of BHV such as porcine valves or pericardial bovine valves using the finite element method (FEM) can be generally categorized into four groups: linear isotropic, nonlinear isotropic, linear anisotropic and nonlinear anisotropic that come with varying degrees of accuracy [4]. These studies have demonstrated increasingly sophisticated means to mitigate mineralization and to reduce unwanted biological responses, it was found that a proper design of the supporting stent can significantly reduce the flexural stresses [5].

However, these studies were mainly conducted on stress state of the valves, little attention has been devoted to suture of the BHV, García Páez et al. (2003) compared the mechanical behaviour of biological tissues testing. Lim and Cheong (1994) carried out uniaxial tests on bovine pericardium strips cut along three different axes. They found that suturing reduced the strength of the tissue and that tissue with thicker sutures ruptured at significantly lower stresses [6,7]. A.N. Smuts et al. (2010) performed rupture tests on the tissues used for the prototype valves which also verified that the suture weakens the tissue and reduces the effective load-carrying connection area at the attachments [8]. The above-mentioned researches were conducted by only kind of BHV model. There may be some uncertainties. Gould et al. 1973 had found that the stress of the leaflet is sensitive to geometrical variation of the leaflet [9], thus it is unclear how the results of such studies translate to other types of BHV. These previous results are unsatisfactory.

Therefore, the aim of the present study is to extend A.N. Smuts, Lim and García Páez's analysis of suture density effect on BHV via finite element modeling of the diastole, and to account for the effect of suture on different BHV models not previously considered.

2   Analysis of Bioprosthetic Heart Valve

2.1   Mathematical Modeling of Leaflets with Different Shapes

Bioprosthetic heart valve(BHV) consists of valvular leaflets, supporting stent and sutural ring. The flow field of bioprosthetic heart valve is similar to that of the human heart valve. Its flow pattern is central-like. Although it has been improved in antihemolysis and antithrombotic function, the efficiency of the bioprosthetic heart valve is still not satisfactory. The main objective for the bioprosthetic heart valve designer is to improve its long-term durability which is closely associated with the geometrical design. The geometrical shape of the closed aortic valve in the state of diastolic is rather complicated, depending on the individual as well as the pressure of the valve. The valve design must meet three basic requirements.

(1) Three leaflets intersect with the root of the aortic at the lines which divide the circle into three equational parts.

(2) There should be no leak when the valves close.

(3) Projecting the free edge of valve leaflets at the normal direction, the sum area should be larger than that of the sutural ring at least [10].

Based on three basic requirements, we create the cylindrical and ellipsoidal curved surfaces, which satisfy the actual condition.

BHV includes three leaflets made of proince pericardial. The thickness of the leaflets is 0.5 mm [11]. Edges of the leaflets are sewn on supporting stent firmly. Geometrical shapes of the leaflet's unloaded state are simulated by three-dimension curved surface with cylindrical or ellipsoidal shape. The leaflet's height h is 15.7 mm, the stent's radius r is 13 mm, the stent's angle a is 3° [12].

We construct 3-dimensional model using the Pro/ENGNEER software. Firstly, we create a conic curved surface and a cylindrical curved surface, and then make them intersect. Finally we get intersecting curves which are boundary curves of leaflets, as shown in Fig. 1. Equation (1) is the mathematical description of cylindrical surface leaflet:

$$\left(x\cos\frac{\pi}{4} - z\sin\frac{\pi}{4}\right)^2 + y^2 = 13 \tag{1}$$

$$x^2 + y^2 = \left[13 + \left(13\sqrt{2} + 13 + z\right)\tan a\right]^2$$

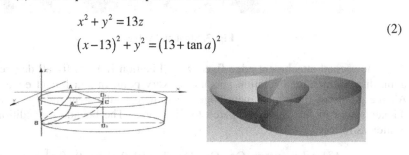

Fig. 1. Effective view of the cylindrical leaflet valve (CLV)

As described above, we can get boundary curves from intersection between the conic curved and the ellipsoidal curved surfaces, as shown in Fig. 2.

Equation (2) is the Equation of ellipsoidal surface leaflet:

$$x^2 + y^2 = 13z \tag{2}$$

$$(x-13)^2 + y^2 = (13 + \tan a)^2$$

Fig. 2. Effective view of the ellipsoidal leaflet valve (ELV)

2.2   Finite Element Model Strategy

Based on geometrical features of leaflets, we create the model with Pro/ENGNEER and save it as IGES file. Then we import the IGES file into ANSYS.

In ANSYS, the explicit finite-element code LS-DYNA was used in conducting the analyses, an explicit code being much more efficient and appropriate than implicit ones in solving problems with large deformations and with only modest computer storage requirements, especially in short time structural dynamics problems. The advantage over implicit is that explicit formulation require no global inversion of the stiffness matrix. It is however necessary to introduce a time-step which is small enough to reduce problems of numerical instability. The thickness of the finite element model is 0.5 mm.   Every element has five integration points with six degrees of freedom per node and five integration points are assumed to be through shell thickness. The Belytschko-Leviathan shell elements with a lagrangian formalism is selected. After meshing the models in ANSYS finite element package, we translate the model into LS-DYNA.

2.3   Boundary Condition of Attachment Edge

(1) BHVs are seamed to the stent in the attachment edge as showed in Fig. 4. In order to investigate the effect of suture density on BHV, we assume two attachment edge fixation ways, which stand for different suture densities.

The first kind of attachment edge fixed way (Fixation I) is that all displacement of the attachment edge is constrained, all the rotation is ignored. This allows points in the attachment edge some degree of rotation. This kind of fixation is assumed to represent a type of low density suture. Its mathematical expression is as follows.

$$\{\delta\} = \{\,u\,,v\,,w\,,Q_x\,,Q_y\,,Q_z\,\}^T = \{0\,,0\,,0\,,Q_x\,,Q_y\,,Q_z\,\}^T \tag{3}$$

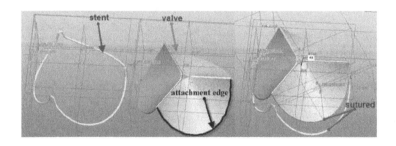

Fig. 3. Stent and valve

In the second attachment edge fixed way (Fixation II), we fix all degree of freedom, displacement and rotation vectors of every point in attachment edge are zero. All the points of the attachement edge are sutured to the stent tightly. It represents thicker suture of the valve compared to Fixation I. The boundary condition can be written as follow.

$$\{\delta\} = \{\,u\,,v\,,w\,,Qx\,,Qy\,,Qz\,\}T = \{0\,,0\,,0\,,0\,,0\,,0\,\}^T \tag{4}$$

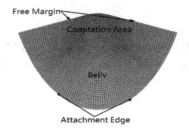

Fig. 4. Front view of the BHV

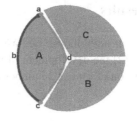

Fig. 5. Aortic side of the BHV

(2) The restraint circumstance of free margin adc (Fig. 4) and its bind area is comparatively complicated. Free margin adc (Fig. 4) is a joint brim of valve leaf B and C (Fig. 5). Nodes are restricted there and only move along vertical direction. With load increasing, the junction area of leaflets increases. Then some nodes will enter the juncture area. So we must restraint these nodes again. When we analyze finite elements, we load step by step. As we load, we should judge if some nodes enter or leave the junction area. Boundary condition of the bind area's every point displacement in a coordinate can be expressed as:

$$\{\delta\} = \{u, v, w, Q_x, Q_y, Q_z\}^T = \{0, 0, w, 0, 0, 0\}^T \tag{5}$$

(3) The elastic modulus in this study has been taken to be 2 MPa for the leaflets. A Poisson's Ratio of 0.3 is chosen to overcome numerical difficult encountered at values near 0.5, the density of the leaflets is taken to be 1.1g/ml.

2.4 Pressure Loading Pattern

It is known that the highest stresses occur during the closing phase (diastole) of the valve, which is one of the main causes of valves failure [13], and in order to achieve a good compromise between numerical precision and time of calculation. Thus we simulate the model only during the diastole. To represent loading during the BHV closing, the following pressure-time relationship is assumed in this work. The pressure on the BHV is modeled as to ramp, indicating an increase of pressure from 0 to 20 mmHg. The complete cycle is shown in Fig. 6.

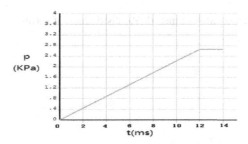

Fig. 6. Pressure loading curve for BHV

3   Results

We focus our attention on two aspects of the BHV function: (1) the peak von-Mises stress, and (2) the development of von-Mises stress in the leaflet with time. The stress with evolution of time at a number of locations is presented in Fig. 7.

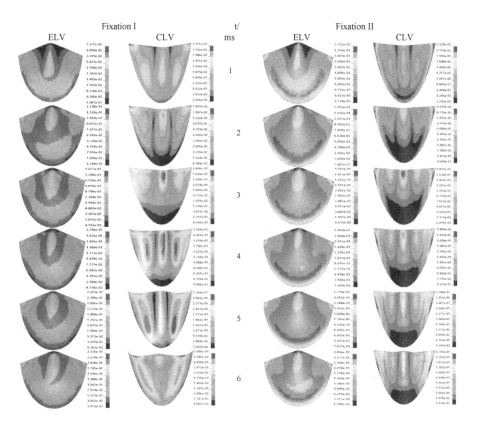

Fig. 7. Von-Mises Stress (MPa) distribution of valves leaflets

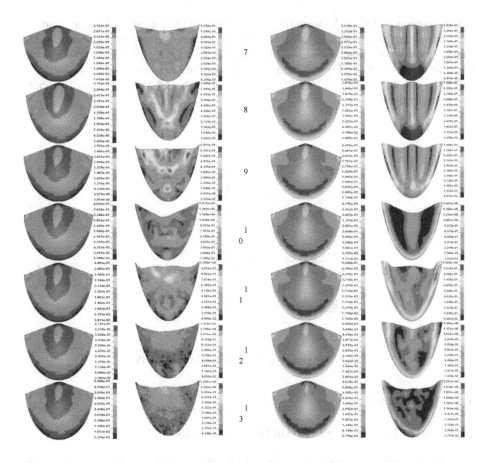

Fig. 7. (*Continued.*)

As seen in the above figures (in Fig. 7), on Fixation I, with the development of physiological pressure, the stress value of the ELV develops steady, the stress distribution of the ELV maintains uniform. During this stage, the peak stress value is located near the top edge of the attachment edge. However, the stress distribution of the CLV is quite different from that of the ELV, in the CLV model, the stress increases notably. From 1ms to 2ms, the peak stress appears near the top edge of the attachment edge. From 2ms to 3ms, the belly of the CLV has a sudden stress increase, the local stress concentration occurs. From 3ms to 4ms, there are three local stress concentration areas locating in the belly. After 5ms, the stress increases seriously. There are many local stress concentration areas appearing in the belly. As presented in Fig. 8, it can be seen that the peak stress values in the ELV and CLV are 0.473MPa, 1.437MPa, respectively. In the CLV, the maximum stress value increases by about three fold.

On Fixation II, the peak stress is also located near the top edge of the attachment edge, the stress distribution is still uniform, but there is an apparent difference, the attachment edge is subjected to high stress level state. The stress is mainly concentrated in the belly. From Fig. 8, it can be seen that the peak stress values of the ELV and CLV are 0.562MPa, 2.252MPa, respectively. The CLV' peak stress is about 300% higher than the ELV's.

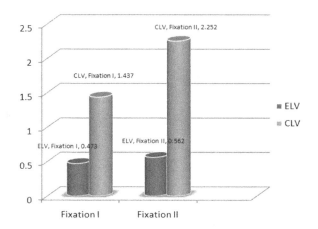

Fig. 8. The peak von-Mises stress (MPa) of BHV

4   Discussion

4.1   The Influence of the Different Geometrical Models

We compare the ELV under two different boundary conditions. On Fixation I, the bottom of the attachment edge in a state of low stress. But on Fixation II, the attachment edge in high stress level, the peak stress values on the Fixation I and II are 0.473MPa, 0.562MPa, respectively. The peak stress on Fixation II is 20% higher than that on Fixation I. To the CLV model, the bottom attachment edge on Fixation I is in low stress level, which on Fixation II is in a state of high stress level. On Fixation I, the stress concentration mainly appears in the belly, on Fixation II, stress concentration mainly occurs in the attachment edge, which can affect the long term durability of leaflets. The peak stress on Fixation I (1.437MPa) is much lower than that on Fixation II (2.252MPa).

Through the above analysis, it can be seed that density suture has a direct effect on the stress state of leaflet. It may lead not only to different stress peak values, but also to different stress distribution. On Fixation I, the peak stress is lower. The stress concentration mainly occurs in belly not in the attachment edge. Previous studies have indicated that local stress concentration at the stent interface is important for the BHV' failure [14], thus, the BHV on Fixation II may fail early. In addition, the Fixation I contribute to better mechanical behavior of leaflet. Fixation I represent low density of the attachement edge sutured to the stent. These results are consistent with Lim and García Páez's analysis, which suture density has a significant effect on the long term durability of the value.

Table 1. Stress concentration areas of the BHV appeared during the diastole

		Attachment edge	Belly	Coaptation area
Fixation I	ELV	✓	✗	✗
	CLV	✓	✓	✓
Fixation II	ELV	✓	✗	✗
	CLV	✓	✗	✓

✓ represents stress concentration   ✗ represents uniform stress distribution

By making a comparison of the ELV and CLV under the same condition, we can clearly see that, The CLV shows markedly increased stress values in all of the investigated leaflet regions when compared to the ELV. The ELV is superior to the CLV in mechanical properties. The ELV has the following advantages over the CLV, lower peak von-Mises stress, smaller stress concentration area, and relatively uniform stress distribution.

4.2   Effect of Suture Density on the Dynamic Behavior of the Valves

The thicker suture of the CLV makes the peak stress increase almost 57%. It also causes additional stress concentration areas appearing in the belly of the valve. In the ELV model, that change is only a peak stress increase of 19%, the stress still concentrates in the attachment edge. The CLV model is more sensitive to the density of suture. Thicker suture makes the mechanical behavior of the CLV inferior. This conclusion accords with that the suture weakens the tissue and reduces the effective load-carrying connection area at the attachments [8], which is argued by A.N. Smuts, et al (2010). But to the ELV model, the influence of suture density is just reflected in stress increase. Besides, the influence of the degree of stress increase (19%) to the valve behavior is not clear,.   In ELV, the degeneration to the mechanical properties of BHV is not explicit, needing further research. Gould et al. (1973) had put forward that the stress of leaflet is sensitive to geometrical variations of the leaflets [6], this conclusion is widely confirmed and accepted. It is verified again in this study. In addition, the influence of suture density in the stress sate of the leaflet also differs with the geometries of the model. The degree of influence of the suture density in the BHV may be dependent on the geometries of the valves. Thus the conclusion raised by A.N. Smuts, Lim and García Páez et al. may remain some uncertainties. That is whether other kinds of valve models are affected by the suture density and how much it influence. Hence further studies are still necessary to reveal effect of suture density on the dynamic behavior of the valve.

The above results described herein need careful interpretation, since the FE model is affected by some limitations: In the FEA the leaflets are subjected to a uniform pressure load on the aortic side during the valve closing phase. Fluid flow patterns may vary in different regions, particularly in the vicinity of the valve leaflets [4, 15]. Hence, spatially non-uniform pressure can be induced on the surface of the leaflets during the closing phases. In addition, the load applied on the stress-free leaflets during the BHV closing is hard to measure. It is easy to apply that kind of boundary conditions of the BHV. Therefore, a more realistic fluid-structure interaction analysis of the BHV during the cardiac cycle is required to study the effect of suture density. The BHVs were modelled as homogeneous, linear, elastic and isotropic materials. In fact, the BHVs have a non-linear and anisotropic response since they consist mainly of an elastin matrix reinforced by collagen fibres that have a preferential direction within the matrix and a locally variable concentration [16]. Orthotropy can significantly affect the mechanical behavior of the valve [15, 5]. However, these simplifications alter stress distribution, they are not likely to affect the conclusions based on the comparison of the simulated conditions.

In spite of these limitations, this study can clearly indicate that the degree of influence of the suture density in the BHV relates with geometrical variations of the leaflets. The main purpose of this study is to test the reliability of theory that suture density influences in valve behavior during valve operation. From above discussion, we can see that further studies are still necessary to reveal effect of suture density on the dynamic behavior of the valve.

5   Conclusions

This paper constructs the bioprosthetic valve leaflets' parametric model via computer aided design, a series of accurate parameters of the bioprosthtetic heart valve, the height of the supporting attachment edge and the inclination of the supporting attachment edge, are determined. We use numerical simulation to determine the effect of different shape designs and suture density of the attachment edge on the mechanical performance of the valve. The mechanical behavior of the bioprosthetic valve leaflet during diastolic phase is analyzed; the biomechanics of the valve is assessed in term of peak von-Mises stress, local stress concentration and stress location.

By comparing the mechanical behavior of the cylindrical leaflet valve with that of the ellipsoidal leaflet valve on the same boundary condition, it can be concluded that the stress distribution of the ellipsoidal leaflet valve is comparatively reasonable. The ellipsoidal leaflet valve has the following advantages over the cylindrical leaflet valve, lower peak von-Mises stress, smaller stress concentration area, and relatively uniform stress distribution. In addition, above analysis clearly shows that Fixation I can act to reduce the pressure and make the stress distribution reasonable. Low density suture of the valve can act to reduce the pressure and make the stress distribution reasonable.

What's more important, we find that the ellipsoidal leaflet valve is very sensitive to the suture, when doing suture density test. Thicker suture seduces the peak stress of valve increasing deadly, and apearing additional local stress concentration located in the belly of the valve. But that kind of change is not accordant with the ellipsoidal leaflet valve. The change in suture density of the ellipsoidal leaflet valve only causes the peak stress of the valve increasing. The increased peak stress is just third of that in ellipsoidal leaflet valve. The influence of suture density in the bioprosthetic heart valve is of some degree dependent on the geometries of the bioprosthetic heart valve model. Further researches are still needed to reveal the effect of suture density on the bioprosthetic heart valves. These researches may contribute to the choice of the final suture density to reduce tearing of the leaflet, thereby prolong the lifetime of the bioprosthetic heart valve.

References

1. Schoen, F.J., Gimbrone, M.A.: Ramzi S. Cotran, MD, 1932-2000. Cardiovascular Pathology 10(3), 107–108 (2001)
2. Sacks, M.S., Mirnajafi, A., et al.: Effects of cyclic flexural fatigue on porcine bioprosthetic heart valve heterograft biomaterials. Journal of Biomedical Materials Research Part A 94A(1), 205–213 (2010)
3. Sacks, M.S., Iyengar, A.K.S., et al.: Dynamic in vitro quantification of bioprosthetic heart valve leaflet motion using structured light projection. Annals of Biomedical Engineering 29(11), 963–973 (2001)
4. Mohammadi, H., Bahramian, F., Wan, W.: Advanced modeling strategy for the analysis of heart valve leaflet tissue mechanics using high-order finite element method. Medical Engineering & Physics 31(9), 1110–1117 (2009)
5. Broom, N.D.: The stress/strain and fatigue behaviour of glutaraldehyde preserved heart-valve tissue. Journal of Biomechanics 10(11-12), 707-724 (1977)
6. Garcıa Páez, J.M., Jorge Herrero, E., et al.: Comparison of the mechanical behaviors of biological tissues subjected to uniaxial tensile testing: pig, calf and ostrich pericardium sutured with Gore-Tex. Biomaterials 24(9), 1671–1679 (2003)
7. Lim, K.O., Cheong, K.C.: Effect of suturing on the mechanical properties of bovine pericardium — implications for cardiac valve bioprosthesis. Medical Engineering & Physics 16(6), 526–530 (1994)
8. Scheffer, C., Smuts, A.N., et al.: Application of finite element analysis to the design of tissue leaflets for a percutaneous aortic valve. Journal of the Mechanical Behavior of Biomedical Materials 4(1), 85–98 (2011)
9. Gould, P.L., Cataloglu, A., et al.: Stress analysis of the human aortic valve. Computers & Structures 3(2), 377–384 (1973)
10. Zilla, P., Human, P., et al.: Bioprosthetic heart valves: the need for a quantum leap. Biotechnology and Applied Biochemistry 40(1), 57–66 (2004)
11. Vongpatanasin, W., Hillis, L.D., et al.: Prosthetic Heart Valves. New England Journal of Medicine 335(6), 407–416 (1996)
12. Gillinov, A.M., Blackstone, E.H., et al.: Prosthesis-patient size: Measurement and clinical implications. Journal of Thoracic and Cardiovascular Surgery 126(2), 313–316 (2003)
13. Sacks, M.S., Eckert, C.E., et al.: In Vivo Dynamic Deformation of the Mitral Valve Annulus. Annals of Biomedical Engineering 37(9), 1757–1771 (2009)
14. Vesely, I.: The evolution of bioprosthetic heart valve design and its impact on durability. Cardiovascular Pathology 12(5), 277–286
15. Franz, T., Koch, T.M., et al.: Aortic valve leaflet mechanical properties facilitate diastolic valve function. Computer Methods in Biomechanics and Biomedical Engineering 13(2), 225–234 (2010)
16. Luo, X.Y., Li, J., et al.: A nonlinear anisotropic model for porcine aortic heart valves. Journal of Biomechanics 34(10), 1279–1289 (2001)

An Analysis on Risk Factors
of Chronics Diseases Based on GRI

Zhuoyuan Zheng, Ye Li, and Yunpeng Cai

Key Laboratory for Biomedical Informatics and Health Engineering,
Chinese Academy of Sciences, Institute of Biomedical and Health Engineering
in Shenzhen Institutes of Advanced Technology, Shenzhen 518055
{zy.zheng,ye.li,yp.cai}@siat.ac.cn

Abstract. Chronics diseases have become the major cause of the death for human all over the world and every country had to pay a heavy price for it in past years. It is of great significance for researchers to find out the risk factors that affect the onset, maintenance and prognosis of a variety of chronic diseases. In this research we aim to find out the risk factor of chronics from questionnaire data in Pizhou city by GRI. We develop some customized preprocessing methods according to the characteristics of questionnaire data and discover some significant results in conformance with medical conclusion. The result shows that obesity, smoking and lack of sleeping are three vital risk factors which could cause some chronic diseases.

Keywords: Chronic Diseases, Risk Factors, Questionnaire, Data Mining, Generalized Rule Induction.

1   Introduction

According to WHO, chronics have become the major cause of the death for human all over the world. In the next decade, the mortality from chronics will increase by 17%. It is of great significant for the prevention, control, cure and recover of chronic to carry out research on risk factors about it.

In the fields of research on chronic risk factors, a lot of data were acquired through questionnaire of random sampling. For example, L.Nikolajsen and N.J.Talley [1, 2] make use of questionnaire to do their research works. Generally, researchers adopt the classic statistical analysis methods [3, 4] to analysis data obtained. With the emergency and development of data mining, more and more researchers applied it to medical areas for data analysis and knowledge discovery. S.E.Brossette [5] etc. developed a data mining system which uses novel data mining techniques to discover unsuspected, useful patterns of nosocomial infections and antimicrobial resistance from the analysis of hospital laboratory data. Jiuyong Li [6] etc. make use of the anti-monotone property of risk pattern sets and present an algorithm to find patterns associated with an allergic event for ACE inhibitors. Lihua Lia [7] etc. select feature by means of genetic algorithms. In their study, cross validation with receiver operating characteristic (ROC)

Y. Zhang et al. (Eds.): HIS 2014, LNCS 8423, pp. 40–46, 2014.

curve is used for evaluation and comparison of cancer detection performance. The results showed that the classification algorithm using features can detect ovarian cancer with a reasonably high performance.

In data mining, association rules are used to describe interesting associations and correlations between different factors in data. Apriori [8] is an algorithm for extracting association rules from data. It constrains the search space for rules by discovering frequent itemsets and only examining rules that are made up of frequent itemsets. Generalized Rule Induction [9] (GRI) generates rules to summarize patterns in the data using a quantitative measure for the interestingness of rules. This measure provides a method for ranking competing rules and allows the system to constrain the search space for useful rules, as well as identifying the best or most interesting rules describing a database. GRI is based on the ITRule [10] algorithm and extends that algorithm with added functionality. Comparing with Apriori, the prominent advantages of GRI is that GRI can deal with continuous data and the discretization is unnecessary. In our research, GRI is employed to analysis the questionnaire data from Pizhou city so as to find out some rules pertaining to risk factors of chronic diseases.

The material of the paper is organized as follows. Section 2 introduces materials, method and algorithms used in the paper as well as some results mined. In section 3 the results are analyzed and some conclusions are arrived.

2   Materials and Method

2.1   Subject

Questionnaire data involve 6564 residents (3231 males and 3333 females) in four towns of Jiangsu province. Their age is 42.39±14.64, the oldest is 70 and the youngest is 16.

In the questionnaire, a total of 11 big items (personal information, living condition, health care, chronic history, familial chronic history, smoking, drink, alcohol use, eating habits, daily living & physical exercise, woman menstruation & birth history) and 221 subitems. Among chronics, emphasis will be placed on high blood pressure, coronary heart disease, stroke, diabetes and malignant tumors. The statistic information is shown as following Table 1.

Table 1. Chronics statistics

chronics	number of cases	percent
high blood pressure	198	3.02%
coronary heart disease	37	0.56%
stroke	41	0.62%
diabetes	21	0.32%
malignant tumors	13	0.20%

The total numbers of chronic are 310, which account for 4.72 of all respondents.

2.2   Preprocessing

Real world data are generally incomplete inconsistent dirty data. Using these raw data, people are always incapable either to carry out data mining directly or to mine a satisfying result. Data preprocessing techniques can improve data mining quality and reduce mining time. Preprocessing include data cleaning, data integration, data transformation and so on.

Aiming at the complexity of questionnaire data, four major preprocessing methods as show below are employed.

2.2.1   Data Transformation

Most of data from questionnaire are numbers of some options. For example, species of tumors are inquired in the sub-questionnaire of cancer, and these options include stomach cancer =01, esophagus cancer =02, liver cancer =03, lung cancer =04, colorectal cancer =05, breast cancer =06, cervical cancer =07, leukemia cancer =08 and others =88. In order to transform these data to form which suit to be mined, this field must be divided. And every possible value should be a new field. The value of this new field is either "true" or "false" ("T" or "F", "1" or "0"). The value "true" ("T" or "1") means the corresponding option is picked out, and the value "false" ("F" or "0") means the corresponding option is not picked out. For example, a record numbered 50324 in Table 2 can be transformed into the record shown in Table 3.

Table 2. Original record

number	species of tumors
50324	01, 07

Table 3. Record transformed

number	Stomach cancer	esophagus cancer	liver cancer	lung cancer	colorectal cancer	breast cancer	cervical cancer	leukemia cancer	others
50324	T	F	F	F	F	F	T	F	F

2.2.2   Data Normalization

In questionnaire, the choice of "01" means a positive response while "02" is a negative one. So in the process of preprocessing, the choices of "01" and "02" must be modified into "true" ("T" or "1") and "false" ("F" or "0") respectively. Some fields have the values of 00, 01, ..., and 09. these values must be changed to 0, 1, ..., and 9. In addition, due to some inputting mistakes, there are some insignificant values such as "0." and ".". These values can be changed to value "0".

2.2.3   Blank Handling

Because of the carelessness of investigators or typist, there are some missing values in some fields. For different fields, the methods handling missing values are different.

For instance, the missing value about age can be filled by average of age, while the missing value like alcohol intake can be filled by zero.

2.2.4   Removing Void Value

Some attributes like number, name, address and phone number are insignificant for risk factors mining and should not be considered in data mining. Besides, there is only one value for all records in some fields, and these fields can not show the discrepancy of different records. So these fields should be excluded from the range of mining.

2.3   Feature Selection

Feature selection can generate the minimal subsets of attributes for specific application without loss of data value and remove the irrelevant and redundant attributes. What's more, feature selection can also improve the quality of data, speed up the data mining and bring the rule discovered more comprehensible.

2.4   Generalized Rule Induction

Generalized Rule Induction (GRI) generates rules to summarize patterns in the data using a quantitative measure for the interestingness of rules. This measure provides a method for ranking competing rules and allows the system to constrain the search space for useful rules, as well as identifying the best or most interesting rules describing a database. GRI is based on the ITRule algorithm and extends that algorithm with added functionality. The J measure maximizes the simplicity/goodness-of-fit trade-off by utilizing an information theoretic based cross-entropy calculation.

A rule in GRI takes the form:

If $Y=y$ then $X=x$ with probability p.

Where X and Y are two fields (attributes) and x and y are values for those fields. The consequent (the "then" part of the rule) is restricted to being a single value assignment expression while the antecedent (the "if" part of the rule) may be a conjunction of such expressions, for example If $Y=y$ and $Z=z$, then $X=x$ (with probability p). The complexity of a rule is defined as the number of conjuncts appearing in the rule's antecedent.

The quantitative interestingness measure J is defined as:

$$J(x/y) = p(y)\left(p(x/y)\log\frac{p(x/y)}{p(x)} + (1-p(x/y))\log\frac{1-p(x/y)}{1-p(x)} \right)$$

Where $p(y)$ is the probability of the rule's antecedent matching an example from the data set, $p(x)$ is the probability of the rule's consequent matching an example from the data set, and $p(x/y)$ is the conditional probability of the rule's consequent conditioned on the antecedent.

2.5   Data Mining

The flow chart of data mining in Clementine is shown as Figure 1:

The node "pizhou.xls" in Figure 1 is data source node which can provides data source such as database, excel files, SPSS files and so on. The node "Type" is field option, by which we can choose the necessary fields and set the output fields. The node "FeatureSelection" selects these fields which could reflect the features of data. The node "SelectedFeatures" is the result of "FeatureSelection" and "ChronicDisease" is for the purpose of the extraction of rules.

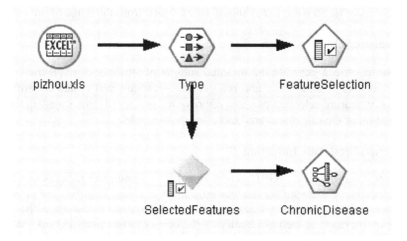

Fig. 1. The flow chart of data mining in Clementine

Some results of association rules (3-items set) mined in Clementine are shown as Table 4.

Table 4. Results of association rules mining

Antecedent	consequent	support
no passive smoking and SBP < 128.500 and WC< 83.875	healthy	42.76
male and no passive smoking and HC < 82.750	healthy	7.89
male and drinking well water and no smoking	healthy	16.47
no passive smoking and WC < 78.875 and eating bean products more than three times per month	healthy	23.83
no passive smoking and HC < 82.750 and literate	healthy	14.69
male and passive smoking and DBP >120.350	suffer from chronic	0.05
drinking groundwater and 4 to 6 hours of sleep time every day and no leisure entertainment	suffer from chronic	0.02
drinking groundwater and 4 to 6 hours of sleep time every day and exercise less than once a week	suffer from chronic	0.12

Due to the small number (4.7%) of these who suffer from chronic disease, the support is set in a low level (0.01%). For healthy and non-healthy people, the lowest confident are set to 95% and 85% respectively. The results discovered are some association rules and only some representative rules are presented in Table 4.

3   Conclusions

From the result discovered we can see that healthy (without any chronic disease) people's WC (waist circumference) or HC (hip circumference) are less than some level. Actually, WC or HC is an indicator of one person on degree of obesity. This shows that if one person is overweight, he/she will take more risks of suffering from chronic ills.

Meanwhile, among rules in table 4, for the healthy, the antecedents include the item either "no passive smoking" or "no smoking". This says that "no passive smoking" or "no smoking" is good for people to keep a healthy body. This can explain from another aspect that "passive smoking" or "smoking" is likely to induce chronic diseases.

In one hundred rules whose consequent is "suffer from chronic" and minimum confident is 70%, there are 49 rules which include the antecedents "4 to 6 hours of sleep time every day". This result shows that insufficient sleep is a risk factor which could induce chronic diseases.

From what discussed above, we can conclude that overweight, smoking (passive smoking) and insufficient sleep are major risk factors which can induce chronic diseases. According to this conclusion, in order to prevent and curb the happening and aggravating of chronic disease, it is suggested that local residents should control the weight, give up smoking and assure enough sleep. This will be great significant directive for local medical treatment decision organization.

Acknowledgments. This work is supported in part by the Country Science and Technology Supporting Plan (No.2008BAI65B16), by the CAS Key Projects Deployment (Low-cost Health Engineering).

References

1. Nikolajsen, L., Brandsborg, B., Lucht, U., Jensen, T.S., Kehlet, H.: Chronic pain following total hip arthroplasty: a nationwide questionnaire study. Acta Anaesthesiol Scand. 50, 495–500 (2006)
2. Talley, N.J., Newman, P., Boyce, P.M., Paterson, K.J., Owen, B.K.: Initial validation of a bowel symptom questionnaire and measurement of chronic gastrointestinal symptoms in Australians. Internal Medicine Journal 25(4), 302–308 (1995)
3. Masson, L.F., MCNeill, G., Tomany, J.O., Simpson, J.A., Peace, H.S., Wei, L., Grubb, D.A., Bolton-Smith, C.: Statistical approaches for assessing the relative validity of a food-frequency questionnaire: use of correlation coefficients and the kappa statistic. Public Health Nutrition 6, 313–321 (2003)

4. Hagströmer, M., Oja, P., Sjöström, M.: The International Physical Activity Questionnaire (IPAQ): a study of concurrent and construct validity. Public Health Nutrition 9, 755–762 (2006)
5. Brossette, S.E., Sprague, A.P., Jones, W.T., Moser, S.A.: A Data Mining System for Infection Control Surveillance [J]. Methods of Information in Medicine 39, 303–310 (2010)
6. Li, J., Fu, A.W., He, H., Chen, J.: Mining Risk Patterns in Medical Data. In: International Conference on Knowledge Discovery and Data Mining KDD 2005, pp. 770–775 (2005)
7. Lia, L., Tanga, H., Wu, Z., Gong, J., Gruidl, M., Zou, J., Tockman, M., Clark, R.A.: Data mining techniques for cancer detection using serum proteomic profiling. Artificial Intelligence in Medicine 32, 71–83 (2004)
8. Agrawal, R., Srikant, R.: Fast Algorithms for Mining Association Rules. In: Proceedings of the 20th International Conference on Very Large Databases, pp. 487–499 (1994)
9. Clementine 11.1, Clementine Algorithms Guide, Integral solutions Limited (2007)
10. Smyth, P., Goodman, R.M.: An information theoretic approach to rule induction from databases. IEEE Transactions on Knowledge and Data Engineering, 310–316 (1992)

A Study on the Nonlinearity Relationship between Quadriceps Thickness and Torque Output during Isometric Knee Extension

Xing Chen[1,2], Xin Chen[2], Jizhou Li[1], and Yongjin Zhou[1,*]

[1] Shenzhen Institutes of Advanced Technology, Chinese Academy of Sciences, China
[2] Shenzhen University, Shenzhen 518060, China
y.zhou.cn@ieee.org

Abstract. The quadriceps femoris is a large muscle group which is crucial in walking, running, jumping and squatting. Therefore, study on quadriceps muscle activity is of realistic significance. As one of architectural parameters, muscle thickness has been investigated in many aspects for various purposes. However, there are few studies on quantitating the relationship between quadriceps muscle thickness and torque output. In this study a coarse-to-fine method based on a compressive tracking algorithm is used for real-time estimation of muscle thickness during isometric contraction on ultrasound images. Ultrasonography is a convenient and widely-used technique to look into the muscle contraction as it is non-invasive and real-time. The relationship between quadriceps muscle thickness and torque output are investigated with data from 13 subjects. The experimental result showed that the change of muscle thickness in cross-sectional plane is similar to its torque during muscle contraction, but the relationship between them is nonlinear.

Keywords: Muscle thickness(MT), Isometric knee extension, Quadriceps muscle(QM), Sonomyography.

1 Introduction

The quadriceps femoris is a major muscle group, which includes the four prevailing muscles (rectus femoris, vastus lateralis, vastus medialis, and vastus intermedius) on the front of the thigh. All four quadriceps are powerful extensors of the knee joints which are crucial in walking, running, jumping, squatting and stabilizing the patella and the knee joint during gait [1]. Therefore, this study on quadriceps muscle (QM) activity is not only a exploreation of human body, but also expected to show its realistic significance with follow-up works. Nowadays, various techniques have been introduced in measuring muscle activities from different aspects, such as electromyography (EMG), mechanomyography (MMG) and ultrasonography (US), etc. To the best of our knowledge, as the most commonly used method [2], EMG has its own inherent limitations, such as the difficulty in collecting signals from single section of muscle or looking into the change of deep muscles when using the surface EMG.

---

* Corresponding author.

Y. Zhang et al. (Eds.): HIS 2014, LNCS 8423, pp. 47–54, 2014.

Similarly, MMG can be influenced by many factors of muscle morphology and the physical milieu. Ultrasonography is widely used in measuring morphology changes of skeletal muscles since it is low-cost, noninvasive and able to record instantaneous activities from the deeper muscles without cross-talk between adjacent ones [3]. So far, sonography has been used to measure the changes in muscle thickness[3,4,5,6], pennation angle [7,8,9,10], muscle fascicle length [3], [10,11,12], and muscle cross-sectional area [13,14,15] during isometric and dynamic contractions. As is know to all, these architectural parameters have a close relationship with the muscle functions [16], they can be potentially used to characterize muscle activities during its contraction. Among these morphological parameters, muscle thickness has the potential to be the most direct determinant factor in many aspects. For example, in [17] muscle thickness was introduced to estimate the muscle volume of the quadriceps femoris, while in [18] it was employed to quantify the muscle strength of people with severe cerebral palsy (CP). However, few studies focused on the relationship between quadriceps muscle thickness (QMT) and its torque output during isometric contraction.

Hodges *et al.* [3] reported that architectural parameters significantly changed with contractions up to 30% maximal voluntary contraction (MVC) but changed less at higher levels of contraction. To specify their relationship, a method to automatically detect muscle thickness is necessary, especially when the number of subjects is more than one. Recently, a coarse-to-fine method for real-time estimation of muscle thickness based on a compressive tracking algorithm had been proposed[19], which was proved to be sensitive and efficient. The more subjects there are, the more obvious its advantage is.

In this study, the details of this nonlinearity relationship between QMT changes during muscle contractions and synchronized torque signals are investigated with the application of the method mentioned above. The quantitating relationship can help provide more details to the muscle contraction mechanism.

2   Method

2.1   Subjects and Experiment Protocol

Thirteen healthy male subjects (mean ± SD, age=28.6 ± 0.6 years; body weight 67.0 ± 1.7 kg; height=1.72 ± 0.01 m) volunteered to participate in this study. None of them had a history of neuromuscular disorders, and all were aware of experimental purposes and procedures. Human subject ethical approval was obtained from the relevant committee in the authors'institution, and informed consent of each subject was obtained prior to the experiment.

The testing position of the subject was in accordance with the Users Guide of a Norm dynamometer (Humac/Norm Testing and Rehabilitation System, Computer Sports Medicine, Inc., Massachusetts, USA). Each subject was required to put forth his maximal effort of isometric knee extension for a period of 3 seconds with verbal encouragement provided. The MVC was defined as the highest value of torque recorded during the entire isometric contraction. The MVC torque was then calculated by averaging the two recorded highest torque values from the two tests. The subject was instructed to generate a torque waveform in ramp shape, up to 90% of his MVC, using isometric knee extension in prone position. The torque was measured by the aforementioned dynamometer and the reason for choosing 90% MVC as the highest value was to avoid muscle fatigue.

2.2   Data Acquisition and Data Processing

The sonography of muscle thickness was obtained using a real-time B-mode ultrasonic scanner (EUB-8500, Hitachi Medical Corporation, Tokyo, Japan) with a 10 MHz electronic linear array probe (L53L, Hitachi Medical Corporation, Tokyo, Japan). The long axis of the ultrasound probe was arranged perpendicularly to the long axis of the thigh on its superior aspect, 40% distally from the knee (measured from the anterior superior iliac spine to the superior patellar border). The ultrasound probe was fixed by a custom-designed foam container with fixing straps, and a very generous amount of ultrasound gel was applied to secure acoustic coupling between the probe and skin during muscle contractions, as shown in Fig.1. The probe was adjusted to optimize the contrast of muscle fascicles in ultrasound images. Then the B-mode ultrasound images were digitized by a video card (NI PCI-1411, National Instruments, Austin, USA) at a rate of 25 frame/s for later analysis. A total of 13 (subjects)×300 (frames) ultrasound images were acquired and all the images were cropped to keep the image content only. Ultrasound images and torque signals were simultaneously collected and stored by custom-developed software for the ultrasonic measurement of motion and elasticity (UMME, http://www.tups.org) for further analysis. All data were processed off-line using programs written in Matlab (Version 7.12, MathWorks, Inc., Massachusetts, USA).

2.3   Muscle Thickness Detection

In this study, a novel coarse-to-fine method based on a compressive-tracking algorithm was developed to detect the continuous MT changes in the ultrasound image sequence automatically. The method is carried out in two steps: coarse locating and fine-tuning. In the first image of each trial, two initial tracking windows are selected manually along the top of the rectus femoris muscle and femur, respectively. A representative example is shown in Fig. 2. The thickness of QM is defined as the minimum vertical distance between window A and window B. The location of window A is determined by the center-based method while window B is determined by the edge-based method. More details can be seen in our previous work [19].

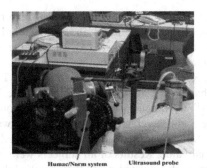

Fig. 1. Experimental setup for collecting ultrasound images from the subject's right quadriceps muscle during isometric contraction. The ultrasound probe was aligned perpendicularly to quadriceps muscle belly using a multi-degree adjustable bracket.

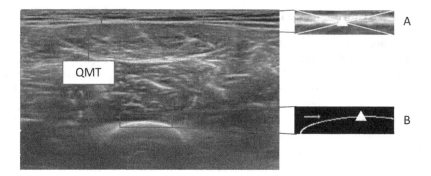

Fig. 2. Illustration of MT definitions. Two initial tracking windows A and B are selected to obtain QMT. B have been handled by the Canny edge detector and the maximal connected components search technology while A is determined by the center-based method. The triangles point out the locations of the selected window A and window B, respectively.

3   Results

3.1   Relationship between Thickness and Torque

A representative example of normalized QMT and torque is shown in Fig.3. Generally speaking, in contraction phase, QM thickness grew larger as the torque increased, while in relaxation phase, thickness also became smaller with the decrease of the torque. In this study, more attention was paid to the contraction phase. Moreover, the rising trend of muscle thickness is more gentle at higher level than that of torque. The nonlinearity relationship exists between them, which well agreed with a previous report [3]. The results of other subjects showed similar trends. Both torque and thickness are normalized to range of (0-1) in following sections.

3.2   Quantification of the Nonlinearity Relationship

To quantify the relationship between QM thickness and its torque output, 20 frames from each side of maximal torque were taken and the standard deviation (std) of this data set was calculated, as shown in Fig.3. Compared the result to the standard deviation of normalized QM thickness from same position, the flatter the curve is, the smaller the std would be. Results of all subjects were listed in Table 1.

Another method to characterize their relationship was the lag. When the muscle struggled to reach its MVC, the measured thickness is found to do not always simultaneously reach the same level. That is to say, there was a time discrepancy between the occurrence time of torque output and measured thickness when they reached their own maximal value. Results of all subjects were listed in Table 2. In the same way, time discrepancy also existed when they reached their own 50% maximal values, as shown in Table 3. Time discrepancy was calculated as:

$$time(s) = (f_T - f_Q)/25 \qquad (2)$$

where f_T was the frame that torque reached its maximal or 50% MVC and f_Q was the frame that QM thickness arrived at its highest level or 50% level during contraction. 25 (frame/s) is the rate of US. As shown in Table 3, the arrival of measured thickness at its 50% maximal value is earlier than that of the torque output (Table 3), while such relationship is not as obvious for 100% maximal value (Table 2). The temporal resolution is up to 0.04 seconds for all these time discrepancy, limited by the scanning frame rate of US.

Table 1. Normalized Std of QMT and torque output from forty frames of data which were taken from each side of the maximal torque equally

Subject	QMT Std	Torque Std
1	0.048	0.254
2	0.038	0.161
3	0.106	0.141
4	0.098	0.285
5	0.047	0.211
6	0.055	0.153
7	0.069	0.136
8	0.029	0.165
9	0.046	0.164
10	0.036	0.135
11	0.033	0.056
12	0.047	0.110
13	0.060	0.075
Mean	0.055	0.157

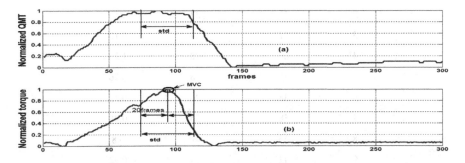

Fig. 3. (a) and (b) represent the normalized QMT and its torque output, respectively. Use torque as reference, 20 frames of each side of its MVC was taken. Std of this piece of data of both torque and QMT was calculated to quantitate their relationship.

Table 2. Time discrepancy of SMG and torque reaching their own maximum

Subject	Maximal torque(frame)	Maximal QMT(frame)	Time delay(s)
1	105	115	-0.4
2	88	87	0.04
3	86	96	-0.4
4	101	89	0.48
5	94	85	0.36
6	74	87	-0.52
7	81	89	-0.32
8	70	38	1.28
9	78	59	0.76
10	82	48	1.36
11	61	67	-0.24
12	84	85	-0.04
13	61	62	-0.04
Std	13.5	21.3	0.630
Mean	81.9	77.5	0.178

Table 3. Time discrepancy of SMG and torque reaching their 50% maximum

Subject	50% torque(frame)	50% QMT(frame)	Time delay(s)
1	47	33	0.56
2	51	37	0.56
3	47	44	0.12
4	60	28	1.28
5	57	38	0.76
6	38	20	0.72
7	58	36	0.88
8	26	6	0.8
9	42	19	0.92
10	38	15	0.92
11	16	5	0.44

Table 3. (*Continued.*)

12	43	27	0.64
13	19	13	0.24
Std	14.2	12.7	0.31
Mean	41.7	24.7	0.68

4   Discussion

In this study, two approaches are used to quantify the nonlinearity relationship between quadriceps thickness and its generated torque. Experimental results showed generally similar trends in QM thickness and torque output, that is, during contraction phase, both torque and thickness struggled to reach their maximal while in relaxation phase they went back to the original state slowly. From Table 1, std of torque was as several times as that of thickness, that means at higher levels QM thickness changed much less than its torque output. Another method we used to quantify the nonlinearity was named time discrepancy (100% maximum and 50% maximum), which were shown in Table 2 and Table 3. Hodges *et al.* [3] reported that architectural parameters changed markedly with contractions up to 30% maximal voluntary contraction. To evaluate the critical point, time discrepancy when they reached their own 30% maximal values was also calculated. The average of all subjects was 0.26 ± 0.20s. That means the nonlinearity relationship had already existed at 30% maximal value, but not as obvious as its 50% MVC. From Table 2 and 3, nonlinearity was validated for the disproportion of time discrepancy. Moreover, during relaxation phase, torque is always earlier to get back to its original state than thickness. Details of this phenomenon can be further investigated.

5   Conclusion

In conclusion, we applied a coarse-to-fine method based on the compressive tracking algorithm to US sequences of thirteen subjects to automatically detect thickness changes of QM during isometric knee extension. The results demonstrated the feasibility to disclose details about that nonlinearity existed between quadriceps thickness and torque with temporal resolution up to 0.04 seconds. Future studies are also necessary to investigate the relaxation phase of the muscle contractions.

Acknowledgement. The project is supported partially the next generation communication technology Major project of National S&T (2013ZX03005013), the Low-cost Healthcare Programs of Chinese Academy of Sciences, the Guangdong Innovative Research Team Program (2011S013, GIRTF-LCHT), International Science and Technology Cooperation Program of Guangdong Province (2012B050200004).

References

[1] Kisner, C., Colby, L.A.: Therapeutic Exercises, 5th edn., pp. 692–693 (2002)
[2] Mobasser, F., Eklund, J., Hashtrudi-Zaad, K.: Estimation of elbow-induced wrist force with EMG signals using fast orthogonal search. IEEE Trans. Biomed. Eng. 54, 683–693 (2007)

[3] Hodges, P., Pengel, L., Herbert, R., Gandevia, S.: Measurement of muscle contraction with ultrasound imaging. Muscle & Nerve 27, 682–692 (2003)

[4] Shi, J., Zheng, Y.-P., Chen, X., Huang, Q.: Assessment of muscle fatigue using sonomyography: Muscle thickness change detected from ultrasound images. Medical Engineering & Physics 29(4), 472–479 (2007)

[5] Thoirs, K., English, C.: Ultrasound measures of muscle thickness: intra-examiner reliability and influence of body position. Clinical Physiology and Functional Imaging 29(6), 440–446 (2009)

[6] Zheng, Y.-P., Chan, M., Shi, J., Chen, X., Huang, Q.: Sonomyography: Monitoring morphological changes of forearm muscles in actions with the feasibility for the control of powered prosthesis. Medical Engineering & Physics 28(5), 405–415 (2006)

[7] Zhou, Y., Zheng, Y.-P.: Estimation of muscle fiber orientation in ultrasound images using revoting hough transform (RVHT). Ultrasound in Medicine & Biology 34(9), 1474–1481 (2008)

[8] Zhou, Y., Zheng, Y.-P.: Longitudinal enhancement of the hyperechoic regions in ultrasonography of muscles using a gabor filter bank approach: A preparation for semi-automatic muscle fiber orientation estimation. Ultrasound in Medicine & Biology 37(4), 665–673 (2011)

[9] Zhou, Y., Li, J.-Z., Zhou, G., Zheng, Y.-P.: Dynamic measurement of pennation angle of gastrocnemius muscles during contractions based on Ultrasound imaging. BioMedical Engineering OnLine 11(63), 1–10 (2012)

[10] Maganaris, C., Baltzopoulos, V., Sargeant, A.: Repeated contractions alter the geometry of humanskeletal Muscle. Journal of Applied Physiology 93(6), 2089–2094 (2002)

[11] Narici, M., Binzoni, T., Hiltbrand, E., Fasel, J., Terrier, F., Cerretelli, P.: In vivo human gastrocnemius architecture with changing joint angle atrest and during graded isometric contraction. J. Physiology 496, 287–297 (1996)

[12] Fukunaga, T., Ichinose, Y., Ito, M., Kawakami, Y., Fukashiro, S.: Determination of fascicle length and pennation in a contracting human muscle invivo. J. Appl. Phys. 82, 354–358 (1997)

[13] Reeves, N., Maganaris, C., Narici, M.: Ultrasonographic assessment of human skeletalmuscle size. Eur. J. Appl. Physiol. 91, 116–118 (2004)

[14] Guo, J., Zheng, Y.-P., Xie, H., Chen, X.: Continuous monitoring of electromyography (EMG), Mechanomyography(MMG), sonomyography (SMG) torque output during rampand step isometric contractions. Medical Engineering & Physics 32(9), 1032–1042 (2010)

[15] Chen, X., Zheng, Y.-P., Guo, J.-Y., Zhu, Z., Chan, S.-C., Zhang, Z.: Sonomyographic responses during voluntary isometric ramp contraction of the human rectus femoris muscle. Eur. J. Appl. Physiol. 112, 2603–2614 (2012)

[16] Liber, R.L.: Skeletal muscle structure, function, and plasticity. Lippincott Williams & Wilkins (2002)

[17] Miyatani, M., Kanehisa, H., Kuno, S., Nishijima, T., Fukunaga, T.: Validity of ultrasonograph muscle thickness measurements for estimating muscle volume of knee extensors in humans. Eur. J. Appl. Physiol. 86(3), 203–208 (2002)

[18] Ohata, K., Tsuboyama, T., Ichihashi, N., Minami, S.: Measurement of muscle thickness as quantitative muscle evaluation for adults with severe cerebral palsy. Physical Therapy 86(9), 1231–1239 (2006)

[19] Li, J., Zhou, Y., Lu, Y., Zhou, G., Wang, L.: The sensitive and efficient detection of quadriceps muscle thickness changes in cross-sectional plane using ultrasonography: a feasibility investigation. IEEE J. Biomedical and Health Informatics (2013) (to be published), doi: 10.1109/JBHI2013.2.275502

A Comparative Study of Improvements Filter Methods Bring on Feature Selection Using Microarray Data

Yingying Wang, Xiaomao Fan, and Yunpeng Cai[*]

Research Center for Biomedical Information, Shenzhen Institutes of Advanced Technologies,
Chinese Academy of Sciences, Shenzhen, China
{yywang,xm.fan,yp.cai}@siat.ac.cn

Abstract. Feature selection techniques have become an apparent need in biomarker discoveries with the development of microarray. However, the high dimensional nature of microarray made feature selection become time-consuming. To overcome such difficulties, filter data according to the background knowledge before applying feature selection techniques has become a hot topic in microarray analysis. Different methods may affect final result greatly, thus it is important to evaluate these filter methods in a system way. In this paper, we compare the performance of statistical-based, biological-based filter methods and the combination of them on microRNA-mRNA parallel expression profiles using L1 logistic regression as feature selection techniques. Four types of data were built for both microRNA and mRNA expression profiles. Results showed that with similar or better AUC, precision and less features, filter-based feature selection should be taken into consideration if researchers need fast results when facing complex computing problems in bioinformatics.

Keywords: comparative study, feature selection, microarray.

1   Introduction

During the last decade, feature selection techniques have become an apparent need in biomarker discoveries [1]. With the development of experimental molecular biology, scientists could detect the expression of molecular on omics scale using microarray. Probes were often designed based on messenger RNA (mRNA) transcripts and/or microRNAs (miRNAs, a class of small, non-coding RNAs that play important regulation roles by targeting hundreds or even thousands of target genes) thus made analyses of mRNA and/or miRNAs expression profiles become one of the most widely used basic techniques in geneome-wide RNA microarray analyses studies. Microarrays detecting thousands of miRNAs have become a new hot topic in many fields such as biomarker discovery, etc. The microarray technology could help improving disease classification and diagnosis at molecular levels. However, the high dimensional nature of microarray made feature selection become time-consuming processes.

---

[*] Corresponding author.

Y. Zhang et al. (Eds.): HIS 2014, LNCS 8423, pp. 55–62, 2014.
© Springer International Publishing Switzerland 2014

To overcome such difficulties, filter some features according to the characteristics of data before applying feature selection techniques become a kind of popular methods. Researchers often pay attention to statistics significance and/or biological functions of analyses results. Thus, many filter methods had been proposed based on statistical or biological considerations as follows: (1) statistical-based filter methods: using statistical methods to find out the differential expressed molecular among different conditions. Differential expression molecular identifications are often the first step of microarray and are also one of the most commonly used filter methods. In such kind of procedure, statistical test: such as t-test are usually chosen due to their stability and easy operability. (2) biological-based filter methods: using enrichment analysis based on biological function and/or pathway information to find out potential disease-related molecular. Gene Ontology (GO) is widely used in molecular function analyses while biological pathways are used to exhibit the structure of some biological processes in a systematic way.

However, it is unclear to us that how much improvements these filter methods could bring on the feature selection results. In this paper, we compare the performance of these two kinds of filter methods and the combination of them on 4 miRNAs and 10 mRNA microarray datasets, all the class labels of these samples were known. L1 logistic regression was used as feature selection and 5-fold cross validation was adopted as results evaluation. Our results showed that both of the two kinds of filter methods could increase classification precision slightly while the combination of them could increase the AUC (Area Under Curve) of ROC (Receiver Operating Characteristic) curve slightly.

2   Materials and Methods

2.1   Microarray Dataset

miRNA and mRNA expression profiles of human hypertrophic cardiomyopathy (HCM) were downloaded from NCBI GEO (GSE36961and GSE36964). Samples with both miRNA and mRNA taken from a same person were collected from 106 HCM patients and 20 healthy donors. The raw miRNA microarray data contained 1145 probes which could be mapped to 819 mature miRNAs. The raw mRNA microarray data contained 37846 probes which could be mapped to 18756 Ensembl genes.

2.2   Construction of mRNA Dataset

4 types of mRNA data were built as follows (See Figure 1 for details)

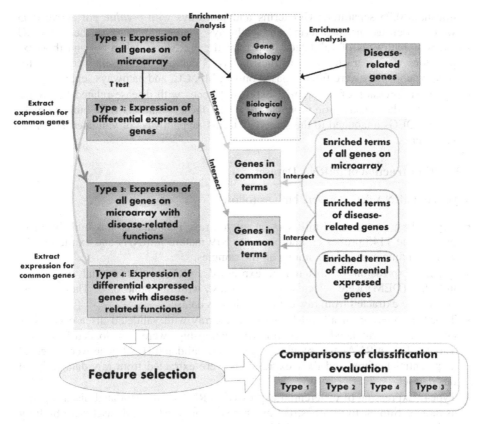

Fig. 1. Framework of mRNA analysis in this study. Tangles filled with different colors represented the 4 types of mRNA datasets (dark green for type1, light green for type2, purple for type3, and pink for type4) while lines with different colors represent 3 kinds of analysis (light and dark orange for intersect, purple and pink for extracting expression for common genes, and black for enrichment analysis).

- Type1: Expression of all genes on microarray. This dataset was built by mapping all the 37846 probes on microarray to 18756 Ensembl genes and extracting the corresponding expressions among all the samples.
- Type2: Expression of differential expressed genes. Differential expression genes (DEG) were selected based on t-test, with threshold 0.05. Their expressions were extracted from raw data to build this dataset.
- Type3: Expression of all genes on microarray with disease related functions. 372 validated HCM related genes were collected from GeneCards [2] and GAD [3]. The terms of 3 domains of GO (Gene Ontology) [4] were included in this study: 5140 biological process (BP) terms, 2782 molecular function (MF) terms, and 851 cellular component (CC) terms. 2999 biological pathways were downloaded from several online databases including BioCarta[5], KEGG[6], Pathway Interaction Database[7], Reactome[8]. The 372 genes and all genes on microarray were annotated to GO and pathways by enrichment analysis using hypergeometric test with

threshold 0.05 separately. GO terms and pathways with *p-value* not above 0.05 were chosen as enriched terms and pathways. Genes annotated to the same GO terms or pathways of validated HCM related genes were picked out and their expressions were extracted to construct the type3 datasets. 4 datasets were built for such type for they were filtered based on BP, MF, CC, and pathways separately.

- Type4: Expression of differential expressed genes with disease-related functions. Similar to the construction processes of type3, these 4 datasets were built by picking out DEGs annotated to the same GO terms or pathways of validated HCM related genes.

2.3   Construction of miRNA Dataset

4 types of miRNA datasets were built as follows:

- Type1: Expression of all miRNAs on microarray. This dataset was built by mapping all the 1145 probes on microarray to 819 mature miRNAs and extracting the corresponding expressions among all the samples.
- Type2: Expression of differential expressed miRNAs. Differential expression miRNAs (DEM) were selected based on t-test, with threshold 0.05. Their expressions were extracted from raw data to build this dataset.
- Type3: Expression of all miRNAs on microarray with validated disease genes as targets. 19550 validated miRNA-mRNA relationships were downloaded from mirTarBase [9]. miRNAs that regulate at least one validated HCM gene were selected as potential features and their expressions were extracted from raw data to build this dataset.
- Type4: Expression of differential expressed miRNAs with validated disease genes as targets. Similar to the construction processes of type3, this dataset were built by picking out the expression of DEMs that had at least one validated HCM genes as target.

2.4   Feature Selection

We used L1 logistic regression to perform the feature selection procedures due to its ability to dispose the high dimensional data [10]. The model describes are as follows:

Let $D = \{x^n, y_n\}_{n=1}^{N}$ denotes the dataset, where $x_n \in R^N$ is the n-th feature and $y_n \in R$ is the label of the n-th observer. We used (w, b) as the coefficients and intercept of *L1* logistic regression. The following is the problem of the *L1* logistic regression model:

$$\min_{w,b} f(w,b) = \frac{1}{N} \sum_{n=1}^{N} L(y_n, w^T x^{(n)} + b) + \lambda \sum_{j} |w_j|$$

where $L(.)$ is the loss function and λ is a regularization parameter which has the ability to dispose high dimensional data.

2.5   Evaluation of Classification Results

5-fold cross validation was used to analyses the classification results of L1 logistic regression on all the 14 datasets (10 mRNA datasets and 4 miRNA datasets). AUC value, precision, and computing time were computed and compared for these test datasets.

3   Results and Discussion

3.1   Effects of Filter Methods on Reducing Feature Dimension

4 types of datasets were built for the mRNA expression profiles. The detailed information for the number of raw variables in each set could be found in Table 1. Statistical-based filter methods (Type2) could reduce the dimension of raw data (Type1) which can be found in Table 1 (Type1 contained 18756 features while this number decreased to 3604 after t-test). Compared with this, biological-based filter methods reduce some features while the combination of the two methods reduces about 8/9 of the features in mRNA expression profiles.

Table 1. Dataset built for mRNA expression profile

	Type1	Type2	Type3				Type4			
			BP	MF	CC	Pathway	BP	MF	CC	Pathway
Raw variables	18756	3604	10542	11149	10678	13603	2116	2232	2135	2808
Selected features	8465	168	60	270	628	248	416	131	239	482

For 4 datasets of miRNA, both the statistical-based and biological-based filter methods could reduce the number of features greatly while the combination of them could extract 8 miRNAs from all the 819 mature ones (See Table 2 for details).

Table 2. Data set built for miRNA expression profile

	Type1	Type2	Type3	Type4
Raw variables	819	114	37	8
Selected features	23	46	23	3
AUC	0.5990566	0.5698113	0.5216981	0.4358491
Precision	0.6031746	0.6190476	0.4761905	0.3968254
Computing time(second)	61.424	26.986	26.972	12.911

3.2   Effects of Filter Methods on Classification Performance

Our results showed that for mRNA expression profiles, the filter methods could increase the classification precision (See Fig.2 for details). These indicated that filter methods may improve the performance of feature selection techniques on samples' positive prediction levels. However, only combined filter methods increased the AUC values slightly (from 0.5764151 to 0. 5933962).

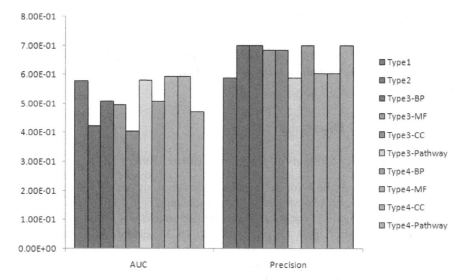

Fig. 2. Comparison of AUC and classification precision of 4 types of mRNA data. The bars in the graph are clustered in two groups: the left group marked as "AUC" on the x-axes means the height of the bars stand for the AUC values of each dataset while the right group marked as "Precision" on the x-axes means the height of the bars stand for the precision values of each dataset. The 10 datasets are represented with 10 different colors as shown in the figure legend.

The performance of filter methods on miRNA expression profile did not show similar results with mRNA (See Table 2 for details). All the filter methods did not show improvements on AUC which may partly due to the small number of features Type2-4 contain. Only Type2 could improve the precision slightly (from 0.6031746 to 0.6190476).

3.3   Effects of Filter Methods on Computing Time

All the computing time were shortened after all the filter methods used in this paper (See Table 2 and Fig.3 for details). These indicated us that a dramatically advantage of applying filter methods before feature selection is the shortening of computing time. With similar or better classification improvements and less features, filter-based feature selection should be taken into consideration if researchers need fast results when facing complex computing problems in bioinformatics.

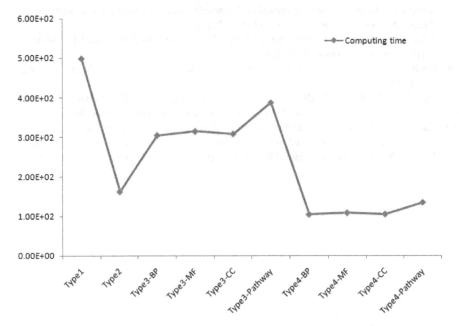

Fig. 3. Comparison of computing time for 4 types of mRNA data. The points stand for the computing time of all the 4 types of mRNA data which including 10 datasets.

4 Conclusion

Feature selection techniques are often time-consuming when applied on microarray datasets without filters. Our results showed that filter methods could reduce the computing time of the procedure while keeping or improving precision compared with the results of feature selection based on raw dataset.

Acknowledgment. This work was supported by National Natural Science Foundation of China (Grant No. 31022995) and the development funds for Key Laboratory in Shenzhen (Grant No. CXB201104220026A).

References

1. Saeys, Y., Inza, I., Larranaga, P.: A review of feature selection techniques in bioinformatics. Bioinformatics 23(19), 2507–2517 (2007)
2. Rebhan, M., et al.: GeneCards: integrating information about genes, proteins and diseases. Trends Genet. 13(4), 163 (1997)
3. Becker, K.G., et al.: The genetic association database. Nat. Genet. 36(5), 431–432 (2004)
4. Ashburner, M., et al.: Gene ontology: tool for the unification of biology. The Gene Ontology Consortium. Nat. Genet. 25(1), 25–29 (2000)
5. Nishimura, D.: BioCarta. Biotech Software & Internet Report 2(3), 117–120 (2001)

6. Kanehisa, M., et al.: Data, information, knowledge and principle: back to metabolism in KEGG. Nucleic Acids Res. 42(1), 199–205 (2014)

7. Schaefer, C.F., et al.: PID: the Pathway Interaction Database. Nucleic Acids Res. 37(Database issue), D674–D679 (2009)

8. Croft, D., et al.: The Reactome pathway knowledgebase. Nucleic Acids Res. 42(1), D472–D477 (2014)

9. Hsu, S.D., et al.: miRTarBase: a database curates experimentally validated microRNA-target interactions. Nucleic Acids Res. 39(Database issue), D163–D169 (2011)

10. Cai, Y., et al.: Fast Implementation of l1 Regularized Learning Algorithms Using Gradient Descent Methods. In: Proceedings of the 10th SIAM International Conference on Data Mining (SDM 2010), Columbus, Ohio, USA, pp. 862–871 (2010)

Real-Time Estimation of Tibialis Anterior Muscle Thickness from Dysfunctional Lower Limbs Using Sonography

Xiaolong Li[1,2], Huihui Li[1], Jizhou Li[1], Yongjin Zhou[1,*], and Jianhao Tan[2]

[1] Shenzhen Institutes of Advanced Technology, Chinese Academy of Sciences, China
[2] Hunan University, China
y.zhou.cn@ieee.org

Abstract. Muscle thickness is an important parameter related to musculoskeletal functions and has been studied in many ways and for various purposes. In recent years, ultrasound imaging has been widely used for measuring muscle properties of human muscles non-invasively, with the advantages of real time and low cost. The muscle thickness is usually measured manually, which is subjective and time consuming. In addition, there are few studies on automatic estimation of muscle thickness during dynamic contraction. In this study, an automatic estimation method based on compressive tracking algorithm is proposed to detect the thickness changes of tibialis anterior muscle during dynamic contraction on ultrasound images. The performance of the proposed method is compared to manual detection using clinical images from tibialis anterior muscles of ten patients. As a result, we found that the proposed method agrees well with the manual measurement, and it was able to provide an accurate and efficient approach for estimating muscle thickness during human motion.

Keywords: Muscle thickness, Ultrasound image, Tibialis anterior, Compressive tracking.

1 Introduction

Ultrasound imaging has been widely adopted to investigate morphology changes of skeletal muscles as it has many advantages, such as being stable, easy to use, low cost, and able to provide real time images and to view the deeper muscle fiber dynamics during contraction [1]. Recently, ultrasound imaging has been introduced to qualify the muscle changes during contractions [2] [3], such as in muscle thickness [4], pennation angle [5], fascicle length [6] and other properties [7] [8]. As these architectural parameters are directly related to the mechanical properties of the muscle during dynamic contraction. They are able to provide a valid method for revealing the intrinsic muscle characteristic [9][10].

Muscle thickness is a very important parameter related to musculoskeletal functions; it is probably the most direct determinant to quantify muscle activity in the

---

[*] Corresponding author.

Y. Zhang et al. (Eds.): HIS 2014, LNCS 8423, pp. 63–71, 2014.

cross-sectional plane among these morphological parameters [4] [11]. In most cases, muscle thickness was conventionally detected manually in ultrasound images of muscles, for example [12] [13], but with the increasing amount of ultrasound images, it is time-consuming to manually obtain or measure these muscle architecture parameters. Subsequently this greatly affects the wider applications of these parameters, particularly for the study of dynamic muscle contraction.

Recently, a number of studies have been reported for the automatic estimation of muscle thickness or other related parameters using normalized cross-correlation algorithm (NCC) [3] [14]. However, the NCC method has several drawbacks, such as too sensitive to the size of tracking window. In this study, we applied an automatic tracking algorithm to achieve the continuous and quantitative measurement for muscle thickness of tibialis anterior (TA) in ultrasound images. The core concept of this algorithm is to manually select two initial windows in ultrasound image and adopt the compressive tracking strategy in [15] to automatically track the window location in the next frame. In addition, center-based method [4] was used to obtain more precise results.

2   Method

2.1   Method Overview

Ten patients who had cerebral surgery in the physical therapy rehabilitation center for post Intracerebral Hemorrhage rehabilitation were recruited to participate in the study, and consent forms were obtained from the patients and his/her authorized legal representatives. Human subject ethical approval was granted by the authors_institution.

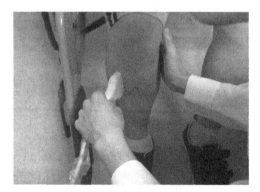

Fig. 1. Experimental setup for collecting ultrasound images from the subject's TA

The patients were in the seat position on an anchored wheel chair and performed ankle joint dorsiflexion under the direction of examiner. In this process, tibialis anterior muscle contraction was recorded using ultrasound imaging and a motion capture system simultaneously. The ultrasound device was used with a linear array ultrasound (US) transducer (Sonostar Technologies Co., Ltd., Zhuhai, Guangdong, China). The transducer was held properly by examiner to ensure consistent image acquisition in the test. Subject activity was controlled by cadence so that examiner could hold the position of probe on target. Besides, adequate coupling gel was used on transducer to guarantee sound wave well travel through the skin. Frequency of US transducer was at

7.5 (MHz) with 70 (mm) depth detection, as shown in Fig.1. Then the images were collected from the patients on the tibialis anterior muscle under the relaxed condition. A total of 10 (subjects) ×128 (frames) ultrasound images with 251×431 pixels were acquired and all the images were cropped to keep the image content only. All data were processed using programs written in matlab (Version R2011b) on a PC equipped with Windows 7, Intel (R) Core T6570 2.10 GHz processors and 2GB RAM.

2.2   Tracking Strategy

The proposed method of this study for continuously detecting the muscle thickness changes includes two steps: coarse locating and exact distance extraction. The first step of the method is to extract coarse location using the compressive tracking algorithm [10] [16]. For each subject's ultrasound image sequence, we manually select two initial tracking windows along the top and bottom of tibialis anterior muscle in the first frame. As shown in Fig.2. For each incoming frame, these results from previous frame could be used as prior knowledge to track the boundary of tibialis anterior muscle. The classifier will be updated in this process in real time, and some samples around the current target location are drawn to predict the object location in the next frame, and the one with the maximum classification score is treated as the expected location [4]. The main steps of compressive tracking are briefed as follows:

Input: t-th image frames.

- For a series of images, $D^{\gamma} = \left\{ z \middle| \| l(z) - l_{t-1} \| < \gamma \right\}$ where l_{t-1} is the tracking location at the (t-1)-th frame, and extract the features with non-adaptive low dimensionality based on compressive sensing theories.
- For each sample $z \in R^m$, its low-dimensional representation is $v = (v_1, ..., v_n)^T \in R^n$ with $m \gg n$. All elements in v are assumed independently distributed. A naive Bayes classifier H is used in each feature vector

$$H(v) = \log \left(\frac{\prod_{i=1}^{n} p(v_i \mid y=1) p(y=1)}{\prod_{i=1}^{n} p(v_i \mid y=0) p(y=0)} \right) = \sum_{i=1}^{n} \log \left(\frac{v_i \mid y=1}{v_i \mid y=0} \right) \tag{1}$$

Where $p(y=1) = p(y=0)$, $y \in \{0, 1\}$ is a binary variable which represents the sample label. The conditional distributions $p(v_i \mid y=1)$ and $p(v_i \mid y=0)$ in the classifier $H(v)$ are assumed to be Gaussian distributed with four parameters $(\mu_i^1, \sigma_i^1, \mu_i^0, \sigma_i^0)$ where

$$p(v_i \mid y=0) \sim N(\mu_i^0, \sigma_i^0), \ p(v_i \mid y=1) \sim N(\mu_i^1, \sigma_i^1) \tag{2}$$

and the maximal classifier response is used to find the tracking location l_t.

- Sample two sets of image patches, $D^{\gamma} = \left\{ z \middle| \| l(z) - l_t \| < \alpha \right\}$ and $D^{\varsigma, \beta} = \left\{ z \middle| \varsigma < \| l(z) - l_t \| < \beta \right\}$ with $\alpha < \varsigma < \beta$.

- Extract the Haar-like features with these two sets of samples and the scalar parameters in (2) are incrementally updated by

$$\begin{cases} \mu_i^1 \leftarrow \lambda\mu_i^1 + (1-\lambda)\mu^1 \\ \sigma_i^1 \leftarrow \sqrt{\lambda(\sigma_i^1)^2 + (1-\lambda)(\sigma^1)^2 + \lambda(1-\lambda)(\mu_i^1 - \mu^1)^2} \end{cases} \tag{3}$$

Output: Tracking location l_t and classifier parameters.

The main components of compressive tracking algorithm are shown in Fig.2 and more implementation details can be found in [16].

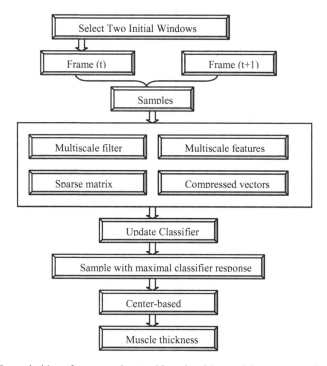

Fig. 2. The main idea of compressive tracking algorithm and the coarse-to-fine method

2.3   The Detection of Muscle Thickness

Now that we have tracked the target location and got the exact positions, muscle thickness can be calculated from the vertical distance between the two windows, i.e., the thickness of tibialis anterior muscle is the distance between window A and window B, and the distance between window A and B will be calculated as the center-based distance as proposed in [4].

For each frame, the windows distance is calculated as the vertical distance between the centers of window A and window B, which is distinctly illustrated in Fig.3.

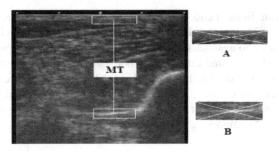

Fig. 3. Illustration of muscle thickness definitions. Two initial tracking windows A and B are selected to obtain muscle thickness (MT). The intersections point out the locations of the selected window A and window B respectively.

3   Results

The manual detection is accomplished by one clinical expert, the operation is repeated for three times and the results are averaged to obtain the final results.

Tracking result comparison between two methods are shown in Fig.4 and Table 1. Blue and red lines in Fig.4 represent results from the proposed method and manual measurement respectively, and the Mean in Table 1 represents the mean difference and standard deviation of all frames from ten subjects.

Table 1. The difference between manually detection and proposed method

Subject	Mean Difference (mm)	Standard Deviation
1	-0.89	0.84
2	0.29	0.74
3	-0.37	0.70
4	0.77	1.17
5	-0.56	0.33
6	-0.46	0.82
7	1.01	0.41
8	-0.28	0.85
9	-0.05	0.54
10	-0.07	0.64
Mean	-0.24	0.90

It is not hard to see from the curves in Fig.4 that two results are close to each other. As shown in Table 1, results from the proposed method agree very well with those from the manual measurement, and for data from individual subject, the maximum mean difference of two methods is 0.89 mm, and the mean difference is within 1.01 mm and less than 0.50 mm in most cases. For all of the image frames of the ten subjects, the mean difference is -0.24 mm and the standard deviation is 0.90 mm. Furthermore, we used the SPSS software to analysis the difference between results from manual detection and proposed method. It's found that they are not statistically significantly different and the differences fit the normal distribution well, as shown in Fig. 5. It can be concluded that the proposed method is both robust and accuracy, and the accuracy can be further improved by selecting the appropriate initial window. Certainly, the detecting results could be more precise by improving the quality of acquired images.

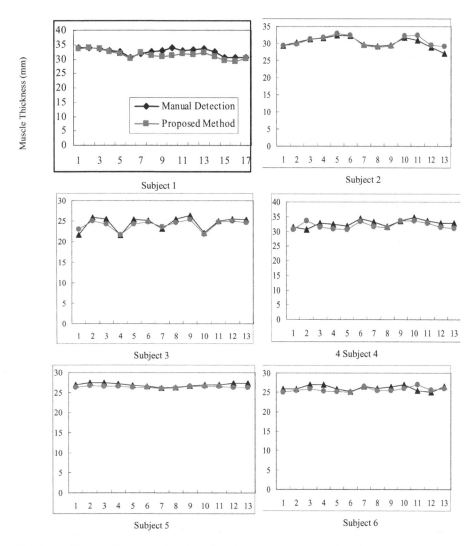

Fig. 4. Tracking results comparison between the proposed method (red line) and manual measurement (blue line). The x-axis represents the muscle thickness and the y-axis the t-th image frame.

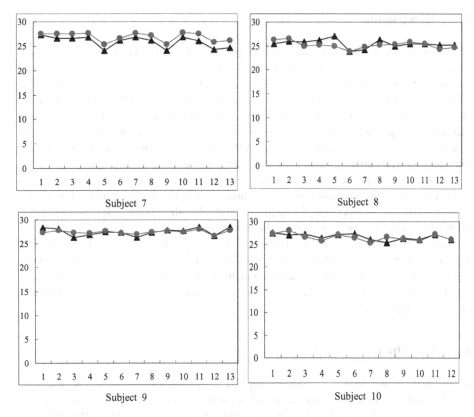

Subject 7

Subject 8

Subject 9

Subject 10

Fig. 4. (*Continued.*)

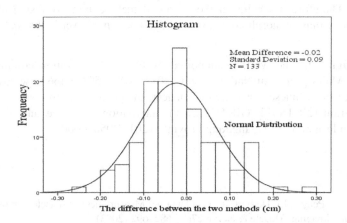

Fig. 5. Histogram and the Normal Distribution for the differences between results from the proposed method and manual measurement

4   Discussion

This proposed a method for automatic estimation of TA thickness during dynamic contraction for dysfunctional lower limbs. The comparison between the results using the proposed method and those using manual measurement showed that the proposed method can detect the muscle thickness efficiently and results for thickness estimation of TA is not statistically significantly different from those using the conventional manual drawing. Meanwhile, the efficient automatic estimation of TA thickness also enabled the continuous monitoring of TA morphology during ankle exercises with fine temporal resolution, limited only by the frame rate of ultrasonography.

It was found from the experiment that the compressive tracking algorithm can be inaccurate when the boundary of tibialis anterior muscle in the original ultrasound images is indistinct (especially for aged patients). In other words, the performance of the method is occasionally limited by the image quality.

Despite these limitations, the findings of this study - that ultrasound measures of muscle thickness can be obtained both accurately and in real-time, once further validated in clinical settings, this measurement method will provide the necessary measurement tool to investigate changes in skeletal muscle mass in acutely ill people and to evaluate appropriate interventions.

5   Conclusions

In this article, we have successfully applied a method of automatically detecting muscle thickness in a huge amount of ultrasound images of tibialis anterior muscles from dysfunctional lower limbs. The preliminary results obtained using the proposed methods agree well with those obtained using manual measurement but with much less labor. Therefore it's believed the proposed method is a promising alternative means to study muscle morphology, even for dysfunctional lower limbs such as TA.

Acknowledgment. The work is supported by the next generation communication technology Major project of National S&T (2013ZX03005013), the Low-cost Healthcare Programs of Chinese Academy of Sciences, the Guangdong Innovative Research Team Program (2011S013, GIRTF-LCHT), International Science and Technology Cooperation Program of   Guangdong Province (2012B050200004).

References

1. Hodges, P., Pengel, L., Herbert, R., Gandevia, S.: Measurement of muscle contraction with ultrasound imaging. Muscle & Nerve 27(6), 682–692 (2003)
2. Han, P., Chen, Y., Ao, L., Xie, G., Li, H., Wang, L., Zhou, Y.: Automatic thickness estimation for skeletal muscle in ultrasonography: evaluation of two enhancement methods. BioMedical Engineering OnLine 12(6) (2013), doi:10.1186/1475-925X-12-6

3. Thoirs, K., English, C.: Ultrasound measures of muscle thickness: intra-examiner reliability and influence of body position. Clinical Physiology and Functional Imaging 29(6), 440–446 (2009)
4. Li, J., Zhou, Y.J., Zheng, Y.-P., Wang, L., Guo, J.-Y.: Sensitive and Efficient Detection of Quadriceps Muscle Thickness Changes in Cross-sectional Plane using Ultrasonography: A Feasibility Investigation. IEEE Journal of Biomedical and Health Informatics (2013), doi:10.1109/JBHI.2013.2275002
5. Zhou, Y., Zheng, Y.-P.: Longitudinal enhancement of the hyperechoic regions in ultrasonography of muscles using a gabor filter bank approach: A preparation for semi-automatic muscle fiber orientation estimation. Ultrasound in Medicine & Biology 37(4), 665 – 673 (2011)
6. Loram, I.D., Maganaris, C., Lakie, M.: Use of ultrasound to make noninvasive in vivo measurement of continuous changes in human muscle contractile length. Journal of Applied Physiology 100(4), 1311–1323 (2006)
7. Muramatsu, T., Muraoka, T., Kawakami, Y., Shibayama, A., Fukunaga, T.: In vivo determination of fascicle curvature in contracting human skeletal muscles. Journal of Applied Physiology 92, 129–134 (2002)
8. Guo, J., Zheng, Y.-P., Xie, H., Chen, X.: Continuous monitoring of electromyography (EMG), mechanomyography (MMG), sonomyography (SMG) and torque output during ramp and step isometric contractions. Medical Engineering & Physics 32(9), 1032–1042 (2010)
9. Kass, M., Witkin, A.: Analyzing oriented patterns. Comput. Vis. Graph, Image Process 37, 362–397 (1987)
10. Li, J., Zhou, Y.J., Ivanov, K., Zheng, Y.-P.: Estimation and visualization of longitudinal muscle motion using ultrasonography: A feasibility study. Ultrasonics 54(3) (2014), doi:10.1016/j.ultras.2013.09.024
11. Chen, X., Zheng, Y.-P., Guo, J.-Y., Zhu, Z., Chan, S.-C., Zhang, Z.: Sonomyographic responses during voluntary isometric ramp contraction of the human rectus femoris muscle. European Journal of Applied Physiology 112(7), 2603–2614 (2012)
12. Berg, H.E., Tedner, B., Tesch, P.A.: Changes in lower limb muscle crosssectional area and tissue fluid volume after transition from standing to supine. Acta Physiol. Scand. 148, 379–385 (1993)
13. Zheng, Y.-P., Chan, M., Shi, J., Chen, X., Huang, Q.H.: Sonomyography: Monitoring morphological changes of forearm muscles in actions with the feasibility for the control of powered prosthesis. Med. Eng. Phys. 28, 405–415 (2006)
14. Guo, J., Zheng, Y.-P., Huang, Q., Chen, X., He, J., Lai-Wa Chan, H.: Performances of one-dimensional sonomyography and surface electromyography in tracking guided patterns of wrist extension. Ultrasound in Medicine & Biology 35(6), 894–902 (2009)
15. Chen, X., Zheng, Y.-P., Guo, J.-Y., Shi, J.: Sonomyography (SMG) control for powered prosthetic hand: A study with normal subjects. Ultrasound in Medicine & Biology 36(7), 1076–1088 (2010)
16. Zhang, K., Zhang, L., Yang, M.-H.: Real-time compressive tracking. In: Fitzgibbon, A., Lazebnik, S., Perona, P., Sato, Y., Schmid, C. (eds.) ECCV 2012, Part III. LNCS, vol. 7574, pp. 864–877. Springer, Heidelberg (2012)

A Prosthesis Control System
Based on the Combination of Speech
and sEMG Signals and Its Performance Assessment

Zheng Wei[1,2], Peng Fang[1,2,*], Lan Tian[1], Qifang Zhuo[1,2], and Guanglin Li[1,2]

[1] Shenzhen Institutes of Advanced Technology,
Chinese Academy of Sciences, Shenzhen, China
[2] University of Chinese Academy of Sciences, Beijing, China
{zheng.wei,peng.fang,lan.tian,qf.zhuo,gl.li}@siat.ac.cn

Abstract. Surface electromyographic (sEMG) signals from the residual limb muscles after amputation have been widely used for prosthesis control. However, for the amputees with high-level amputations, there usually exists a dilemma that the sEMG signal sources for prosthesis control are limited but more limb motions need to be recovered, which strongly limits the practicality of the current myoelectric prostheses. In order to operate prostheses with multiple degrees of freedom (DOF) of movements, several control protocols have been suggested in some previous studies to deal with this dilemma. In this paper, a prosthesis control system based on the combination of speech and sEMG signals (*Strategy 1*) was built up in laboratory conditions, where speech commands were applied for the prosthesis joint-mode switching and sEMG signals were applied to determine the motion-class and execute the target movement. The control performance of the developed system was evaluated and compared with that of the traditional control strategy based on the pattern recognition of sEMG signals (*Strategy 2*). The experimental results showed that the difference between *Strategy 1* and *Strategy 2* was insignificant for the control of a 2-DOF prosthesis, but *Strategy 1* was much better in the control of a prosthesis with more DOFs in comparison to *Strategy 2*. In addition, the positive user experience also demonstrated the reliability and practicality of *Strategy 1*.

Keywords: sEMG, Speech, Prosthesis control, Pattern recognition, Limb Amputee.

1   Introduction

Multifunctional prostheses are very useful for amputees to recover the lost body functions and improve their life quality. Up to now, most modern motorized prostheses are controlled with the surface electromyographic (sEMG) signals from muscles of residual limbs, and several methods have been developed to realize possible practical control of myoelectric prostheses [1-4]. Conventionally, sEMG signals from a pair of

---

* Corresponding author.

Y. Zhang et al. (Eds.): HIS 2014, LNCS 8423, pp. 72–82, 2014.
© Springer International Publishing Switzerland 2014

residual muscles are applied to control one degree of freedom (DOF) of movements [5]. However, in the case of high-level amputations, the residual muscles are usually limited and cannot supply sufficient sEMG signals for the control of multifunctional prostheses with multiple DOFs. In order to control multiple DOFs with a pair of residual muscle (a muscle pair), a so-called "mode switching" [6] procedure is used for the switching among different joints, which is mostly realized by simultaneous co-contractions of a muscle pair. Take a 3-DOF-prosthesis as example: it has three joint-modes of "hand", "wrist" and "elbow", and sEMG signals recorded from the muscle pair of bicep-tricep determine the motion-classes of each joint. The switching among the three joint is performed by the co-contraction of bicep-tricep muscle pair as well. The predetermined switching order is "hand-wrist-elbow..." and the current mode is "hand". If the user wants to do an elbow movement, he/she has to conduct the co-contraction of the muscle pair twice to switch the joint-mode from "hand" to "wrist" and from "wrist" to "elbow", and then contracts either the bicep or the tricep to execute an elbow movement. In this way, users have to take a lot of time and efforts in the mode switching and always remember the current joint-mode. As a result, the control method based on the sequential mode switching is strongly limited and commonly rejected by most of the users.

To improve the control performance of the current myoelectric prostheses, a control strategy based on the pattern recognition of sEMG signals has been proposed [7-8]. Here, a pattern recognition algorithm is applied to classify the target motion-classes by decoding the sEMG signals from residual muscles. However, the pattern recognition method is still not much practical if there are not enough residual muscles, especially after high-level amputations. In addition, the signal quality, the operation flexibility, and the real-time patter recognition algorithm are also big challenges which prevent the further improvement of this method.

Some extra non-sEMG signals have been taken into account to overcome the problem of insufficient sEMG signal sources in the present prosthesis control, and one of the possible candidate control information may be the human speech [9]. Speech is a native ability for most people except for the language disabled, and is also independent off the limb functions and amputation conditions. In our pilot study [9], the speech signals were used as additional information and combined together with the sEMG signals for the control of a multifunctional myoelectric prosthesis. A PC-based control system was built up and the primal results demonstrated the practicality of the proposed strategy.

In order to further investigate the performance of the recently proposed control strategy for its practical application, in this work, an embedded myoelectric-prosthesis control system was built up in laboratory conditions by the combination of speech and sEMG signals (*Strategy 1*). For comparison purpose, another system based on the pattern recognition of sEMG signals was also set up. The control performances of both systems were evaluated and compared. The outcomes of this study could make an important progress of the proposed method toward developing a practical prosthesis control system for clinical use.

2   Method

2.1   Subjects

In this study, three able-bodied subjects (marked as *A1*, *A2* and *A3*) and one unilateral transradial amputee (marked as *B1*) were recruited. The demographic information of the subjects is summarized in Table 1. All subjects had full language competence. The protocol of this research was approved by the Institutional Review Board of Shenzhen Institutes of Advanced Technology, Chinese Academy of Sciences. All subjects gave written informed consent and provided permission for publication of photographs for a scientific and educational purpose.

Table 1. Demographic information of the subjects recruited in the study

Subjects	Gender	Age	Body situation	Test side
A1	Male	22	Able-bodied	Right
A2	Male	31	Able-bodied	Right
A3	Male	24	Able-bodied	Right
B1	Male	24	Right forearm amputated	Right

2.2   Control Strategies

In the experiments, a commercial myoelectric prosthesis from *Shanghai Kesheng MH32, China* was used. This prosthesis has three joint-modes of "hand", "wrist", and "elbow", and each joint-mode involves two motion-classes as "hand closing/opening", "wrist pronation/supination", and "elbow flexion/extension". Two control systems based on different strategies were built up and examined in the study:

(1) *System 1(Strategy 1)*: Prosthesis control based on the combination of speech and sEMG signals

In *Strategy 1*, the joint-mode switching was firstly conducted according to the user's speech commands, and then the sEMG signals from a muscle pair were used to determine one of two motion-classes involved in the selected joint-mode and execute the target movement, as shown in Fig 1.

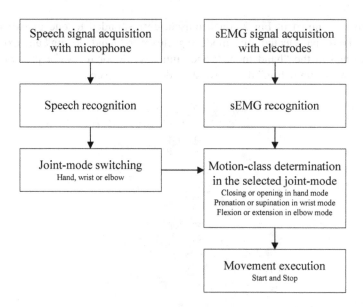

Fig. 1. *Strategy 1:* Prosthesis control based on the combination of speech and sEMG signals

In an office environment (background noise of 55±5 dB), speech signals were acquired with a commercial throat microphone that was attached to the subject's larynx near the vocal folds. Different from normal microphones, the throat microphone only recorded the speech signals transferred through the larynx and was insensitive to the background noise, which might improve the recognition accuracy [10]. Practically, any words could be used as the speech commands depending on users' preference. In this study, three single Chinese characters as shown in brackets, "hand (手)", "wrist (腕)", and "elbow (肘)", were used as the keywords to represent each of the three joint-modes in *Strategy 1*. To avoid the recognition failure due to the dialect or accent of different subjects, an individual recognition template was created for each subject instead of a preset standard speech bank. The speech-signal processor used in this work was SPCE061A (*SUNPLUS Technology*). After amplification, second-order butterworth band-pass filtration (passing band of 340-3700 Hz), and A/D conversion, the speech signals were recognized with the dynamic time warping (DTW) algorithm [11]. In addition, instead of the linear prediction coefficients (LPC) [12], the mel-frequency cepstral coefficients (MFCC) [11] based on auditory mode was used to extract the speech characteristic parameters to improve recognition precision. The acquired speech signals were compared to each template with the DTW algorithm, and the template that had a minimum Euclidian distance to the speech signals was considered as the most matching one and its corresponding keyword was considered as the recognition result to represent the desired joint-mode.

For sEMG signal acquisition, the muscle pair of flexor-extensor was used as the signal source, and each muscle was attached with a bipolar sEMG electrode respectively, as shown in Fig 2. Each muscle corresponded to one of two motion-classes involved in a selected joint-mode, e.g. flexor to "hand closing" and extensor to "hand opening" in the "hand mode", and similarly, flexor to "wrist pronation" and extensor to "wrist supination" if the "wrist mode" was chosen.

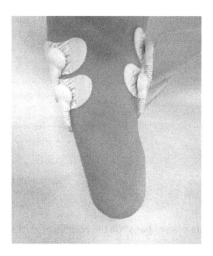

Fig. 2. Position of bipolar electrodes on the residual forearm of the transradial amputee in *Strategy 1*

In the embedded system, MC9S12XEP100 (*Freescale semiconductor company, USA*) was used as the micro-controller and responsible for the signal processing and the prosthetic arm driving. sEMG signals were acquired through the bipolar electrodes with a sampling rate of 1000 Hz. After amplification, 50 Hz notch filtration, and A/D conversion, the sEMG signals were transmitted to the micro-controller. The mean absolute value (MAV) was used as the characteristic parameter of the sEMG signals and the K-nearest neighbors (KNN) algorithm was applied for the sEMG signal decoding [13]. Compared to other algorithms, the KNN algorithm is one of the simplest machine learning algorithms with high performance [14]. In this work, it was found that K=3 could achieve the real-time processing and relatively high accuracy.

The control system was composed of five parts as micro-controller, sEMG acquisition module, speech acquisition module, speech recognition module, and motor driver, as shown in Fig 3. The hardware realization is shown in Fig 4.

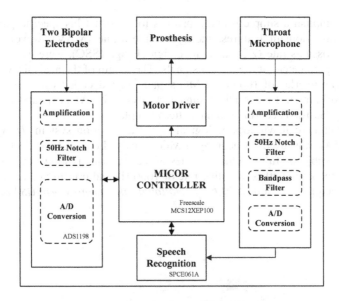

Fig. 3. Diagram of the control system based on the combination of speech and sEMG signals

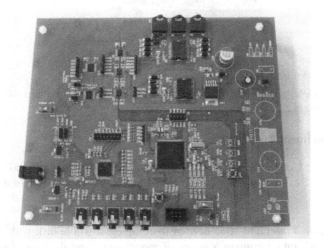

Fig. 4. Hardware realization of the system shown in Fig 3

(2) *System 2* (*Strategy 2*): Prosthesis control based on the pattern recognition of sEMG signals

For a comparison purpose, a control system based on the pattern recognition of sEMG signals was also developed. In this study, it was not necessary to recover the elbow movements for the transradial amputee and therefore the joint-mode of elbow was excluded in *Strategy 2*. Five motion-classes, "hand opening", "hand closing", "wrist pronation", "wrist supination", and "no-movement", were defined. Each subject was asked to accomplish a simple training process to construct his specific pattern template. Four time-domain features, mean absolute value (MAV), waveform length (WL), zero-crossings rate (ZC), and slope sign change (SSC), were extracted as the characteristic parameters of the sEMG signals. The length of the analysis window was 150 ms with an overlap of 100 ms. sEMG signals were decoded with the pattern recognition algorithm of Linear Discriminant Analysis (LDA) [15], and the motion-classes were classified according to the pattern template.

Here, a commercial wireless biological signal acquisition system (*Delsys Trigno Wireless, USA*) was used to acquire sEMG signals. Four sEMG electrodes were placed on the subjects' full/residual muscles of the forearm, as shown in Fig 5. sEMG signals were recorded with a sampling rate of 1000 Hz and transmitted to the computer via a data acquisition card (*USB-6218, National Instruments Corp, USA*).

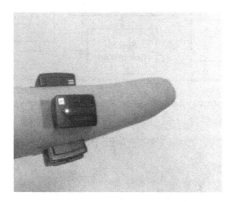

Fig. 5. Four bipolar sEMG electrodes were placed on the residual forearm of the transradial amputee in *Strategy 2*

2.3   Experiment Protocol

To evaluate and compare the control performance of *Strategy 1* and *Strategy 2*, a measure of *task execution time* was proposed and two different functional tasks were designed.

***Task Execution Time*:** The time needed to complete a whole task without any misoperation. A task might contain a series of movements, and the procedure to finish a single movement included the joint-mode switching (in *Strategy 1*) and the movement execution (start and stop, in both strategies).

***Task 1* (Three Joint-Modes Applied):** Subjects were required to complete a task of "water pouring" continuously without any misoperation, which included a series of following movements: "hand-closing" to hold a cup with water inside, "elbow-flexion" to lift up the cup, "wrist-pronation" to pour the water out, and then "wrist-supination", "elbow-extension", and "hand-opening" to return. Since it was not possible to execute elbow movements with *Strategy 2*, only *Strategy 1* was tested in this task.

***Task 2* (Two Joint-Modes Applied):** Similar to *Task 1* but the elbow-joint movements were excluded, i.e. "hand-closing" to hold a cup with water inside, "wrist-pronation" to pour the water out, and then "wrist-supination" and "hand-opening" to return. Both strategies were tested in this task.

All the tests were repeated at least five times and the results were calculated as the average values over the repeated measurements.

3   Results

In *Task 1* where three joint-modes were applied, all the able-bodied subjects and the transradial amputee could complete the specified "water pouring" successfully with *Strategy 1*, and the *task execution time* of each subject is summarized in Table 2. As can be seen, the able-bodied subjects *A1*, *A2* and *A3* spent 19.4, 21.7, and 21.9 s to complete the task, respectively. The transradial amputee *B1* spent similar time of 21.2 s to complete the same task as the able-bodied subjects did.

Table 2. *Task execution time* to complete *Task 1* with *Strategy 1* for all the subjects

Subjects	Task execution time (s)
	Strategy 1
A1	19.4±1.3
A2	21.7±0.5
A3	21.9±1.0
B1	21.2±2.8

In *Task 2* where two joint-modes were applied, all the subjects could also complete the required movement series successfully, and the *task execution time* is shown in Table 3. With *Strategy 1*, the able-bodied subjects *A1*, *A2* and *A3* spent 10.8, 10.5, and 11.4 s to complete the task, respectively, and the *task execution time* for the transradial amputee *B1* was 11.8 s. With *Strategy 2*, the time was 11.1, 10.3 and 9.2 s for the able-bodied subjects, respectively, and 9.5 s for the transradial amputee *B1*. The average value of *task execution time* for *Strategy 2* was slightly less than that for *Strategy 1*. Fig 6 shows the comparison of the statistical analysis for the *task execution time* with different control strategies.

Table 3. *Task execution time* to complete *Task 2* with *Strategy 1* and *Strategy 2* for all the subjects

Subjects	Task execution time (s)	
	Strategy 1	Strategy 2
A1	10.8±0.8	11.1±0.6
A2	10.5±1.2	10.3±2.4
A3	11.4±0.9	9.2±1.0
B1	11.8±0.4	9.5±0.7
Average	11.1	10.0

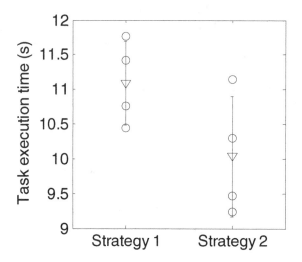

Fig. 6. Comparison of *task execution time* for *Strategy 1* and *Strategy 2* in *Task 2*, where the circles represent the value of each subject, and the triangles represent the calculated average value

4   Discussion

In *Strategy 1*, only a pair of muscles was applied to control the prosthesis with multiple DOFs, which was quite suitable for the amputees without sufficient residual muscles. With *Strategy 1*, the burden from the frequent muscle-pair co-contraction used in the traditional control strategy may be released. What is more, the speech-based joint-mode switching is very flexible and it will be possible to control more DOFs by just adding more speech commands to the system. In *Strategy 2*, high quality sEMG signals and long training process were required for accurate motion-class classification. In addition, it was found that during the experiments the subjects always became tired just after the execution of a few movements. With *Strategy 2*, it will be difficult if more DOFs are required since a more sophisticated recognition algorithm is needed. It should be noted that the transradial amputee still owned the elbow joint, and thus the prosthetic movements of elbow were actually not necessary for them. In the experiments, the joint-modes of "hand", "wrist", and "elbow" were just used to represent a 3-DOF experimental prosthesis to assess the control performance. In the case of transhumeral amputation, the users can still control a 3-DOF prosthesis (e.g. hand, wrist, and elbow) by the residual muscles of upper arm (e.g. bicep and tricep) with *Strategy 1*. However, with *Strategy 2*, the transhumeral amputees cannot conduct any hand or wrist movements because no sEMG signals from forearm can be acquired.

With *Strategy 1*, the able-bodied subjects and the transradial amputee achieved similar experimental results of *task execution time* in both *Task 1* and *Task 2* since they all had full language competence. Generally speaking, in *Task 2*, the average *task execution time* with *Strategy 1* is slightly longer than that of *Strategy 2*. This is because the pronunciation and recognition of speech signals took some time. Compared with *Strategy 2*, *Strategy 1* does not have obvious advantage for the control of prostheses with less DOFs. Nevertheless, *Strategy 1* can be easily expanded for more DOFs and complicated tasks, but *Strategy 2* will be strongly limited.

5   Conclusion

In this study, a myoelectric-prosthesis control system based on the combination of speech and sEMG signals was built up. Its control performances were evaluated through practical operations and compared with the system based on the pattern recognition of sEMG signals. The strategy of the combination of speech and sEMG signals is flexible and easy to use, which has been approved by the positive user experiences. In addition, it can be expanded in the case that more DOFs are required. The strategy based on the pattern recognition of sEMG signals is practical only if sufficient residual muscles can be obtained and less DOFs are needed. The control systems designed in this work is practical and stable and can be embedded into the present myoelectric prostheses for applications.

Acknowledgments. This work was supported in part by the National Natural Science Foundation of China under Grant (#61203209), the Shenzhen Governmental Basic Research Grand (#JC201005270295A), the Shenzhen Governmental Basic Research Grand (#JCYJ20120617114419018), and the Guangdong Innovation Research Team Fund for Low-cost Healthcare Technologies.

References

1. Graupe, D., Cline, W.K.: Functional separation of EMG signals via ARMA identification methods for prosthesis control purposes. IEEE Transactions on Systems, Man, and Cybernetics 5(2), 252–259 (1975)
2. Zardoshti-Kermani, M., Wheeler, B.C., Badie, K., Hashemi, R.M.: EMG feature evaluation for movement control of upper extremity prostheses. IEEE Transactions on Rehabilitation Engineering 3(4), 324–333 (1995)
3. Tenore, F., Ramos, A., Fahmy, A., Acharya, S., Etienne-Cummings, R., Thakor, N.V.: Towards the control of individual fingers of a prosthetic hand using surface EMG signals. In: 29th Annual International Conference of the IEEE EMBS, Lyon, pp. 6145–6148 (2007)
4. Castellini, C., van der Smagt, P.: Surface EMG in advanced hand prosthetics. Biological Cybernetics 10, 35–47 (2009)
5. Parker, P.A., Scott, R.N.: Myoelectric control of prostheses. Critical Reviews in Biomedical Engineering 13(4), 283 (1986)
6. Williams III, T.W.: Practical methods for controlling powered upper-extremity prostheses. Assistive Technology 2(1), 3–18 (1990)
7. Young, A.J., Smith, L.H., Rouse, E.J., Hargrove, L.J.: Classification of simultaneous movements using surface EMG pattern recognition. IEEE Transactions on Biomedical Engineering 60(5), 1250–1258 (2013)

8. Li, G., Li, Y., Yu, L., Geng, Y.: Conditioning and sampling issues of EMG signals in motion recognition of multifunctional myoelectric prostheses. Annals of Biomedical Engineering 39(6), 1779–1787 (2011)

9. Fang, P., Wei, Z., Geng, Y., Yao, F., Li, G.: Using speech for mode Selection in control of multifunctional myoelectric prostheses. In: 35th Annual International Conference of the IEEE EMBS, Osaka, pp. 3602–3605 (2013)

10. Mubeen, N., Shahina, A., Khan, A.N., Vinoth, G.: Combining spectral features of standard and throat microphone signal for speaker recognition. In: 2012 International Conference on Recent Trends in Information Technology (ICRTIT), Chennai, pp. 119–122 (2012)

11. Muda, L., Begam, M., Elamvazuthi, I.: Voice recognition algorithms using mel frequency cepstral coefficient (MFCC) and dynamic time warping (DTW) techniques. Journal of Computing 2(3) (2010)

12. Paul, A.K., Das, D., Kamal, M.M.: Bangla speech recognition system using LPC and ANN. In: 7th International Conference on Advances in Pattern Recognition, Kolkata, pp. 171–174 (2009)

13. Al-Faiz, M.Z., Ali, A.A., Miry, A.H.: A k-nearest neighbor based algorithm for human arm movements recognition using EMG signals. In: 1st International Conference on Energy, Power and Control (EPC-IQ), Basrah, pp. 159–167 (2010)

14. Bay, S.D.: Combining nearest neighbor classifiers through multiple feature subsets. In: ICML, vol. 98, pp. 37–45 (1998)

15. Chen, L., Geng, Y., Li, G.: Effect of upper-limb positions on motion pattern recognition using electromyography. In: 4th International Congress on Image and Signal Processing (CISP), Shanghai, vol. 1, pp. 139–142 (2011)

Detecting Adolescent Psychological Pressures from Micro-Blog

Yuanyuan Xue[1,2], Qi Li[1], Li Jin[1], Ling Feng[1],
David A. Clifton[3], and Gari D. Clifford[3]

[1] Dept. of CS&T, Tsinghua University, Beijing, China
[2] Dept. of CT&A, Qinghai University, Xining, China
[3] Institute of Biomedical Engineering, University of Oxford, London, U.K.
{xue-yy12,liqi13,l-jin12g}@mails.tsinghua.edu.cn,
fengling@mail.tsinghua.edu.cn,
davidc@robots.ox.ac.uk, gari.clifford@eng.ox.ac.uk

Abstract. Adolescents are experiencing different psychological pressures coming from study, communication, affection, and self-recognition. If these psychological pressures cannot properly be resolved, it will turn to mental problems, which might lead to serious consequences. Traditional face-to-face psychological diagnosis and treatment cannot meet the demand of relieving teenagers' stress completely due to its lack of timeliness and diversity. With micro-blog becoming a popular media channel for teenagers' information acquisition, interaction, self-expression, emotion release, we envision a micro-blog platform to sense psychological pressures through teenagers' tweets, and assist teenagers to release their stress through micro-blog. We investigate a number of features that may reveal teenagers' pressures from their tweets, and then test five classifiers (Naive Bayes, Support Vector Machines, Artificial Neural Network, Random Forest, and Gaussian Process Classifier) for pressure detection. We also present ways to aggregate single-tweet based detection results in time series to overview teenagers' stress fluctuation over a period of time. Experimental results show that the Gaussian Process Classifier offers the highest detection accuracy due to its robustness in the presence of a large degree of uncertainty that may be encountered with previously-unseen training data on tweets. Among the features, tweet's emotional degree combining negative emotional words, emoticons, exclamation and question marks, plays a primary role in psychological pressure detection.

Keywords: Teenager, psychological pressure, pressure category, pressure level, detection, micro-blog.

1 Introduction

With the coming of information age and the rapid development of society, growing teenagers have to experience various adolescent psychological pressures, coming from study, communication, affection, self-recognition, etc. Too much stress will result in psychological health problems. When these mental issues are too

Y. Zhang et al. (Eds.): HIS 2014, LNCS 8423, pp. 83–94, 2014.

serious and do not get resolved promptly and properly, adolescents with some mental problems will turn to hurt either themselves or others for stress release. For instance, at the primary school shooting event in Connecticut, USA on December 14, 2012, 20 children and 6 adults were killed by a gunman named Adam Lanza, who is suspected suffering from the mental disease - autism [1]. Statistics from [2, 3] show that over 17% of 1000 college students from over 10 universities in Chongqing Province of China feel stressful and have suicidal thoughts or behaviors. Therefore, close attention to and proper treatment of teenagers' pressures is critical to further development of our society. However, because most teenagers' psychological pressures cannot timely be found out, plus teenagers usually hesitate to share and talk with others about their mental issues, the traditional psychological guidance mode, which is via face-to-face instruction, cannot meet the demand of relieving teenagers' stress alone for its lack of timeliness and diversity.

With micro-blog becoming the most popular information broadcast and communication media nowadays, more and more teenagers go to micro-blog for information acquisition, self-expression, emotion release, and personal interaction due to its instantiation, interactivity, unique equality, freedom, fragmentation, and individuality characteristics. This makes the detection of teenagers' pressures through their tweets on micro-blog feasible. For instance, in the previous examples, if we could detect the psychological disorder from Adam Lanza's twitter and take appropriate actions, we might be able to avoid the tragedy. Micro-blog, as a new kind of social communication mode, could play positive roles to some extent. To those pessimistic adolescents, if we could discover psychological pressures from their micro-blog (if they have micro-blog) timely and guide them to think in a positive and optimistic way, we may hopefully save more lives.

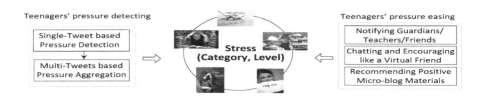

Fig. 1. A micro-blog platform for detecting and easing adolescent psychological stress

In this study, we envision a micro-blog platform [4] solution for detecting and easing adolescent psychological pressures, as shown in Figure 1. It is comprised of two components. The first *pressure detecting component* analyzes and detects from a teenager's tweets whether s/he has some stress, and the stress category and stress level. Based on the detected stress category and level, the second *pressuring easing component* encouragingly recommends relevant materials, chats like a virtual friend, or brings guardians' attention at the worst case to assist stressful teenagers.

The focus of this work is on the first pressure detection component. In order to timely and effective detect teenagers' psychological pressures, we investigate a number of such features that may reveal some adolescent psychological pressures, including tweet's content, emoticons, punctuation, post time and frequency, content of re-tweeted tweet posted by other user, and music that the teenager posts. Based on the extracted and analyzed features, we examine the performance of five classifiers (Naive Bayes, Support Vector Machines, Artificial Neural Network, Random Forest, and Gaussian Process Classifier). We also present ways to aggregate single-tweet based detection results in time series, which is helpful in predicting implicit stress tendency, dealing with stress overlooked by individual tweet's detection, and getting an overview of stress fluctuation over a period of time. Experimental results show that the Gaussian process classifier offers the highest detection accuracy compared to other popularly used approaches. Among the features, tweet's emotional degree combining negative emotional words, emoticons, exclamation and question marks, plays a primary role in psychological pressure detection.

The contributions of the paper are: (1)Propose to exploit the micro-blog platform for detecting and easing adolescent psychological pressures from teenager's tweets. (2)Construct four teenagers' stress-related linguistic lexicons on micro-blog, and select a number of tweet features that may reveal teenager's psychological pressures and test five classifiers for pressure detection. (3)Provide two methods to aggregate single-tweet based detection results from one or multiple teenagers' tweets in time series to get an overview of teenagers' stress fluctuation and variation over a certain period of time.

2 Related Work

Research into micro-blog contents most relevant to this study is sentiment analysis. Most previous work on sentiment analysis aims to extract people's opinions and sentiments polarity, which is mainly classified into two polarities: positive and negative, and sometimes including neutral.

There are rich works on sentiment analysis. Both natural language processing and machine learning are popularly used in sentiment analysis. [5–7] employed the lexicon-based strategy to obtain the overall polarity of a document by computing the number of positive words and negative words in blogs or reviews. [8] also developed a syntactic parser and sentiment lexicon to discover the semantic relationship between target and expression. [9] collected 40 emoticon classes found in Yahoo! blog articles, and utilized sentences containing these emoticons to automatically detect user's emotions from messenger logs. [10] researched the performance of three machine learning methods over movie reviews, including Naive Bayes, Maximum Entropy, and Support Vector Machines. Their experimental result showed that the performance of SVM classifier with unigram presence features is superior to others.

Most of sentiment analysis on micro-blog also makes use of [11, 12]. [13] used emoticons as labels to reduce dependency in machine learning techniques for sentiment classification. [11] employed Twitter hashtags and smileys to enhance sentiment learning. [14] built a graph model for sentiment classification at the hashtag level in Twitter, where three approximate classification algorithms were investigated. [15] presented a two-staged SVM classifier for robust sentiment detection from biased and noisy data on Twitter.

In terms of application areas, most research in sentiment analysis aims at offering techniques to business domains by detecting users' opinions towards a product or proposal. But recently, there has been a few researches in using twitter as a tool for depression detection. [16, 17] built a statistical classifier to estimate whether individuals are in the risk of depression before been reported onset by analyzing users behavioral attributes on twitter. Similarly, [18] proposed a two-stage supervised learning framework to detect whether the user is suffering from depression currently by evaluating content and temporal features of postings on BBS.

To our knowledge, this paper is the first to detect and analyze adolescents' psychological pressures from micro-blog, aiming to combine traditional adolescent mental education with micro-blog media and turn micro-blog into a new kind of adolescent mental education mode and platform.

3   Problem Definition

Considering the characteristics of teenagers micro-blog, we give our single-tweet based adolescent pressure detection problem statement as follows.

Let $\mathcal{C}_{ategory}$={NULL, academic, interpersonal, affection, self-cognition} be the set of pressure categories. We use NULL to denote an unknown category.

Let $\mathcal{L}_{evel}$={none, very light, light, moderate, strong, very strong} be the set of pressure levels, where none means no pressure level.

Given a tweet t, the pressure detection result from t is either null (meaning no pressure detected) or a few tuples $PressureDetect(t) = \langle(C_1, L_1), \cdots, (C_n, L_n)\rangle$, where $C_i \in \mathcal{C}_{ategory}$ and $L_i \in \mathcal{L}_{evel}$ $(1 \leq i \leq n)$ correspond to the detected pressure category and pressure level.

4   Detecting Pressures from a Teenager's Tweet

We first extract and analyze eight features from a teenager's tweeting and forwarding behavior, and then classify a tweet's revealed pressure level in $\mathcal{L}_{evel}$.

4.1   Tweet's Feature Space

Linguistic Association between Pressure Category and Negative Emotion Words. We construct four teenagers' stress-related linguistic lexicons on micro-blog, including stress-category lexicon, negative-emotion lexicon, degree lexicon and negation lexicon. For each sentence in a tweet, we apply a graph-based Chinese parser [19, 20] to find out associated word pairs. The discovered associated word pairs form a directed word-association tree, where each node denotes a word token, and each edge between two nodes denotes a word association. If there exists a path between a stress-category-related word node and a negative emotion word node and no negation lexicon word in between, a stress in the corresponding category is detected. A Chinese word-association tree example is given in Figure 2. It is derived from a Chinese sentence, translated into English as *"My world is really bad-terrible grade, hypocritical friendship."*. Two word pairs, (*grade, terrible*) and (*friendship, hypocritical*), reveal more or less the pressure in the stress categories of *study* and *interpersonal*. The path length is the number of edges in the path, showing the linguistic tightness between the two words. In the example, both path lengths are 2.

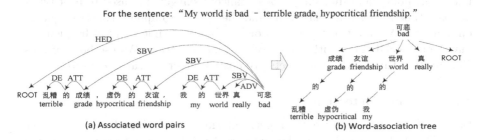

Fig. 2. Identifying associated-word pairs and generating a word-association tree from a Chinese sentence, translated into English *"My world is bad - terrible grade, hypocritical friendship"*

Number of Negative Emotion Words. Negative emotion words may reveal teenagers' negative emotions, and the number of negative emotions is a good indicator to pressure level. We use this feature to judge whether teenagers feel negative emotions.

Numbers of Positive and Negative Emoticons. Teenagers are keen on express feelings and emotions by posting emoticons on micro-blog. Negative and positive emoticons usually indicate one's bad or good mood. We use this feature to make up the ambiguity of natural language.

Numbers of Exclamation and Question Marks. Special marks such as exclamation and question marks are most commonly used by teenagers in their tweets to express their emotions. Exclamation marks are used to indicate extreme emotions such as angry, whiny, etc., and question marks are used to imply confused emotions.

Emotional Degree. Emotional degree denotes the intensity of emotion in a tweet. For example, "I hate so much!!!" owns a high level of emotional intensity because of "so much" lexicon and three exclamation marks. We consider 5 elements including negative-emotion word, adverb of degree, negative emoticon, exclamation mark and question mark. We firstly separately count the numbers of these elements in a tweet, and then, we use formula $ED = (N_{NegEmoticon} + N_{NegEmotionWord} + N_{AdvDegree} + 1)*(N_{Exclamation} + N_{Question} + 1)$ to compute the tweet's emotional degree. Where ED denotes the emotional degree, and $N_{NegEmoticon}, N_{NegEmotionWord}, N_{AdvDegree}, N_{ExclamationMark}, N_{QuestionMark}$ denote the number of emoticons, negative emotion words, adverb of degree, exclamation, and question marks, respectively.

Shared Music Genres. Sad music conveys sorrow emotion and many teenagers who sink into stress are attracted to share it through micro-blog to express their low moods. We regard it as a feature for detecting teenagers' depression.

(Un)usual Post Time and Post Frequency. In macroscopic view, the posting time and posting frequency of tweets are quite random. After observing about 1000 teenagers' tweets, we find that each teen posts tweets on relative fixed time points and frequency. For instance, teenagers are used to post tweets at spare time rather than class time and they prefer to update tweets frequently on holidays. When a tweet is posted on an abnormal time point of frequency, it may be a special tweet with probably a strange emotion. We use both of these features to estimate whether tweets are posted under a strange emotion.

4.2   Pressure Detection

Based on the features, we then perform single-tweet based pressure detection. The task is to classify the pressure level to one category in $CSet = \{C_1, \cdots, C_n\}$ ($n=6$ in the study), corresponding to none, very light, light, moderate, strong, very strong pressure level. We test five different classifiers, which are Naive Bayes, Support Vector Machines, Artificial Neural Network, Random Forest, and Gaussian Process Classifier.

5   Aggregating Single-Tweet Based Pressure Detection Results

Aggregating sensed stress from a sequence of tweets posted by one or multiple teenagers is helpful in predicting implicit stress tendency, dealing with stress overlooked by individual tweet's detection method, and getting an overview of stress fluctuation over a period of time. One challenge here is that most teenagers write tweets using an informal language, and some stress category related and/or degree words may be missing from a tweet. Detecting pressures from a tweet sequence needs to cope with such incomplete elements.

Considering that a teenager's stress may last for a while (say, during an exam period), we take neighbor tweets' stress category as the implicit one. Also, stress from neighbor tweets affects the current tweet due to the continuity of emotions. We fill in the missing stress levels based on the previous tweets' stress levels, and the closest tweet has the highest influence.

Given a tweet sequence $\langle t_1, t_2, \cdots, t_n \rangle$, without loss of generality, different aggregation operations (like Avg, Sum, Count, Max, Min) can be enforced. For instance, let $\langle (C, L_1), \cdots, (C, L_x) \rangle$ be a sequence of sensed stress in category C from a teenager's 1-week tweets, then we can get the average stress as $Avg(C, \langle (C, L_1), \cdots, (C, L_x) \rangle) = (C, \sum_{i=1}^{x} L_i / x)$.

6 Evaluation

6.1 Experimental Settings

Tweets of 459 middle-school students (of age 14-20) are collected from Chinese Sina micro-blog from the first time they launched micro-blog to July 7, 2013. All of the students label themselves with a micro-blog tag named "The Generation After 90s". This tag is the clue via which we find out these teenagers. We randomly pick up 23 teenagers' tweets as our experimental data. Each of the 23 teenagers posted around 300-1000 tweets with a total number of tweets to 10,872, and an average number to 473 per teenager.

Three experiments are conducted on this data set, aiming to examine: 1) the single-tweet based pressure detection performance of five different classifiers, including Naive Bayes, SVM, ANN, Random Forest, and Gaussian Process classifier; 2) the impact of different features on micro-blog pressure detection; and 3) aggregation performance, showing teenager's emotion fluctuation within a certain period of time.

From each tweet *tweet*, we preprocess and obtain its pressure category, together with its eight features. We compare the stress detection results obtained from the classification experiments with the ones given by volunteers.

6.2 Experiment 1: Performance of Single-Tweet Based Pressure Detection

Pressure Category-Independent Detection Performance. Firstly, we randomly select 80% data from 23 teenagers tweets for training, and the rest 20% for testing without distinguishing tweets revealed pressure categories. The results in Table 1 show that Gaussion Processing performs the best with high precision and recall rates over 0.8, while Naive Bayes performs the worst whose precision and recall rates are lower than 0.8. The result verifies the good robustness of GP classifier in the presence of the large degree of uncertainty, which may be encountered with previously-unseen training data.

Table 1. Pressure Category-Independent Detection by Five Classification Methods

Pressure Level	NB (Pre. Rec.)		RF (Pre. Rec.)		SVM (Pre. Rec.)		ANN (Pre. Rec.)		GP (Pre. Rec.)	
None	0.817	0.920	0.944	0.913	0.907	0.924	0.875	0.927	0.947	0.917
Very Light	0.608	0.364	0.693	0.737	0.677	0.659	0.720	0.690	0.707	0.732
Light	0.495	0.569	0.614	0.633	0.609	0.528	0.619	0.602	0.618	0.646
Moderate	0.543	0.504	0.539	0.574	0.515	0.590	0.630	0.459	0.543	0.583
Strong	0.574	0.502	0.540	0.540	0.604	0.560	0.615	0.500	0.580	0.639
Very Strong	0.753	0.741	0.712	0.717	0.763	0.797	0.773	0.744	0.767	0.739
Avg.	0.720	0.734	0.818	0.812	0.796	0.798	0.794	0.802	0.826	0.820

Impact of the Number of Pressure Levels. Considering that six pressure levels might be too fine-grained, we collapse the two pressure levels `very light` and `light` into `light`, and `strong` and `very strong` into `strong`, thus only four pressure levels (`none, weak, moderate, strong`) are taken as the classifier output domain. Table 2 shows that the performance of five classifiers are improved, indicating the influence of classification grain in classification.

Table 2. Collapsing Pressure Levels from 6 to 4

Pressure Level	NB		RF		SVM		ANN		GP	
	(Pre. Rec.)		(Pre. Rec.)		(Pre. Rec.)		(Pre. Rec.)		(Pre. Rec.)	
None	0.810	0.897	0.940	0.899	0.920	0.899	0.924	0.892	0.943	0.905
Light	0.720	0.587	0.783	0.853	0.786	0.817	0.785	0.814	0.800	0.867
Moderate	0.555	0.504	0.553	0.562	0.525	0.512	0.511	0.562	0.586	0.479
Strong	0.807	0.793	0.815	0.788	0.778	0.804	0.795	0.821	0.772	0.849
Avg.AfterCollapse	0.769	0.775	0.862	0.857	0.847	0.845	0.849	0.845	0.867	0.866
Avg.BeforeCollapse	0.720	0.734	0.818	0.812	0.796	0.798	0.794	0.802	0.826	0.820

Pressure Category-Dependent Detection Performance. We conduct this experiment to find out pressure level from teenager's tweet under different stress categories (`unknown, academic, interpersonal, affection, self-cognition`). Firstly, we divided data into 5 subsets according to five stress categories. The tweet number of each data set is 3143 (interpersonal category), 1518 (self-cognition category), 433 (academic category), 217 (affection affection category), and 5527 (unknown stress category), respectively. Then 5 category-specific classification models are trained and tested, with 80% data for training and 20% data for testing in each category. Table 3 shows the classification result for `interpersonal` stress category. Comparing these results with the first experimental results in Table 1, the difference is not much. Most precision and recall rates(on average)reach a high value around 0.8, except for the Naive Bayes method, indicating that the specific category condition increases the classification performance.

6.3 Experiment 2: Impact of Tweet's Features on Pressure Detection Performance

We use *information gain* to measure the impact of tweet's features on the detection result based on the entropy and conditional entropy.

Table 3. Category-Dependent Pressure Detection(in Interpersonal Category)

Pressure Level	NB (Pre. Rec.)		RF (Pre. Rec.)		SVM (Pre. Rec.)		ANN (Pre. Rec.)		GP (Pre. Rec.)	
None	0.796	0.912	0.930	0.917	0.938	0.915	0.943	0.912	0.936	0.923
Very Light	0.600	0.315	0.703	0.726	0.695	0.718	0.682	0.726	0.702	0.742
Light	0.446	0.597	0.578	0.597	0.563	0.581	0.540	0.548	0.655	0.581
Moderate	0.412	0.233	0.467	0.467	0.432	0.533	0.485	0.533	0.514	0.633
Strong	0.519	0.583	0.609	0.583	0.667	0.667	0.583	0.583	0.619	0.542
Very Strong	0.810	0.654	0.846	0.846	0.909	0.769	0.885	0.885	0.889	0.923
Avg.Dependent	0.694	0.707	0.813	0.811	0.817	0.809	0.814	0.808	0.828	0.825
Avg.Independent	0.720	0.734	0.818	0.812	0.796	0.798	0.794	0.802	0.826	0.820

$$InfoGain(C|f) = H(C) - H(C|f), \ where$$

$$H(C) = -\sum_{i=1}^{n} P(C = C_i)logP(C = C_i);$$

$$H(C|f) = \sum_{j=1}^{m} P(f = f_i)H(C|f_j) =$$

$$\sum_{j=1}^{m} P(f = f_j) \sum_{i=1}^{n} P(C = C_i|f = f_j)logP(C = C_i|f = f_j)$$

Information gain represents the change of information amount when bringing in feature f. The bigger the value of information gain is, the more important the feature is. Thus the impact degree of features on the detection performance can then be evaluated. Based on the training tweets, we compute the information gain of different features, shown in Table 4. In the test, we treat positive and negative emoticons, as well as question and exclamation marks, separately.

Table 4. Impact of Different Tweet's Features on Pressure Detection Performance

Rank	Feature	InfoGain	Rank	Feature	InfoGain
1	emotional degree	0.285675	6	positive emoticons	0.048038
2	negative emotion words	0.279034	7	question Marks	0.036773
3	linguistic association	0.212512	8	(un)usual post time	0.023496
4	exclamation marks	0.208379	9	(un)usual post frequency	0.010988
5	negative emoticons	0.137678	10	shared music genre	0.000319

Among the features, tweet's emotional degree combining negative emotional words, negative emoticons, exclamation and question marks, plays the most significant role.This result demonstrates features related to tweets content are important to the pressure level detection.

Next, we test the classification performance with features ranked top 2, top 3, top 4, and top 5, respectively with Gaussian process method, and found out the more features we use, the more accurate detection performance we can achieve, as illustrate in Table 5. However, such performance increasing trend becomes slowly when more features are added in. For instance, when only top 2 features are considered, we get a low precision rate 0.378, and the precision increases abruptly to 0.615 when top 3 features are used. This verifies the importance of features with big information gain.

Table 5. Features utilized by Gaussian Process Classifier

Pressure Level	Top2Features (Pre. Rec.)	Top3Features (Pre. Rec.)	Top4Features (Pre. Rec.)	Top5Features (Pre. Rec.)
None	0.634 0.986	0.778 0.861	0.773 0.883	0.790 0.884
Very Light	0.000 0.000	0.323 0.265	0.536 0.324	0.553 0.319
Light	0.000 0.000	0.368 0.357	0.473 0.578	0.524 0.598
Moderate	0.327 0.694	0.544 0.463	0.527 0.479	0.556 0.612
Strong	0.000 0.000	0.489 0.431	0.494 0.373	0.567 0.500
Very Strong	0.000 0.000	0.613 0.494	0.565 0.506	0.629 0.727
Avg.	0.378 0.598	0.615 0.638	0.663 0.682	0.688 0.704

6.4 Experiment 3: Aggregating Single-Tweet Based Pressure Detection Results

We focus on category-dependent pressure detection, and try to find out how a teenager's emotion fluctuates within a certain time period. We randomly select 244 tweets posted from 2011/8/31 to 2013/7/18 (172 days and 17 months) by one teenager. To get a global view of his emotional fluctuation, we search for topics in each tweet according to the constructed stress category lexicon, perform GP classification to obtain single-tweet based pressure levels, and aggregate these results by months, as shown in Figure 3.

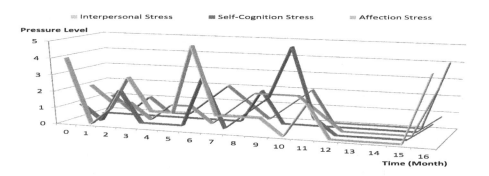

Fig. 3. The average stress level on a monthly basis

7   Conclusion

Adolescent mental health cannot be ignored, and psychological pressure is one of the prominent problems of current teenagers. Micro-blog, as the most important information exchange and broadcast tool, is becoming an important channel for teenagers information acquisition, inter-interaction, and self-expression. In this paper, we propose a pressure detection strategy on micro-blog to timely detect teenagers psychological pressures status and psychological pressures changes. we first extract and analyze features from teenagers tweets, then test five popular classification algorithms for timely and effective detection of teenagers psychological pressures status and changes. Going one step further, we aggregate multi-tweets in a time series to find out the variation of teenagers pressures. Experiment results show that the Gaussian Process Classifier has the highest detection accuracy, and among the features, tweets synthesized emotional degree, negative emotional words, emoticons, exclamation and question marks, plays important roles in pressure detection.

We are currently implementing the micro-blog based strategies for assisting teenagers to relieve the stress. 1) Considering teenagers in the growth many times hesitate to express their feelings to their parents and teachers, when a teenager is detected to have a strong consistent stress, the micro-blog platform will notify his/her guardians and friends to care for his/her psychological change and issue helps immediately to avoid tragedy. 2) For a teenager experiencing a moderate stress, the micro-blog platform can chat and encourage him/her like a personal virtual friend. 3) For a teenager experiencing a weak stress, the micro-blog platform can search and recommend relevant encouraging messages or micro-bloggers of positive attitudes to him/her.

Acknowlegement. The work is supported by National Natural Science Foundation of China (61373022, 61073004), and Chinese Major State Basic Research Development 973 Program (2011CB302203-2).

References

1. Sohu news (2012), http://learning.sohu.com/s2012/shoot/
2. Sohu news (2013), http://learning.sohu.com/20130402/n371458123.shtml
3. Sohu news (2012), http://learning.sohu.com/20120316/n337991511.shtml
4. Xue, Y., Li, Q., Feng, L., et al.: Towards a micro-blog platform for sensing and easing adolescent psychological pressures. In: Proc. of the 15th ACM International Joint Conference on Pervasive and Ubiquitous Computing (UbiComp), pp. 215–218 (2013)
5. Andreevskaia, A., Bergler, S.: Mining wordnet for fuzzy sentiment: Sentiment tag extraction from wordnet glosses. In: Proc. of the 11th Conference of the European Chapter of the Association for Computational Linguistics (EACL), pp. 209–216 (2006)
6. Ku, L.W., Wu, T.H., Lee, L.Y., et al.: Construction of an evaluation corpus for opinion extraction. In: Proc. of the Intl. Conf. on NTCIR, pp. 513–520 (2005)

7. Turney, P.: Thumbs up or thumbs down? semantic orientation applied to unsupervised classification of reviews. In: Proc. of the 40th Annual Meeting on Assoc. for Computational Linguistics, ACL (2002)

8. Nasukawa, T., Yi, J.: Sentiment analysis: Capturing favorability using natural language processing. In: Proc. of the 2nd International Conference on Knowledge Capture (K-CAP), pp. 70–77 (2003)

9. Ku, L., Sun, C.: Calculating emotional score of words for user emotion detection in messenger logs. In: Proc. of the 13th IEEE Intl. Conf. on Information Reuse and Integration: Workshop on Empirical Methods for Recognizing Inference in Text II (EM-RIT), pp. 138–143 (2012)

10. Pang, B., Lee, L., Vaithyanathan, S.: Thumbs up? sentiment classification using machine learning techniques. In: Proc. of the Intl. Conf. on Empirical Methods in Natural Language Processing (EMNLP), pp. 79–86 (2002)

11. Davidov, D., Tsur, O., Rappoport, A.: Enhanced sentiment learning using twitter hashtags and smileys. In: Proc. of the 23rd International Conference on Computational Linguistics, pp. 241–249 (2010)

12. Go, A., Bhayani, R., Huang, L.: Twitter sentiment classification using distant supervision. Stanford University, Tech. Rep. (2009),
http://www.stanford.edu/alecmgo/papers/TwitterDistantSupervision09.pdf

13. Read, J.: Using emoticons to reduce dependency in machine learning techniques for sentiment classification. In: Proc. of the 43rd Meeting of the Association for Computational Linguistics, ACL (2005)

14. Wang, X., Wei, F., Liu, X., Zhou, M., Zhang, M.: Topic sentiment analysis in twitter: A graph-based hashtag sentiment classification approach. In: Proc. of the 20th ACM Conf. on Information and Knowledge Management (CIKM), pp. 1031–1040 (2011)

15. Barbosa, L., Feng, J.: Robust sentiment detection on twitter from biased and noisy data. In: Proc. of the 23rd Intl Conf. on Computational Linguistics (COLING), pp. 36–44 (2010)

16. Choudhury, M., Gamon, M., Counts, S., Horvitz, E.: Prediction depression via social media. In: Proc. of the 7th Intl AAAI Conf. on Weblogs and Social Media (CWSM), pp. 128–137 (2013)

17. Choudhury, M., Counts, S., Horvitz, E.: Social media as a measurement tool of depression in populations. In: Proc. of the ACM Web Science, pp. 47–56 (2013)

18. Shen, Y.-C., Kuo, T.-T., Yeh, I.-N., Chen, T.-T., Lin, S.-D.: Exploiting temporal information in a two-stage classification framework for content-based depression detection. In: Pei, J., Tseng, V.S., Cao, L., Motoda, H., Xu, G. (eds.) PAKDD 2013, Part I. LNCS, vol. 7818, pp. 276–288. Springer, Heidelberg (2013)

19. Che, W., Li, Z., Li, Y., Guo, Y., Qin, B., Liu, T.: Multilingual dependency-based syntactic and semantic parsing. In: Proc. of CoNLL, pp. 49–54 (2009)

20. Che, W., Li, Z., Liu, T.: Ltp: a chinese language technology platform. In: Proc. of Coling, pp. 13–16 (2010)

Detecting Abnormal Patterns of Daily Activities for the Elderly Living Alone

Tingzhi Zhao[1], Hongbo Ni[1], Xingshe Zhou[1], Lin Qiang[1],
Daqing Zhang[2], and Zhiwen Yu[1]

[1] School of Computer Science, Northwestern Polytechnic University, China
bmtingzhi@163.com, {nihb,zhouxs,zhiwenyu}@nwpu.edu.cn,
lutlq@sina.com
[2] Handicom Lab., Institut Telecom SudParis, France
daqing.zhang@it-sudparis.eu

Abstract. In order to reduce the potential risks associated with physically and cognitively impaired ability of the elderly living alone, in this work, we develop an automated method that is able to detect abnormal patterns of the elderly's entering and exiting behaviors collected from simple sensors equipped in home-based setting. With spatiotemporal data left by the elderly when they carrying out daily activities, a Markov Chains Model (MCM) based method is proposed to classify abnormal sequences via analyzing the probability distribution of the spatiotemporal activity data. The experimental evaluation conducted on a 128-day activity data of an elderly user shows a high detection ratio of 92.80% for individual activity and of 92.539% for the sequence consisting of a series of activities.

Keywords: Abnormal Pattern, Infrared Tube, Spatiotemporal, MCM.

1 Introduction

The past several decades have witnessed a rapid increase of elderly people in most countries. In China, people aged 60 and above account for 13.26% of the total population in 2010, with an increase of more than 2.93% as compared to that in 2000. Most importantly, more than 50% of the elderly live alone caring for themselves. The potential risks increase greatly which are mainly caused by the degradation of their physical and cognitive ability. Events of morbidity or even mortality occurrences in their own homes were frequently reported. Providing continuous medical attention in nursing homes or hospitals has obvious effects on the elderly's independence and psychological status but it raises the financial burden to both families and society. Intelligent assistive technologies have great potential for persistent understanding of the elderly's daily life and home conditions in an invasive way, making it possible to recognize their physical or psychological change timely. Especially, for the purpose of reducing potential risk of the elderly living alone, it is thus beneficial to provide a service that can automatically detect abnormal signs in the elderly's ADLs (Activities of Daily Living) for preventing it from becoming worsen and providing the elderly with in-time assistive services.

Y. Zhang et al. (Eds.): HIS 2014, LNCS 8423, pp. 95–108, 2014.

Although human behaviors are quite complicated and hard to be defined precisely, humans always execute a sequence of actions in specific spaces and time ranges within each daily life cycle. For the elderly people living alone, they may tend to have a highly periodic set of daily routine that they do perform day to day [1]. Figure 1 depicts a 5 days' data trace of an elderly man in room-level at home, from which we can obviously see that some spatiotemporal patterns exist in their daily activities. Intuitively, activities in 4th day deviate a lot as compared to their neighbors, especially for the sleeping activity in Bedroom 2, some abnormalities in the day can be found from the irregular movement. As mentioned by Lin et al. [2], abnormal patterns can exist in both individual activity and the sequence of activities. For discovering and measuring possible abnormal patterns, some key factors should be taken into consideration when developing a reliable monitoring system (e.g., detecting anomalies reliably without intervening the elderly's normal life): 1) Minimal interference to their daily life; 2) Sensing devices are inexpensive, robust, and simple enough; 3) Detection results should be accurate and exhaustive; 4) Detection method should be machine-readable with high efficiency; and 5) Maximum privacy protection.

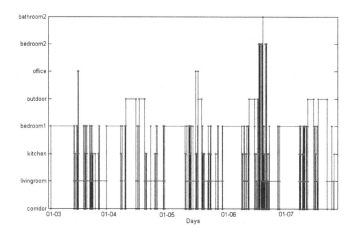

Fig. 1. Daily activity recordings within Five days for an elderly man collected from MSSMP

In this work, we deploy a non-contact mobility sensing and safety monitoring platform (MSSMP) in home setting where sensors consist of simple and cheap infrared sensors tubes, and the inhabitant have no use for wearing sensors. When the monitored person moves from one room to another, we can obtain the room-level trace data of entering in and exiting from door using sensing devices. Focusing on the possible extended duration, the event of an elderly individual remaining at a room too long can be defined as an abnormality in individual activity and can be detected via analyzing its characteristic of small-probability in Gaussian distribution. Based on the temporal features and its relationships with human's activities, the sequences of activities will be converted into spatiotemporal symbols using clustering algorithm, thus the problem that whether an episode of activities is abnormal or not can be formulated as to measure if the sequence of spatiotemporal symbols is more likely belonging to a "abnormal sequence model" rather than a "normal sequence model", with the well-known Markov Chains Model. Finally, the experimental evaluation of the proposed methodology conducted on a real individual dataset that is acquired from home setting of an elderly user shows the effectiveness. In addition, a comparison of the experimental results between our proposed method and the Levenshtein Distance [3] algorithm is also provided, showing a compared performance of the proposed method.

2   Related Work

To improve the autonomy and independence of the elderly at home, intelligent sensing devices at home or worn on the body to collect the time, location, or biometric information for activity recognition[4,5,6,7,8], activity pattern analysis[1,9,10,11], abnormally detection automatically[12,13,14,15] and also forecasting the next activity to facilitate their work in previous work. In pattern detection, the literature [1] presents an automated methodology for extracting the spatiotemporal activity model of a person using a wireless sensor network, Aprior is used for mining frequent patterns, [9] presents a mining method to find natural activity patterns in real life and with those variations, [10] proposes a tree-based mining for discovering patterns of human interaction in meetings, and [11] is trying to recognize sleep patterns in elder assistive environment. When handle the issue of detection of outliers or abnormal patterns as our work, [16] develops IR motion-sensor-based activity-monitorinem, and use SVDD method to classify normal behavior patterns and to detect abnormal behavioral patterns, which is a significant achievement for abnormal patterns detection using three feature value (activity lever, mobility level and non-response interval), however ,when they are lack of consideration on the transition probability in different activities, which is very important to analysis the analysis the sequence of activities . Sequence alignment is also used to detect abnormal signs in a life pattern via changes of a sequence of activities of daily living [17], Jung et al. [18] use a similarity function in a series of events to determine abnormal human behavior, which considers four aspects, sequence of events, the number of common events, time, and duration, however they have to deal the new episode with the dataset one by one leading to inefficiency and hard to determine an appropriate weighs for each individual function.

3   Methodology

3.1   System Overview

As seen in the Fig.2, we can see the deployment of MSSMP, which consists of mobility detecting sensors and an ARM-based data transceiver. For the detecting sensor, we adopted 6 couples of infrared sensing tubes, and each coupled, i.e. the transmitting and receiving infrared tubes are deployed straightly face to face, fixed in both sides of the each doors in the Smart Elderly Assisting Lab. All of the mobility sensors are deployed to monitor the entering and exiting behaviors of the elderly person (we called him Wang) from room to room in the lab. The tubes will be triggered when Wang passes through the door, the direction (entering and getting out of the door) and the sensor's ID will be produced with digital signal '0','1' and transmitted to the ARM-based data transceiver with Bluetooth, which handles digital signal with timestamp into a standard format shown in Table 1 (the duration is the time interval from entering a room to getting out of it). Since the ID of infrared tube and the ID of door share the same number, only a few coupled tubes are needed for the whole house. Furthermore, the formatted data is sent to the sever every two hours with wired or wireless network (i.e. ADSL, 3G,/2G, and WIFI). The server is to not only store formatted data to MySQL database for future analysis but also inform Wang's caregivers when some potential abnormalities occur.

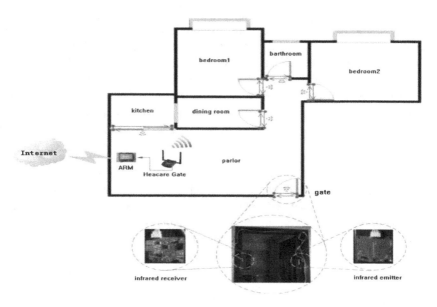

Fig. 2. Five days' tracing data of Wang gaining from MSSMP

Table 1. Examples in the Dataset (the duration accurate to the second)

Room Id	Start time	Duration(s)
1	2013-01-03 11:00:11	381
2	2013-01-03 11:06:56	393
3	2013-01-03 11:13:54	2814
1	2013-01-03 12:01:17	4171
5	2013-01-03 13:10:55	79
2	2013-01-03 13:12:19	66
1	2013-01-03 13:13:40	595
2	2011-01-03 13:23:37	876
1	2011-01-03 13:59:43	221
3	2011-01-03 14:03:26	116
...	...	...

3.2   Definitions

Activity and Activity Sequence: In this paper, we define an activity as a subject (Wang) entering a room and hanging about until exiting the room, which can be represented as a 3-tuple:

$$T = (P, S, D) \tag{1}$$

Where P is the room ID, S is the start time when Wang enters a room, which is recorded as timestamp once the sensors are triggered by Wang, D is the duration of Wang stays in the room (exactly on the second). Thus, moving in different rooms constitute an episode of activities, namely activity sequence.

$$E = < T_1, T_2 ... T_i, T_{i+1} ... T_n > \qquad T_i.s < T_{i+1}.s \tag{2}$$

$T_i.s$ is the start time of activity T_i, the constraint of $T_i.s < T_{i+1}.s$ comes from the fact that Wang just goes out from the prior room could be in a next room, then, any episode of trajectory data can be represented by a time-ordered 3-triples. e.g.: <(2 2013-01-02 06:11:45 414)(1 2013-01-02 06:18:53 1540)>, which describes a moving scene of Wang, who enters the room '2' at time '2013-01-02 06:11:45', remains in this room for 414 seconds, then leaves room '2' and enters room '1' at time '2013-01-02 06:18:53'.

Abnormal Pattern: In our work, abnormal patterns are divided into two groups, one exists in the procedural step inside those individual activity and the other is in sequence of activities. In our scenario, start time and duration are essential characteristic of an individual activity and rational to be the criterion to for abnormal detection, as reflected in the following situation. Wang never goes out around 3:00 in the morning but happened one day possibly on account of something wrong with his physical or mental condition. In addition, if he goes to bathroom at a start time as usual but has stayed more than 30min this time, instead of the common duration (15min), may due to falling down or faint at bathroom. Besides, an activity sequence rarely happened or varied considerably from the daily routines could be thought as abnormal status, despite the right start time and duration. And also if a sequence of activities is similar with some abnormal sequence generated at previous may adumbrate a disease's relapse.

3.3   Abnormal Pattern Detection

It is hard to detect abnormal patterns from activities described with triples (i.e.(2)) directly, depending on the temporal features and relations (e.g. the order of the activities, the start time and the interval) of activity patterns [19], a good solution is to transforms the triples into singletons and lose the original data as little as possible. Then we use the K-means clustering algorithm to analyze the start time and duration data of each room, where the number of the clusters can be set by the parameter K, then we get the clusters relating to start time (Start-time cluster) and so as to the clusters relating to duration (duration cluster). The result on the data of kitchen and bedroom is shown in Fig.3, where the areas with different colors indicate different clusters. (We set the parameter K=3 for kitchen and K=4 for bedroom).

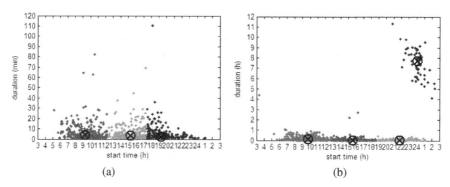

Fig. 3. Clustering results on the data of kitchen (a) and bedroom (b) each dot represents an activity

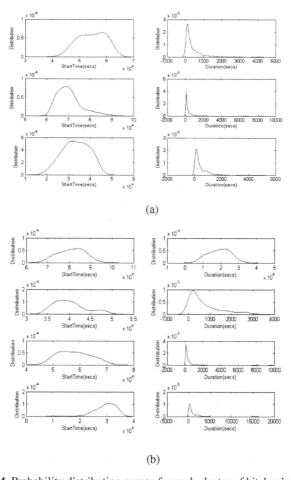

Fig. 4. Probability distribution curves for each cluster of kitchen's data

For each cluster, we use the Matlab to draw the probability distribution curve for each cluster, as presented in Fig.4(a), three subplots in the left depict the probability distribution of start-time clusters of kitchen, and the right subplots depict the same information of duration clusters, and it is worth noting there is one-to-one correspondence between the clusters on the left and the clusters on the right, that is to say, the start time of activities, whose duration contained in the duration clusters, are also contained in the start-time clusters on the left. Fig.4(b) depicts the same information of bedroom. Based on these observations, the distribution probability of each cluster can be approximated expressed by Gaussian functions with appropriate parameters:

$$f(x \mid C^{ij}) = \frac{1}{\sqrt{2\pi}\sigma} \exp\{-\frac{(x-\mu)^2}{2\sigma^2}\} \tag{3}$$

x can be either start-time-cluster or duration cluster, C^{ij} means the jth cluster for the room i,(i=1,2......n; j=1,2,3......K), n is the number of rooms and K is the number of clusters for each room, μ and σ can be automatically acquired from the fitting process.

For an individual activity, we care more about the duration because the elderly man (Wang) may suffer from the fall, faint or some seizures while he stays too long in a room,. Considering the distribution characteristic of an activity, we can use the '$\alpha - quantile$' to detect abnormalities:

$$P(d < d_\alpha) = \int_{-\infty}^{d_\alpha} f(x)d(x) = \alpha \tag{4}$$

After setting an appropriate α, the Gaussian distribution table can be employed to find d_α. Once the duration dx is bigger than d_α (i.e., $dx \in [d_\alpha,+\infty)$), a small probability event happened can be inferred, and we taken it as abnormal activity for granted.

Based on Gaussian distribution characteristic of $P(\mu-2\sigma < X \le \mu+2\sigma)$ =95.45%, we know that activities not falling within the dominant range (i.e.,[μ-2σ, μ+2σ],we called it DR at follows) account for only 4.6% and can be seen as the outliers. In this work, if the start time of an activity does not locate at DR or even belongs to none of the start-time-clusters, the activity can not be regarded as an abnormal activity, because Wang is active at least, but can be taken as deviation, so as to the situations that the duration is too short($dx \in [0, \mu-2\sigma]$) or slightly long($dx \in [\mu+2\sigma, d_\alpha]$).All of them will be taken into account in abnormal sequence detection through defining a new cluster C_{K+1}, that is to say C_{K+1} contains activities that Wang rarely enters a room at the start time or at this start time the duration does not belong to any DR. $C_1, C_2...,C_K$ are be used to represent the activities that both the start time and the duration are located in DR. In this circumstance, only four clusters a_0, a_1, a_2, a_3. can delegate all the triples happened in kitchen: a_0, a_1, a_2 represents normal activities and a_3 is an instance of 'C_{K+1}' involving all the deviations of the activities in kitchen.

The continuous start time of a room can be transformed into discrete sequence of DRs by different clusters:

$$[\mu_1 - 2\sigma_1, \mu_1 + 2\sigma_1], [\mu_2 - 2\sigma_2, \mu_2 + 2\sigma_2], \ldots, [\mu_k - 2\sigma_k, \mu_k + 2\sigma_k] \tag{5}$$

In certain circumstance, overlapped region will emerge into the neighboring DRs, like $\mu_i + 2\sigma_i > \mu_{i+1} - 2\sigma_{i+1}$, means an activity whose start time within $[\mu_{i+1} - 2\sigma_{i+1}, \mu_i + 2\sigma_i]$ could not map to a definite cluster (the activity can locate at both C_i and C_{i+1}), reflecting at the kitchen as shown in Fig.5 ($x1 = \mu_2 - 2\sigma_2$, $x2 = \mu_1 + 2\sigma_1$ and $x1 < x2$). In this work, we set $\mu_i + 2\sigma_i = \mu_{i+1} - 2\sigma_{i+1} = \dfrac{(\mu_i + 2\sigma_i + \mu_{i+1} - 2\sigma_{i+1})}{2}$ to make it possible for representing any activity in a spatiotemporal symbol, namely a cluster label. Then the specific time-division (DRs) of kitchen can be expressed in Table 2.

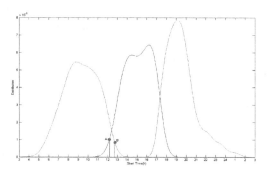

Fig. 5. Overlap in neighboring *DR*s of the start time of kitchen

Table 2. Start time-division of kitchen

Cluster#	Start Time (hh:mm:ss)	Duration(s)	New cluster label
1	[06:03:26,12:18:42]	[0,3611]	b_0
2	[12:18:42,17:41:23]	[0,3214]	b_1
3	[17:45:37,23:55:10]	[0,3477]	b_2
4	others(deviations)	others(deviations)	b_3

In this way each activity can be substituted by a new cluster label, which contains the temporal and spatial information of the activity. Then the dataset in table 1 is represented as a new sequential form:

$$a_0 b_0 c_0 a_1 e_0 b_3 a_1 b_1 a_1 c_1 \ldots \tag{6}$$

where $'a','b','c','d'$ stands for the identification of rooms, and the subscripts '0','1','2'......represents which cluster this activity belongs to. In this way, the sequence of 3-tuples (activities) is formulated as sequence of singletons (cluster labels)

In Biological Sciences, Markov Chains Models is very significant for CpG island finding and we use this model to complete the abnormal sequence detection. To a sequence $S = s_1, s_2 ..., s_l$, how likely it can be generated from the model decided by the transition probability starting from the first state s_1 to s_l successively ($s_1 \rightarrow s_2 \rightarrow ... s_l$).Based on the property of Markov that the probability of s_{i+1} only depends on s_i, the possibility of sequence S can be calculated by:

$$P(S \mid \mathrm{mod}\, el) = p(s_l \mid s_{l-1})p(s_{l-1} \mid s_{l-2})... p(s_2 \mid s_1)p(s_1) \tag{7}$$

For the purpose of utilizing the Markov chains to classify the abnormal sequence, we construct two Markov chains models first. One is for abnormal sequence pattern and the other is for normal sequence pattern. "Normal pattern" is denoted with NP and "abnormal pattern" is denoted with ANP. The concrete steps of the approach are as follows:

1). separate the training dataset into two categories by the marked label (i.e., "normal" and "abnormal")and convert the data into a sequence of cluster labels with the mentioned method.

2). for each category, calculate the probability of any two transferring states and then construct the transition probability matrix. Specifically, for any two states s_a, s_b, count the total occurrence number of the adjacency pairs (s_a, s_b) in dataset as c_{ab}. If there are m states, we will get $m*m$ counts. The transfer probability is defined as:

$$p(s_b \mid s_a) = \frac{c_{ab}}{\sum c_{ij}} \tag{8}$$

$i = 1, 2, ..., m$ and $j = 1, 2, ..., n$ .However, when the pair never appeared in the database, lead to $c_{ab} = 0$ and $p(s_b \mid s_a) = 0$, then the probability of the sequence will be zero even through other pairs in the sequence have high probability, such as $p(s_2 \mid s_1) = 0.99$. In order to solve this problem, we use the Laplace calibration to avoid the zero probability. That is to say, if we add a small figure $'x'$ to all the counts c_{ij}, the variation of probability can be ignored (in the experiment, we set x=0.1).

3). log odds ratio is used to measure whether the sequence is abnormal, which is defined as:

$$LOR = \log \frac{P(S \mid ANP)}{P(S \mid NP)} \tag{9}$$

$P(S|ANP)$ is the probability of S belonging to AM model and $P(S|NP)$ is the probability S belonging to the NM model. Once LOR is bigger than 0, it means the sequence is more likely to match the abnormal sequence model.

4   Experimental Evaluation

The proposed method for abnormal patterns detection was evaluated on a 76-year old man (Wang) who lives alone over the years and has suffered from hypertension disease and mild sleep disorders, and his health condition is checked periodically by the nurses and doctor at a local clinic. We deploy the monitoring system as described in section 3 and get a 128-day tracing data. A 3-day data was taken out because Wang's relatives came to visit him and also a 2 -day data for the neighbors making the rounds. It's hard to affirm abnormal sequences in our own view or with some assumed rules. We get supervised data based on: 1).Wang's own perspective of his health status and interviews with the caregivers. 2).experts' assessments of the tracing data.

Finally, a 9-day data was marked 'abnormal' and the rest are marked 'normal'. To the parameter K, we find the method can work well when we just set K=3 for the kitchen, living room, bedroom, bathroom1, office, and the outer and K=2 for the bathroom2.

4.1   Abnormal Activities Detection

In individual abnormal activity detection, we randomly select 45-day data (nearly 1800 activities) to evaluate our methods. We set α =0.83, 0.84...0.98, and the result is shown in Fig.6.

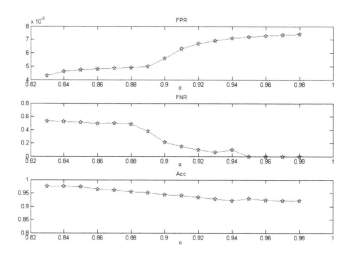

Fig. 6. Experiment result graph of FPR, FNR, and Acc with different α

False Positive Rate (FPR) is to evaluate the poor judgment of the abnormal detection in treating the normal as abnormal.

False Negative Rate (FNR) is to estimate the degree of missing the real abnormal activities.

$$FPR = \frac{TrueNegative}{TrueNegative + FalseNegative}$$

$$FNR = \frac{FalseNegative}{TruePositive + FalseNegative}$$

$$Accuracy(Acc) = \frac{TruePositive + TrueNegative}{Total}$$

Fig.6. shows that with the increase of α, FPR is increasing and FNR is decreasing gradually, and also the Acc lowers slowly leveling near 0.932. When α is 0.93, the method shows best performance, where FPR is 0.69%, FNR is 6% and accuracy is 92.8%, the result contains 7 individual abnormal activities with two activities happening in the bathroom, three activities in bedroom and two in the kitchen. Only an activity in kitchen and the second in bedroom are truly abnormal. But it is crucially important that we had detected hypertensive attacks twice despite of the other fake judgments. Moreover, it is easily accepted for Wang to break the fake by moving through any room when the alarm sounds off at home, because the triggered sensors can generate new data to verify the safety of him, then the alarm will be canceled automatically. Unless the alarm makes sounds for several times indicating that Wang is incapable to eliminate the alarm, we assume that Wang is in terrible situation and needs to be rescued.

4.2   Abnormal Sequences Detection

From the 114 days' normal dataset and the 9 days' abnormal dataset, the k-fold cross-validation is used to evaluate the approach, we set k=7 and the training dataset is selected randomly. Then we repeat the experiment 7 times and calculate the transition probability matrix of ANP and NP on each experiment.

	b_0	b_1	b_2	b_3	c_0	c_1		b_0	b_1	b_2	b_3	c_0	c_1
b_0	0	0	0	0	0.21936	0	b_0	0	0	0	0	0.17912	0.00333
b_1	0	0	0	0	0.00058	0.0114	b_1	0	0	0	0	0.00061	0.01012
b_2	0	0	0	0	0.00242	0	b_2	0	0	0	0	0.00395	0.00020
b_3	0	0	0	0	0.00901	0.00393	b_3	0	0	0	0	0.00711	0.00160
c_0	0.02001	0.00740	0	0.00045	0	0	c_0	0.01919	0.00740	0.00237	0.00745	0	0
c_1	0.01567	0.00068	0.00040	0.00013	0	0	c_1	0	0.01410	0.00142	0.01343	0	0

(a)   (b)

Fig. 7. Part of transition probability matrix: (a) Part of matrix for abnormal dataset, and (b) part of matrix for abnormal dataset

Table 3. Experiment result of abnormal sequence detection ('21'means 21st day's activity sequence and the others are same)

Number	Training set	Test set	Real anomalies	Test result
1	105	19	'21'	'21','13'
2	105	18	'73'	'73'
3	105	18	'16', '23', '102'	'13', '16', '102'
4	105	18	'4'	'4' , 28
5	105	18	'41', '76'	'41', '76', '82'
6	105	18	'96'	'15', '96', '64'
7	108	15	null	'12' '55'

Table 3 reveals that all the real anomalies have been detected except '23' in the third experiment, after figuring out the average FPR(4.363%) and FNR(4.7619%). We can see both of them are very small and can be acceptable in real work. The high accuracy, which is up to 92.539%, means we can almost completely distinguish abnormal sequences by MCM

For advantage analysis, a well-known Levenshtein Distance (LD) is used as a baseline. Noting that our method and the baseline share the same goal of capturing abnormal sequences, we still covert the sensing data as (6), and the difference is that LD detect anomalies by calculating the similarities between a test sequence and all the training sequences, the similarity S_α can be calculated by (10)[20].

$$S_\alpha = 1 - \frac{Dis\tan ce}{Max(Length1, Length2)} \tag{10}$$

Actually, normal sequences always contain several same patterns, but the abnormal ones show big difference, thus for the sake of ease, we use a simple solution to have a threshold value to classify sequences. If the average of the smallest M similarities is less than the threshold, it can be implied that the test sequence greatly different from all the normal training sequences.

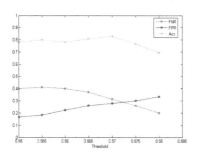 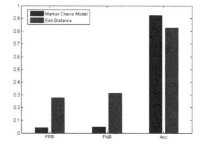

Fig. 8. Experiment result graph of FPR, FNR, and Acc with different threshold

Fig. 9. Accuracy comparison between MCM and LD

We set M=2, threshold =0.55, 0.55... 0.58, respectively. The result is shown in Fig.8, we find that the accuracy is the highest when threshold is 0.57, and then we use this threshold to compare the performance of MCM and LD, accordingly. Fig.9. shows the comparison result between the two algorithms: MCM performs better than LD obviously, and both the FPR and FNR are much smaller than LD.

5   Conclusion

For the purpose of decreasing the potential risks of the elderly living alone at home and assisting their independent living, we propose a mechanism for abnormal pattern detection with several algorithms based on on-contact mobility sensing and safety monitoring platform(MSSMP). The high accuracy on both individual activity and activity sequence in our evaluation reveals that the monitor system and algorithms are very effective. In the future, we hope to involve more elderly people in the research work and collect more diversified information with wearable device, such as smart phone, to improve the system continuously and mine more meaningful patterns from a larger set of data.

Acknowledgement. This work is supported by the National Found of Science of China and Scientific Program Grant of Xi'an.

References

1. Lymberopoulos, D., Bamis, A., Savvides, A.: Extracting spatiotemporal human activity patterns in assisted living using a home sensor network. Universal Access in the Information Society 10(2), 125–138 (2011)
2. Lin, Q., Zhang, D., Li, D., et al.: Extracting Intra-and Inter-activity Association Patterns from Daily Routines of Elders. Inclusive Society: Health and Wellbeing in the Community, and Care at Home, pp. 36–44. Springer, Heidelberg (2013)
3. Levenshtein, V.I.: Binary codes capable of correcting deletions, insertions and reversals. Soviet Physics Doklady 10, 707 (1966)
4. Krishnan, N.C., Panchanathan, S.: Analysis of low resolution accelerometer data for continuous human activity recognition. In: IEEE International Conference on Acoustics, Speech and Signal Processing, ICASSP 2008, pp. 3337–3340. IEEE (2008)
5. Győrbíró, N., Fábián, Á., Hományi, G.: An activity recognition system for mobile phones. Mobile Networks and Applications 14(1), 82–91 (2009)
6. Kwapisz, J.R., Weiss, G.M., Moore, S.A.: Activity recognition using cell phone accelerometers. ACM SIGKDD Explorations Newsletter 12(2), 74–82 (2011)
7. Maurer, U., Smailagic, A., Siewiorek, D.P., et al.: Activity recognition and monitoring using multiple sensors on different body positions. In: Maurer, U., Smailagic, A., Siewiorek, D.P., et al. (eds.) International Workshop on Wearable and Implantable Body Sensor Networks, BSN 2006, vol. 4, p. 116. IEEE (2006)
8. Liang, Y., Zhou, X., Yu, Z., et al.: Energy-Efficient Motion Related Activity Recognition on Mobile Devices for Pervasive Healthcare. Mobile Networks and Applications 1–15 (2013)

9. Rashidi, P., Cook, D.J.: Mining and monitoring patterns of daily routines for assisted living in real world settings. In: Proceedings of the 1st ACM International Health Informatics Symposium, pp. 336–345. ACM (2010)

10. Yu, Z., Yu, Z., Zhou, X., et al.: Tree-based mining for discovering patterns of human interaction in meetings. IEEE Transactions on Knowledge and Data Engineering 24(4), 759–768 (2012)

11. Ni, H., Abdulrazak, B., Zhang, D., et al.: Towards non-intrusive sleep pattern recognition in elder assistive environment. Journal of Ambient Intelligence and Humanized Computing 3(2), 167–175 (2012)

12. Aliakbarpour, H., Khoshhal, K., Quintas, J., Mekhnacha, K., Ros, J., Andersson, M., Dias, J.: HMM-Based Abnormal Behaviour Detection Using Heterogeneous Sensor Network. In: Camarinha-Matos, L.M. (ed.) Technological Innovation for Sustainability. IFIP AICT, vol. 349, pp. 277–285. Springer, Heidelberg (2011)

13. Duong, T.V., Bui, H.H., Phung, D.Q., et al.: Activity recognition and abnormality detection with the switching hidden semi-markov model. In: IEEE Computer Society Conference on Computer Vision and Pattern Recognition, CVPR 2005, vol. 1, pp. 838–845. IEEE (2005)

14. Khan, Z.A., Sohn, W.: Feature extraction and dimensions reduction using R transform and Principal Component Analysis for abnormal human activity recognition. In: 2010 6th International Conference on Advanced Information Management and Service (IMS), pp. 253–258. IEEE (2010)

15. Krishnan, N., Cook, D.J., Wemlinger, Z.: Learning a Taxonomy of Predefined and Discovered Activity Patterns

16. Shin, J.H., Lee, B., Park, K.S.: Detection of abnormal living patterns for elderly living alone using support vector data description. IEEE Transactions on Information Technology in Biomedicine 15(3), 438–448 (2011)

17. Jung, H.Y., Park, S.H., Park, S.J.: Detection abnormal pattern in activities of daily living using sequence alignment method. In: 30th Annual International Conference of the IEEE Engineering in Medicine and Biology Society, EMBS 2008, pp. 3320–3323. IEEE (2008)

18. Park, K., Lin, Y., Metsis, V., et al.: Abnormal human behavioral pattern detection in assisted living environments. In: Proceedings of the 3rd International Conference on PErvasive Technologies Related to Assistive Environments, vol. 9. ACM (2010)

19. Nazerfard, E., Rashidi, P., Cook, D.J.: Discovering temporal features and relations of activity patterns. In: 2010 IEEE International Conference on Data Mining Workshops (ICDMW), pp. 1069–1075. IEEE (2010)

20. Niu, Y., Zhang, C.: Comparison of String Similarity Algorithm. Computer and Digital Engineering 40(3), 14–17 (2012)

Detecting Noun Phrases in Biomedical Terminologies: The First Step in Managing the Evolution of Knowledge

Adila Merabti[1], Lina F. Soualmia[1,2], and Stéfan J. Darmoni[1,2]

[1] CISMeF, TIBS LITIS Laboratory EA 4108, Rouen University Hospital, France
[2] LIMICS, French National Institute for Health, INSERM UMR 1142, Paris, France
{adila.merabti,lina.soualmia,stefan.darmoni}@chu-rouen.fr

Abstract. In order to identify variations between two or several versions of Clinical Practice Guidelines, we propose a method based on the detection of noun phrases. Currently, we are developing a comparison approach to extract similar and different elements between medical documents in French in order to identify any significant changes such as new medical terms or concepts, new treatments etc. In this paper, we describe a basic initial step for this comparison approach i.e. detecting noun phrases. This step is based on patterns constructed from six main medical terminologies used in document indexing. The patterns are constructed by using a Tree Tagger. To avoid a great number of generated patterns, the most relevant ones are selected that are able identify more than 80% of the six terminologies used in this study. These steps allowed us to obtain a manageable list of 262 patterns which have been evaluated. Using this list of patterns, 708 maximal noun phrases were found, with, 364 correct phrases which represent a 51.41% precision. However by detecting these phrases manually, 602 maximal noun phrases were found which represent a 60.47% recall and therefore a 55.57% F-measure. We attempted to improve these results by increasing the number of patterns from 262 to 493. A total of 729 maximal noun phrases were obtained, with 365 which were correct, and corresponded to a 50.07% precision, 60.63% recall and 54.85% F-measure.

Keywords: Biomedical terminologies, medical knowledge evolution, Natural Language Processing, Clinical Practice Guidelines, noun phrases detection, patterns.

1 Introduction

This study was developed in the context of a medical knowledge evolution, and specifically in the context of document evolution such as Clinical Practice Guidelines (CPGs) and Electronics Health Records. It is important for the physician to have a clear perspective of this evolution. As an initial application, we chose to focus on Clinical Practice Guidelines (CPGs), which provide recommendations for the diagnosis and treatment of numerous diseases. These guidelines are

Y. Zhang et al. (Eds.): HIS 2014, LNCS 8423, pp. 109–120, 2014.
© Springer International Publishing Switzerland 2014

a fundamental reference source for physicians [1]. Based on this option, many studies have been proposed to elucidate this problem. However, the methods used remain rather specific to the documents they treat and it is practically impossible to apply the same tools on other types of medical documents. Therefore, we were prompted to propose the implementation of a practical ergonomic tool which is flexible and can manage this evolution in any type of French medical document. This tool will serve as a basis for the evaluation of the proposed approach by comparing our results with those of the other existing methods [2]. This approach involves several steps. The basic step consist of detecting noun phrases by extracting patterns from different medical terminologies. The noun phrases are groups of words constructed around a single noun, which is called the headword of the phrase. We selected specific types of phrases because they represent the general structure of medical terminology which will serve as the basis of our study. Once the various noun phrases are necessarily identified the next step will be a comparison to detect any minor or major changes. For example in the case of chronic diseases that constantly evolve, the physician can use our tool and immediately learn of new practices without necessarily having to search the new CPG. The paper is structured as follow: first we describe the material used in section 2, in section 3 we describe the methods. The step of detecting noun phrases are detailed in section 4, and the evaluation is presented in section 5. In section 6 we present the results of this study. Finally, our conclusions are presented in section 7.

2   Material

To test our approach, we chose the Clinical Practice Guidelines (CPGs) as the basic medical documents to be compared. Medical terminologies are then used to build patterns such as : MeSH (Medical Subject Heading), ICD10(International Classification of Diseases), and an annotating tool Tree Tagger [3]. We there describe the structure of each element.

2.1   Clinical Practice Guidelines

As previously mentioned CPGs contain recommendations for the diagnosis and treatment of numerous diseases. The American Institute of Medicine defines clinical practice guidelines as systematically developed statements to assist practitioner and patient decisions about appropriate health care for specific clinical circumstances [4].

2.2   Biomedical Terminologies

A terminological system links together concepts of a domain and gives their associated terms, as well as their definition and code. It might also provide the designation of terminology, thesaurus, controlled vocabulary, nomenclature, classification, taxonomy or ontology. In [5], a terminology is defined as a set of words.

However, a more precise definition of terminology has been proposed [6]: Terminologies are composed by a list of terms of one domain or a topic representing concepts or notions most frequently used or most characteristic. Therefore, the content and the structure of a terminology depends on its specific function. In a thesaurus the terms are for example organized alphabetically and the concepts may be designed with one or several synonyms. When the terms are associated with definitions, it constitutes a controlled vocabulary.

The main biomedical terminology references are as follow: MeSH, SNOMED Int, MedDRA, ICD10, ATC and FMA. All are annoteted with Tree Tagger [3].

MeSH. The Medical Subject Headings (MeSH) [7] is a biomedical thesaurus, created and updated by the US National Library of Medicine (NLM). It is used for indexing the bibliographic references of MEDLINE/PubMed. Originally in English, the MeSH has been translated into numerous other languages, such as French. It contains 545, 082 concepts (eg: *embryotomy*).

SNOMED Int. The Systematized Nomenclature Of MEDicine International (SNOMED Int) is used essentially to describe electronic health records [8]. It contains 208, 769 terms (eg: *Parkinson's disease*).

MedDRA. The Medical Dictionary for Regulatory Activities (MedDRA) [9] has been designed for the encoding of adverse drug reactions chemically induced. It contains a large set of terms (signs and symptoms, diagnostics, therapeutic indications, complementary investigations, medical and surgical procedures, medical, surgical, family and social history). It contains 45, 663 concepts (eg: *Marfan's syndrome, Asthma*).

ICD10. The International Classification of Diseases (ICD) is the standard diagnostic tool for epidemiology, health management and clinical purposes. This includes the analysis of the general health situation of population groups. It is used fior classifying diseases and other health problems recorded on many types of health and vital records including death certificates and health records. It contain 44, 962 terms (eg: *Turner syndrome*).

ATC. The Anatomical, Therapeutic and Chemical classification (ATC) is an international classification [10] used to classify drugs. The ATC classification is developed and maintained by the Collaborating Centre for Drug Statistics Methodology. In the ATC classification system, the drugs are divided into different groups according to the organ or the system on which they act and their chemical, pharmacological and therapeutic properties. It contains 11, 105 terms (eg : *Acebutolol* and *thiazides*).

FMA. The Foundational Model Anatomy (FMA)is an evolving formal ontology that has been under development at the University of Washington since 1994 [11]. It is the most complete ontology of human "canonical" anatomy. The FMA describes anatomical entities, most of which are anatomical structures composed of many interconnected parts in a complex way. It contains more than $81,000$ classes and 139 relationships connecting the classes, and over $120,000$ terms (eg : *Arm*).

The knowledge terminological ressources MeSH, SNOMED INT, MedDRA, ICD10 and ATC exist in French and in English. FMA terms are currently being translated by CISMeF team(Catalogue et Index des Sites Médicaux de langue Française) [12].

2.3   Tree Tagger

Tree Tagger [3] is a tool for annotating text with part-of-speech (POS) and lemma information. It was developed by Helmut Schmid at the Institute for Computational Linguistics of the University of Stuttgart. The Tree Tagger has been successfully used to tag several languages (German, English, French, etc) and is adaptable to other languages if a lexicon and a manually tagged training corpus are available. It takes as input a text and as output it gives the POS tag (noun, adjective, verb, etc). For example in the Figure 1, the sentence *Carbonate de sodium dihydroxyaluminium* is tagged by carbonate=NOM, de=PRP, etc.

Input: carbonate de sodium dihydroxyaluminium
Output:

word	pos	lemma
carbonate	NOM	carbonate
de	PRP	de
sodium	NOM	sodium
dihydroxyaluminium	NOM	dihydroxyaluminium

NOM = Noun; ADJ = Adjective; VER = Verb

Fig. 1. Example of tagging with a Tree Tagger

3   Methods

Among the works on the Clinical Practice Guidelines, there are Brigitte Seroussi's studies [2], which are based on the formalization of the CPGs in the form of decision tree structure, by comparing the basic CPG which are represented as rules of production, with clinical situations and action plans. In our study we propose a generic method able to manage this evolution on all types of medical documents by ignoring the specificity of the processed document. Our approach includes several steps which are detailed in the Figure 2.

- Step 1: The selection of the CPGs on the same pathology and edited by the same organization with five year published difference for example.
- Step 2: The segmentation of the input text CPGs into sentences.
- Step 3: The correspondence of the sentences of both CPGs which will allow us to obtain the most similar sentences in output. In this step, we used similarity measures (Dice [13], Levenshtein [14] and Stoilos [15]) who calculated the similarity between all the characters that compose sentences of both CPGs.

- Step 4: The extraction of the maximal noun phrases by using a pattern constructed approach on medical terminologies tagged with Tree Tagger.
- Step 5: The comparison of noun phrases extracted from both CPGs based on the context of each phrase (right and left elements) to extract all the possible insertions, deletions and substitutions.

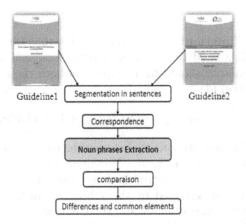

In input: two CPGs on the same pathology with five years difference published.
In output: differences and common elements between the two CPGs.

Fig. 2. Method plan

The following are the equations of the similarity measures used:

1. **Dice's coefficient:** This measure is used in statistics to determine the similarity between two samples X and Y. It is between 0 and 1. In our case, we calculate the coefficient between two sentences. For this, we defined two samples X and Y as the set of bigrams of each respective sentence x and y. A bigram is the union of two letters. The Dice's coefficient is defined by the equation (1).

$$Dice\,(X,Y) = \frac{2 \times |X \cap Y|}{|X| + |Y|} \tag{1}$$

2. **Distance of Levenshtein:** This measure between two sentences x and y is defined as the minimum number of elementary operations that is required to pass from the sentence x to the sentence y. There are three possible transactions: replacing a character with another (*asthma, astmma*), deleting a character (*asthma, astma*) and adding a character (*asthma, asthmma*). This measure takes its values in the interval $[0,\infty[$. The Normalized Levenshtein [16] (*LevNorm*) in the range $[0, 1]$ is obtained by dividing the distance

of Levenshtein $Lev(x, y)$ by the size of the longest string and it is defined by the equation (2).

$$LevNorm(x, y) = 1 - \frac{Lev(x, y)}{Max(|x|, |y|)} \tag{2}$$

LevNorm $(x, y) \in [0, 1]$ because $Lev(x, y) \leq Max(|x|, |y|)$; with $|x|$ the length of the sentence x.

3. **Stoilos similarity function:** is based on the idea that the similarity between two entities is related to their commonalities as well as their differences. Thus, the similarity should be a function of both these features. It is defined by the equation (3).

$$Sim(x, y) = comm(x, y) - Diff(x, y) + Winkler(x, y) \tag{3}$$

Comm(x,y) stands for the commonality between the strings x and y, Diff(x,y) for the difference between x and y, and Winkler(x,y) for the improvement of the result using the method introduced by Winkler in [17]. The function of commonality is determined by the substring function. The biggest common substring between two sentences (MaxComSubString) is computed. This process is further extended by removing the common substring and by searching again for the next biggest substring until none can be identified. The function of commonality is given by the equation (4):

$$Comm(x, y) = \frac{2 \times \sum_i |MaxComSubString|}{|x| + |y|} \tag{4}$$

The function of Difference is defined in the equation (5) where $p \in [0, \infty[$ (usually p= 0.6), $|u_x|$ and $|u_y|$ represent the length of the unmatched substring from the strings sentences and y scaled respectively by their length:

$$Diff(x, y) = \frac{|u_x| \times |u_y|}{p + (1 - p) \times (|u_x| + |u_y| - |u_x| \times |u_y|)} \tag{5}$$

The Winkler parameter Winkler(x,y) is defined by the equation (6):

$$Winkler(x, y) = L \times P \times (1 - Comm(x, y)) \tag{6}$$

Where L is the length of common prefix between the sentences x and y at the start of the sentence up to a maximum of 4 characters and P is a constant scaling factor for how much the score is adjusted upwards for having common prefixes. The standard value for this constant in Winkler's work is P=0.1 [17].

Detection and extraction of noun phrases using patterns based on different medical terminologies and Tree Tagger is the first step in the procedure. Once the detection is accomplished, we procede to the comparison step in an attempt to detect all possible changes. Many studies have been dedicated to the extraction of noun phrases. For example the ACABIT tool [18] is a program that allows a terminological acquisition on a pre-tagged and disambiguated corpus. This acquisition is performed in two steps: 1) a linguistic analysis of the corpus by transducers that produces candidate terms and 2) a statistical filtering step that sorts candidate terms from a reference corpus and valids terms. Another extractor YaTeA (Yet another Term Extractor) [19], is used to assist the process of identifying terms in a French and English, with visualization and configuration interfaces to reduce the complexity of the writing and editing configuration files.

4   Noun Phrases Detection

4.1   Extraction Patterns of Noun Phrases

For the construction patterns of extraction step for noun phrases, we tagged the six biomedical terminologies detailed in section 2, with Tree Tagger. For example: the term *douleur abdominale* (*abdominal pain*) is tagged as follows: douleur **NOM** douleur — abdominale **ADJ** abdomen.

All the corresponding patterns were automatically generated. For example: the corresponding pattern of *douleur abdominale* (*abdominal pain*), is *NOM ADJ* (*NOUN ADJECTIVE*). The duplicates were removed and to reduce the total number of patterns, only some of them were selected. Do do that, we relied on two selection criteria: the length of terms and their relevance. For the first criterion, we performed a statistical study by calculating for every terminology the percentage of terms which length was less than or equal to 1, 2 to 16 words by term, and we found that over 95% of all the terms have a length less than or equal to 8 words. The details are reported in the Table 1.

For the second criterion, which is the relevance of the patterns, we calculated for each pattern, the percentage of words represented by the latter. For example, the pattern *NOM* (*NOUN*) represents 22.16% of the MeSH terminology and *NOM ADJ* (*NOUN ADJ*) represents 13.90%. Therefore 36.06% of the terms may be represented with only these two patterns. Thus we retained the patterns which represent more than 80% of the chosen terminologies. The final list is composed by 262 patterns. Table 2 shows some of the results for the MeSH thesaurus.

4.2   Detection and Extraction of Noun Phrases

The patterns are applied to the CPGs previously labeled with a Tree Tagger to extract the corresponding noun phrases. Since the list of the patterns contains imbricated patterns (e.g.: *NOM* is included in *NOM ADJ* (*NOUN and NOUN ADJECTIVE*)) this implies imbricated noun phrases. (e.g.: the noun phrases *maladie* (*disease*) and *Alzheimer* (*Alzheimer*) are included in the noun phrase *maladie d'Alzheimer* (*Alzheimer's disease*)). To avoid redundancies in noun phrases, we extract them from the maximal noun phrases according to

Table 1. Percentage of length of terms, Nb: Number of terms of length lower or equal to 1, 2 to 9 and the percentage of these terms

	1	2	3	4	5	6	7	8	9
ATC	$Nb = 2,994$	3,568	7,531	8,512	9,683	10,273	10,587	10,823	10,928
	26.97%	32.14%	67.83%	76.67%	87.22%	92.53%	95.36%	97.49%	98.43%
MeSH	$Nb = 33,846$	76,596	103,836	120,717	130,029	135,449	138,204	139,739	140,559
	23.94%	54.17%	73.43%	85.37%	91.96%	95.79%	97.74%	98.83%	99.41%
ICD10	$Nb = 2,661$	9,479	16,370	21,972	25,906	28,856	30,896	32,493	33,720
	5.92%	21.08%	36.41%	48.87%	57.62%	64.18%	68.72%	72.27%	75.00%
FMA	$Nb = 1,817$	7,280	11,495	14,071	15,872	16,872	17,278	17,555	17,675
	10.24%	41.01%	64.76%	79.27%	89.41%	95.05%	97.34%	98.90%	99.57%
SND	$Nb = 27,406$	85,926	123,797	152,553	172,464	185,258	193,508	199,098	202,645
	13.13%	41.16%	59.30%	73.07%	82.61%	88.74%	92.69%	95.37%	97.07%
MDR	$Nb = 4,583$	16,310	26,968	35,540	40,617	43,108	44,350	44,916	45,263
	10.04%	35.72%	59.06%	77.83%	88.95%	94.41%	97.13%	98.37%	99.13%

their positions in the sentence. The process of the algorithm we propose is detailed in the Figure 3.

The position (pos) and the length of each extracted noun phrase is calculated. Then we search for the imbricated noun phrases and see if they have the same position, (i) if this is the case, the smallest noun phrase is deleted. (ii) If not, we verify if the position of the smallest noun phrase is equal to the position of the biggest noun phrase added to the position of the smallest in the largest noun phrase; the smallest noun phrase is then deleted.

For example, by applying this algorithm to the sentence : *Le médecin traitant assure la coordination des soins et la surveillance du patient en ambulatoire en lien avec l'équipe spécialisée*, we obtained: *médecin traitant, coordination des soins, surveillance du patient en ambulatoire, lien* and *équipe spécialisée*.(See Figure 4)

5   Evaluation of Extraction of Noun Phrases

To evaluate this approach, two CPGs were used *Cancer colorectal, Février 2008* and *Cancer colorectal, Janvier 2012* and all the corresponding maximal noun phrases were automatically and manually extracted to be able to calculate: the precision, the recall and the F-measure. These measures are defined as follows:

$$Precision = \frac{Number\ of\ Correct\ maximal\ noun\ phrases\ detected}{Total\ number\ of\ maximal\ noun\ phrases\ detected} \tag{7}$$

$$Recall = \frac{Number\ of\ Correct\ maximal\ noun\ phrases\ detected}{Total\ number\ of\ maximal\ noun\ phrases\ in\ the\ text} \tag{8}$$

Table 2. Patterns compliance. For example : 22.16% of MeSH terms are nouns(NOM), 13.90% are adjectives(ADJ).

Pattern	Percentage of terms	Cumulative percentage of terms
NOM	22.16%	22.16%
NOM ADJ	13.90%	36.06%
NOM NOM	06.24%	42.30%
NOM PRP NOM	04.74%	47.07%
ADJ NOM	03.57%	50.61%
NOM NAM	02.71%	53.32%
NOM PRP : detNOM	02.07%	55.39%

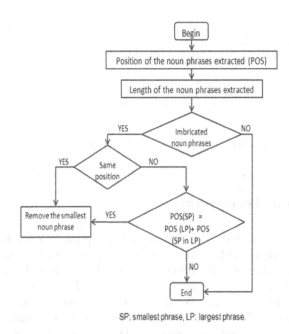

SP: smallest phrase, LP: largest phrase.

Fig. 3. Algorithm for the extraction of maximal noun phrases

$$F - measure = \frac{2 \times Precision \times Recall}{Precision + Recall} \qquad (9)$$

In a first step, we used the list of 262 patterns. This list was built using two criteria which are: the length of the pattern and its relevance. The patterns covers more than 80% of all terms in terminologies. To evaluate the validity of this list, we increased it with 231 new patterns. The new list covered 85% of terms in the six terminologies.

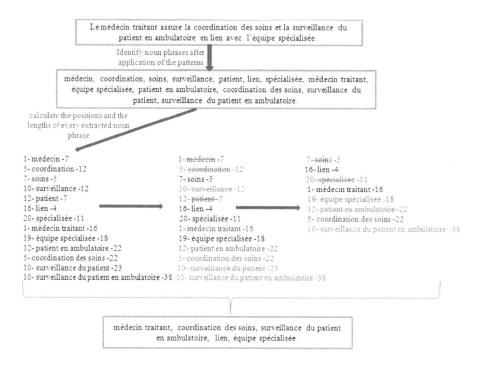

Fig. 4. Example of extraction the maximal noun phrases

6   Results and Discussion

Using a list of 262 patterns, 708 maximal noun phrases were found, among them, 364 were correct which represent a 51.41% precision. However, by detecting these phrases manually, 602 maximal noun phrases were found which represent a 60.47% recall and by consequence a 55.57% F-measure. We attempted to improve these results by increasing a number of patterns from 262 to 493. We obtained a total of 729 maximal noun phrases, with 365 which were correct, which corresponding to a 50.07% precision, 60.63% recall and 54.85% F-measure. These final results are not different from the first results and they comforting the choice of a reduced list of 262 patterns.(see Table 3)

Table 3. Results

Number of Patterns	Precision	Recall	F-measure
262	51.41%	60.47%	55.57%
493	50.07%	60.63%	54.85%

Other options can be tested to improve these results. For example, the use of another tool for tagging (than Tree Tagger), such as GATE Tagger [20]. In another context, we evaluate our approach of detection of noun phrases by applying it to other medical documents such as the Summary of Product Characteristics (SPCs), which are the legal documents approved as part of the marketing authorization for each drug. They are the basis of information for health care professionals on how to use the drug and they are updated throughout the life-cycle of the product as new data emerge. These documents are of interest especially in the comparison step because it exists for each drug, a corresponding SPC which is regularly updated and it will permit us to obtain the documents detailing the same drug but within a 4 or 5 year interval and will give a sense to the comparison and especially to the detection of possible changes.

7 Conclusion

In this paper we presented a useful tool for detection and extraction of noun phrases in order to develop a generic method for comparing medical documents. The method has been used in French but it can easily be applied to other languages. Furthermore, our method is based on the patterns constructed from six medical terminologies (MeSH, ATC, SNOMED INT, FMA, MedDRA and ICD10) that we tagged with a Tree Tagger. These patterns are applied to the CPGs as input to detect and extract the corresponding noun phrases. Then, in the comparison step, we compared different noun phrases and their left and right contexts in order to extract the insertions, additions and substitutions. Finally, a recapitulative file with the differences and the common elements between two or more CPGs inputs is created in order to implement an ergonomic tool to represent knowledge medical evolution. This tool will serve as basis for evaluation of the approach by comparing our results with those of the other existing approaches. The results obtained with hopefully prompt physicians to apply it on other kind of medical documents such as SPCs.

References

[1] Grimshaw, J.M., Russell, I.T.: Effect of clinical guidelines on medical practice: a systematic review of rigorous evaluations. The Lancet. 342(8883), 1317–1322 (1993)

[2] Bouaud, J., Séroussi, B., Brizon, A., Culty, T., Mentré, F., Ravery, V.: How updating uextual Clinical Practice Guidelines impacts Clinical Decision Support Systems: a case study with Bladder Cancer Management. Med. Info., 829–833 (2007)

[3] Schmid, H.: Probabilistic part-of-speech tagging using decision trees. In: Proceedings of International Conference on New Methods in Language Processing, Manchester, UK, vol. 12, pp. 44–49 (1994)

[4] Cheah, T.S.: The impact of clinical guidelines and clinical pathways on medical practice: effectiveness and medico-legal aspects. Annals-Academy of Medicine Singapore 27, 533–539 (1998)

[5] Roche, C.: Terminologie et ontologie. Armand. Colin. 48–62(2005) (in French)

[6] Lefèvre, P.: La recherche d'informations: du texte intégral au thésaurus. Hermes Science (2000) (in French)

[7] Nelson, S.J., Johnston, W.D., Humphreys, B.L.: Relationships in medical subject headings (MeSH). In: Relationships in the Organization of Knowledge, pp. 171–184. Springer (2001)

[8] Cornet, R., de Keizer, N.: Forty years of SNOMED: a literature review. BMC Medical Informatics and Decision Making 8(suppl.1), 1–6 (2008)

[9] Brown, E.G., Wood, L., Wood, S.: The medical dictionary for regulatory activities (MedDRA). Drug Saf. 20, 109–117 (1999)

[10] Skrbo, A., Begović, B., Skrbo, S.: Classification of drugs using the ATC system (Anatomic, Therapeutic, Chemical Classification) and the latest changes. Medicinski. Arhiv. 58(1 suppl. 2), 138 (2004)

[11] Rosse, C., Mejino Jr., José, L.V.: A reference ontology for biomedical informatics: the Foundational Model of Anatomy. Journal of Biomedical Informatics 36(6), 478–500 (2003)

[12] Merabti, T., Soualmia, L., Grosjean, J., Palombi, O., Müller, JM., Darmoni, S.: Translating the Foundational Model of Anatomy into French using knowledge-based and lexical methods. BMC Medical Informatics and Decision Making 11(1), 65 (2011)

[13] Dice, L.R.: Measures of the amount of ecologic association between species. Ecology 26(3), 297–302 (1945)

[14] Levenshtein, V.: Binary codes capable of correcting deletions, insertions and reversals. Soviet Physics-Doklady 10 (1965)

[15] Stoilos, G., Stamou, G., Kollias, S.D.: A string metric for ontology alignment. In: Gil, Y., Motta, E., Benjamins, V.R., Musen, M.A. (eds.) ISWC 2005. LNCS, vol. 3729, pp. 624–637. Springer, Heidelberg (2005)

[16] Yujian, L., Bo, L.: A normalized Levenshtein distance metric. IEEE Transactions on Pattern Analysis and Machine Intelligence 29(6), 1091–1095 (2007)

[17] Winkler, W.E.: The state of record linkage and current research problems. Technical report: Statistics of Income Division, Internal Revenue Service Publication (1999)

[18] Daille, B.: Conceptual structuring through term variations. In: Proceedings of the ACL 2003 Workshop on Multiword Expressions: Analysis, Acquisition and Treatment, vol. 18, pp. 9–16. Association for Computational Linguistics (2003)

[19] Aubin, S., Hamon, T.: Improving term extraction with terminological resources. In: Salakoski, T., Ginter, F., Pyysalo, S., Pahikkala, T. (eds.) FinTAL 2006. LNCS (LNAI), vol. 4139, pp. 380–387. Springer, Heidelberg (2006)

[20] Cunningham, H., Maynard, D., Bontcheva, K., Tablan, V., Aswani, N., Roberts, I., Gorrell, G., Funk, A., Roberts, A., Damljanovic, D., Heitz, T., Greenwood, M.A., Saggion, H., Petrak, J., Li, Y., Peters, W.: Text Processing with GATE, Version 6 (2011) 978-0956599315

Color-Coded Imaging with Adaptive Multiscale Spatial Filtering

Xinhong Zhang[1], Xiaopan Chen[2], Congcong Li[2], and Fan Zhang[2,3,*]

[1] Software School, Henan University, Kaifeng 475001, China
[2] School of Computer and Information Engineering, Henan University, Kaifeng 475001, China
[3] Institute of Image Processing and Pattern Recognition,
Henan University, Kaifeng 475001, China
zhangfan@henu.edu.cn

Abstract. Digital subtraction angiography has become one of the most important approaches to artery disease diagnosis and treatment. Doctors implement diagnose and treatment by subjective analysis of the DSA series, and the results are always dependent on doctors' experience. The application of color-coded imaging technology makes it convenient to identify images and provides additional physiology information auxiliary diagnosis and treatment. Before implementing color-coded imaging technology on DSA series, we preprocess the images with several mutiscale spatial filters to remove noises and enhance vessel structures to make the results readable and clear.

Keywords: Color-coded imaging, Digital Subtraction Angiography, Multiscale Spatial filtering.

1 Introduction

Since 1927 Egaz Moniz introduced angiography according to the theory that different tissues possess different capacities to absorb X-ray, people have utilized the same technology to research the way of blood flow in the brain for almost 100 years. Although the vessel angiography has been improved all the time, doctors still use monochrome images to observe vessel structures in clinical applications.

According to different wave length of lights accepted by eyes, human beings can distinguish different objects. Using intensity factor we can differentiate objects, however, when the intensity varies slightly, color information will always provide another efficient approach for us to distinguish objects. Colors enhance people's consciousness about medicine information because eyes can distinguish wide color series and even catch the very slight change of color signal intensity. As a result, color-coded imaging technology is gaining more and more attention and becomes one of the focuses in the image processing field. However, doctors still diagnose diseases with black and white DSA series. One of the most representative applications of color-coded imaging technology is to reprocess the original DSA images, integrate the DSA

---

* Corresponding author.

Y. Zhang et al. (Eds.): HIS 2014, LNCS 8423, pp. 121–128, 2014.

series into one single image and then color-coded the integrated image. The application can directly display the pathological information and provide more physiological information for doctors. In addition, it is also an objective and quantitative tool for disease diagnose and therapeutic effect evaluation [1,2].

2   Adaptive Multi-scale Spatial Filtering

In order to enhance vessel in DSA image, multi-scale adaptive filtering algorithm is used for DSA vascular enhancement processing. This paper proposes an adaptive multi-scale vessel enhancement filtering algorithm that the filter parameters can be determined adaptively according to image intrinsic characteristics. The main purpose of this algorithm is to improve the visual quality of blood vessel in DSA images.

The purpose of vessel enhancement is to emphasize vascular structures in image, while restrain the non-blood vessel characteristics. So the image recognition will be strengthened. Multi-scale vessel enhancement algorithm is based on multi-scale theory, using eigenvalues characteristics of Hessian matrix. The filter parameters and the scale factor are adapted the vascular structures is enhanced by image filtering. In digital image processing, Hessian matrix is used to extract image orientation feature and to analyze particular shape, while also be used in the curve structure segmentation and reconstruction. Eigenvalues of the Hessian matrix can be used to determine the corner where the density changes rapidly. Therefore the direction and intensity of blood vessels in DSA image can be characterized by Hessian matrix eigenvalues and eigenvectors.

Since the differences of blood vessel diameter and the differences of concentrations of contrast agent, gray value is higher in thick blood vessel of DSA image, and gray value is lower in small blood vessels. Although gray-scale transformation can highlight the great vessels, but it is difficult to distinguish small blood vessels with surrounding tissue, which will affect DSA vascular feature point extraction. In this paper, a Hessian matrix eigenvalue algorithm is used to enhance the blood vessels further. The principle of this algorithm is extracting blood vessels by use of vascular tubular structure. The vessel enhancement is viewed as a filtering process to look for two-dimensional graphical data which is similar as tubular structure [3,4].

The eventual goal of vessel enhancement is to highlight the vessel structures and restrain the non-vessel structures in images. Frangi has proposed an algorithm based on multi-scale spatial filtering and some improved algorithm based on it also arise in recent years.

The idea of Frangi filter and its improved algorithms is to consider the vessel enhancement as a filtering process of locating tubular structures. The analysis of eigenvalues and eigenvectors of Hessian matrix at each pixel point can detect the tubular structures. Since DSA images consist of various sizes of vessels, the enhancements with single scale cannot clearly display vessel structures of different sizes. As a result, multiscale theory is introduced to presents vessel structures of different sizes in these methods.

The theory of Frangi filter is as follows, firstly, the filter obtains the Hessian matrix of the input image by virtue of the convolution of the input image and the four second order deviations of Gaussian function. The eigenvalues of the Hessian matrix point out the directional information of the vessels. The linear model constructed by Gaussian function has the feature that the larger absolute value of eigenvalue indicates the direction along the vessel and the smaller one represents the direction across the vessel. The filter is constructed based on the two eigenvalues of Hessian matrix. Next, according to the multiscale theory, for the linear structure elements, the output of filtering result will be peaked at a scale that approximately matches the size of the vessel to detect. Each point in the image is processed iteratively at different sizes of scales and the maximum filtering result will be the final output of that point. By the algorithm above mentioned, the vessel structures are enhanced and the non-vessel structures are restrained. The filter proposed by Frangi is as follows,

$$
v_o(s) = \begin{cases} 0 & \text{if } \lambda_2 > 0, \\ \exp\left(-\dfrac{R_B^2}{2\beta^2}\right)\left(1 - \exp\left(-\dfrac{S^2}{2c^2}\right)\right) & \end{cases} \tag{1}
$$

where λ_1 and λ_2 are eigenvalues of Hessian matrix at each point, and $|\lambda_2| > |\lambda_1|$; $R_B = |\lambda_2|/|\lambda_1|$, $S = \sqrt{\lambda_1^2 + \lambda_2^2}$, and β and C are respectively proportionality factor of R_B and S.

By iterating scale factor σ at each point of the input image, the values of v_0 are obtained in different scales, and the maximum value of v_0 will be the practical output of that point, that is, $f(x, y) = \max(v_0(x, y; \sigma))$.

The large vessel structures are enhanced after implementation of the Frangi filter, but the enhancements of fine vessel structures are not obvious. Based on Frangi's filter, Cui proposes the following combination of the components to define a vesselness function as follows,

$$
v_o(s) = \begin{cases} 0 & \text{if } \lambda_2 > 0, \\ \exp\left(-\dfrac{D^2}{2\beta^2}\right)\left(1 - \exp\left(-\dfrac{S^2}{2(wC)^2}\right)\right)\left(1 - \exp\left(-\dfrac{|\lambda_2|}{\alpha}\right)\right) & \end{cases} \tag{2}
$$

In this paper, we improve the Frangi filter in the following several ways. In the first, since the region including non-vessel structures is smooth in DSA vessel images and the angle formed by the two eigenvalues and of Hessian matrix approximates to zero, the improved algorithm implements vessel enhancement taking advantage of this angle feature. While is the ratio of the two eigenvalues and of Hessian matrix in formula (1), is the angle formed by the two eigenvalues and of Hessian matrix in formula (2). The value of is as follows, $D = arctg(\lambda_2 / \lambda_1)$.

Next, since the large vessel structures appear when applying the Gaussian convolution with large scale factor, the large vessel structures can be obtained when the corresponding filtering parameter is enlarged. Similarly, the fine vessel structures appear when applying the Gaussian convolution with small scale factor, the small vessel structures can be obtained when the corresponding filtering parameter is diminished.

The parameter of the filter should adapt to the scale factor ∂. The parameter of the filter c in formula (1) is fixed in the iterated process, while the parameter of the filter C adapts to scale factor ∂ in formula (2) in the improved method. C is the module of Hessian matrix in the corresponding scale $C =\parallel H \parallel$.

Then, the adaption of the parameter W of improved filter is realized by the following procedure. The initial parameter W of the improved filter of the input image is related to the histogram distribution bandwidth of the input image. The initial parameter W directly determines the filtering radius of the improved filter and is related to the peak crest width of gray histogram of the input image. The value of the initial parameter W will enlarge when the gray scale histogram distribution bandwidth is large, and the value of the initial parameter W will diminish when the gray scale histogram distribution bandwidth is small. The value of W is defined as follows,

$$w = max(R(P(r_k) < 2d)) - min(R(P(r_k) < 2d))$$

Where the discrete function $P(r_k) = n_k$ corresponds to the normalized histogram of the input image, r_k represents the gray level, and n_k is the probability estimate of the occurrence of gray level r_k. $R(n_k) = r_k$ is the one-to-one mapping between gray level r_k and probability estimate n_k.

Finally, the noises which are magnified in the process of adaption according to the third component of the second row of formula (2) will be removed by the eigenvalues of Hessian matrix. Because the noises usually appear in the non-vessel region where the eigenvalue λ_2 approximates to zero, the last component of the second row of formula (2) removes the noises by virtue of λ_2, where α is the initial parameter.

3   Color-Coded Imaging

Digital subtraction Angiography is a kind of image processing method which implements vessel imaging by virtue of contrast media. In the ordinary X-ray images, the contrast ratio of vessel structures and background tissues is very slight and the vessel structures are hardly visible. In order to increase the contrast ratio, the contrast media is always injected to vessels need to be examined. The angiography theory considers the first few images before the contrast media flow into the vessel as the mask image and the images blood have passed through the vessels of interest are often referred to as contrast images or live images. Subtraction of the mask images from the contrast image can remove the surrounding tissues and bones which remain unchanged in the mask and contrast images. It is one of the ways to obtain visible vessel structures containing contrast materials of low concentrations. The dynamic blood flow can also be observed through the subtracted image series.

Artery angiography was introduced into clinical practice to position tumors and observe the sizes of them. The catheter is inserted into artery observed and inserted the iodine contrast media. The vessel with contrast media passed is projected continuously, and the DSA series of artery vessels are obtained with computer-assisted medical imaging. The DSA series display the anatomy of vessels and the differences between blood flows of before and after treatment, and provide references and foundation for diagnose of artery diseases. However, the passage of contrast media through artery is estimated mainly by human eyes and doctors are requested to overview the whole process of artery contrast media filling vessels with sequence of DSA series which is highly dependent on doctors' experience and subjective feelings, and the data obtained through this approach is lack of objectiveness and comparability. In order to solve the problem, people continuously explore color-coded imaging technology and make the judgments on angiography results rapid and efficient, and obtain quantitative indicator.

Color-coded imaging technology works out time-density curves (TDC) of each point by reprocessing original data of conventional angiography. Two important parameters are calculated in the process, the maximum intensity value and the time when the intensity value achieves peak value of each point. The maximum enhancement of each point is marked by *IMax* and the time when the intensity achieves peak value is marked by *TTP*. They are extracted respectively from the time-density curves of each point by the following method.

$$IMax = Ipeak - IMask$$

Where *IMax* is the maximum enhancement at each point, *Ipeak* is the peak pixel intensity and *IMask* is the pixel intensity in the mask frames.

Based on HSV color model, the two parameters are adapted to the process of color coding. Hue is calculated through *TTP**240/360, saturation is constant, and the intensity value is obtained as *IMax*. By virtue of color coding, the color of each point is determined by *TTP* of contrast media at each point, and the value of each point is determined by the intensity value at that point. HSV value of each point is transported to colors as red, green and blue and so on with different intensity. Thereby, the whole process of contrast media flow through the vessels is displayed in one single image which includes all of the information of the whole DSA series. The information of hemodynamics can be reflected by the single color-coded image. Color convention from warm color to cool color represents the different time cost of contrast media to achieve peak intensity value at each point. In the case that the blood flow is blocked in some part of the vessel and the time cost of contrast media to peak intensity value is delayed, the hue will be cool and is different from surrounding colors which represents poor vascular perfusion. The parameterized vascular perfusion by color-coded imaging technology enhances the data persuasion and makes the perfusion comparable.

4   Experimental Results

The image used in this experiment is a set of brain DSA images. DSA device model is GE LCV plus. DSA images are stored in multi-DICOM files, totally 25 frames. Experiments using computer with hardware configuration as Intel Xeon dual-core CPU, 3.4GHz, 8.0G RAM, 1TB hard drive and 1G graph card. Software environment is Matlab 2012a.

In this section, we choose the cerebral vessel DSA image to conduct experiments. Firstly, Fig.1 shows some results of vessel enhancement filtering in cerebral vessel DSA images with application of the mulitscale spatial theory. By implementing the vessel enhancement algorithm, the vessel structures are improved and the non-vessel structures are restrained. In addition, the results also show that the performance of multiscale adapted algorithm is superior to Frangi filter.

Secondly, in Fig.2, both of the two results can display the blood flow process in one single image by assigning different colors and intensity to each point. The warm color and cool color can clearly reflect different costs of time to achieve peak intensity value of each point. The contrast of the two image shows that the vessel enhancement filter can facilitate removing noise and highlight vessel structures and restrain non-vessel structures.

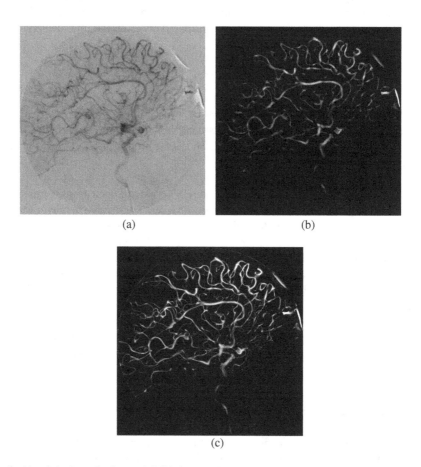

(a)   (b)

(c)

Fig. 1. (a) original cerebral vessel DSA image. (b) vessel enhanced image after implementing Frangi filtering. (c) vessel enhanced image after implementing improved Frangi filter (adapted filtered image with multiscale spatial theory).

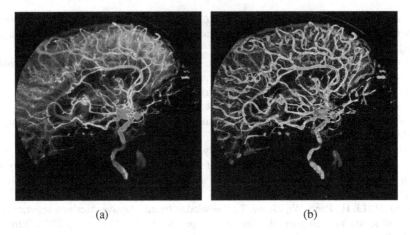

(a)   (b)

Fig. 2. (a) Color-coded image based on the original cerebral vessel DSA image; (b) Color-coded image based on the vessel enhanced image by improved Frangi filter

5   Conclusions

In clinical practice, the color-coded image technology assists doctors in implementing more accurate diagnosis and making more specific medicine treatment scheme especially for junior doctors because the color-coded image can show blood flow changes directly and thoroughly. The preprocessing of original DSA series enhances the vessel structures and restrains non-vessel structures obviously which makes the result more clear and accurate. Since the color-coded imaging technology has not been developed maturely, there are still limitations of this technology. In the future, the combination of additional parameters such as time of maximum increase concentration (TMIC) will improve the practicability of this technology significantly and make it more suitable for clinical application.

Acknowledgements. This research was supported by the Foundation of Education Bureau of Henan Province, China grants No. 2010B520003, Key Science and Technology Program of Henan Province, China grants No. 132102210133 and 132102210034, and the Key Science and Technology Projects of Public Health Department of Henan Province, China grants No. 2011020114.

References

1. Strother, C.M.: Digital Subtraction Angiography Becomes More Colorfuls. AXIOM Innovations, 17–18 (March 2009)
2. Wu, Y.-N., Yang, P.-F., Ye, H., Huang, Q.-H., Liu, J.-M.: Color-coded Imaging Technology and Its Clinical Applications in Cerebral Vessel Disease. China Journal Stroke 8(1), 69–73 (2013)

3. Shang, Y., Deklerck, R., Nyssen, E., Markova, A., de Mey, J., Yang, X., Sun, K.: Vascular Active Contour for Vessel Tree Segmentation. IEEE Transactions on Biomedical Engineering 58(4), 1023–1032 (2011)
4. Frangi, A.F., Niessen, W.J., Vincken, K.L., Viergever, M.A.: Multiscale vessel enhancement filtering. In: Wells, W.M., Colchester, A.C.F., Delp, S.L. (eds.) MICCAI 1998. LNCS, vol. 1496, pp. 130–137. Springer, Heidelberg (1998)
5. Frangi, A.F., Niessen, W.J., Hoogeveen, R.M., van Walsum, T., Viergever, M.A.: Model-based quantization of 3D magnetic resonance angiographic images. IEEE Transactions on Medical Imaging 18(10), 946–956 (1999)
6. Schuldhaus, D., Spiegel, M., Redel, T., Polyanskaya, M., Struffert, T., Hornegger, J., Doerfler, A.: Classification-based summation of cerebral digital subtraction angiography series for image post-processing algorithms. Physics in Medicine and Biology 56(1), 1791–1802 (2011)
7. Sang, N., Li, H., Peng, W., Zhang, T.: Knowledge-based adaptive threshold segmentation of digital subtraction angiography images. Image and Vision Computing 25(8), 1263–1270 (2007)
8. Cebral, R., Castro, A., Appanaboyina, S., Putman, M., Millan, D., Frangi, F.: Efficient Pipeline for Image-Based Patient-Specific Analysis of Cerebral Aneurysm Hemodynamics: Technique and Sensitivity. IEEE Transactions on Medical Image 24(4), 457–467 (2005)

An Architecture and a Platform for Recording and Replaying the Healthcare Information

Yi Ding*, Ji Geng, Zhe Xiao, and Zhiguang Qin

School of Computer Science and Engineering,
University of Electronic Science and Technology of China, 611731, China

Abstract. The hospital domain requires practitioners to retain operational records so as to inspect their day-to-day medical activities in future. Authors' previous research indicated that by employing the Scenario–Oriented ApproaCH (SOACH) equipped with the recording and replaying mechanism, information systems have the ability to record the changing history of information units, and then replay such histories as a flow of information scenarios under users' request.

This paper extends authors' previous research and proposes an architecture and a platform, called Scenario–Oriented PlatForm (SOPF), which is implemented by following the proposed architecture, to demonstrate the applicability of the SOACH. The SOPF aims to manage the scenario in a computerized way so as to support the replaying capability of healthcare information systems. The Microalbuminuria Protocol (MAP) is used as an example in this paper to evaluate the SOPF. Based on experimental results, day-to-day medical activities can be replayed as a continuous and on-the-fly information scenario for a specified duration of time.

Keywords: Scenario, Scenario-Oriented, Replaying, Architecture, Platform.

1 Introduction

The hospital domain requires practitioners to retain operational records so as to inspect their day-to-day medical activities in future, which will incorporate domain knowledge to standardize and enhance their performance. One typical challenge that arises in computerized information systems which are implemented to manage such application domains, is to reproduce the evolution process of certain information units, which not only can treat all the managed information as a whole, but also to show details of any pieces or any dimensions of the specific information cluster. For example, in the hospital domain, doctors not only want to reproduce the whole therapy history of a patient, but also want to review the changing history of one specific test result (e.g. the changing history of the ACR test result) or the reason why the patient took the test.

---

* This project is sponsored by the National Natural Science Foundation of China (Project No. 61300090), the Fundamental Research Funds for the Central Universities (Project No.ZYGX2013J080), and the Scientific Research Foundation for the Returned Overseas Chinese Scholars, State Education Ministry.

Y. Zhang et al. (Eds.): HIS 2014, LNCS 8423, pp. 129–140, 2014.

The concept of *scenario* have been gaining acceptance in both research and practice as a new way of representing the knowledge in many different disciplines[1–3]. The frequent use of scenarios motivated us to investigate its use in the process of *replaying* the healthcare information in the hospital domain. Authors' previous research [4, 5] proposed a $\underline{S}$cenario–$\underline{O}$riented $\underline{A}$pproa$\underline{CH}$ (SOACH) to record and replay the healthcare information within the context of scenario so as to support the information replaying. This approach aims to organize/reorganize related information and knowledge elements, which could constitute a meaningful scenario as a *context* so that medical activities in the real environment can be recorded and then be replayed dynamically later.

This paper extends the previous research and proposes an architecture and a platform, called $\underline{S}$cenario–$\underline{O}$riented $\underline{P}$lat$\underline{F}$orm (SOPF), which is implemented by following the proposed architecture, to demonstrate the applicability of the SOACH. The SOPF utilizes available technologies, such as the database management system (DBMS) and the XML, as a base for implementing the *Scenario-Oriented Language* so as to manage the scenario in a computerized way. One of the benefit of using the SOPF is that users can query and view day-to-day medical activities as a continuous, on-the-fly information scenario through a newly developed REPLAY SCENARIO statement, such as answering the question of "List all activities executed when Julio was inspected for the microalbuminuria from 2008-01-01 to 2010-01-01".

2   Related Work

According to the "Longman Dictionary of Contemporary English" [7], the word 'replay' can be understood as a verb *"to show again on television something that has been recorded"* or as a noun *"a part of a game of sport that has been recorded on video tape or film, and that is shown again, especially in order to examine it more clearly"*. The idea of *replaying the past* has been extensively explored in many fields. Consequently, a number of approaches and methods of supporting the information replaying has emerged. In the research community, many works have been developed to employ the idea of replaying for supporting the debugging or testing programs. For debugging the application, Guo et al. [8] invested and developed a R2 tool to record and replay the application. When an application is running, a record and replay tool records all interactions between applications and its environment (e.g., reading input from a file, receiving a message). Then when a developer wants to track down an error, he/she can replay the application to the given state based on recorded interactions, and investigate how the application reach that state.

Instead of replaying a specific application, a direct way to support legacy applications is to replay the whole system, including the operating system and target applications. VMware [9] offers its new virtual machine with an experimental feature that allows to record and replay the virtual machine activity. This approach captures at the operating system level and its focus is debugging of programs since it allows for the exact duplication of operations and the state of the virtual machine thus enabling deterministic debugging.

The idea of replaying is also adopted in the context of file systems. Joukov et al. [10] designed and implemented the Replayfs, the first system for replaying file system traces at the VFS (Virtual File System) level. File system traces are used to capture all file system operations at the VFS level, which is a layer that abstracts the file system specific interface. These traces are then used to replay the captured activity at different speeds for stress testing.

In order to provide high assurance in determining the impact of changes to a production system before applying these changes, Galanis et al.[11] and Colle et al. [12] presented an Oracle Database Replay, a novel approach for testing changes to the relational database management system component of an information system (software upgrades, hardware changes, etc). Unlike the simple log approach, the Oracle Database Replay adopted a more complex approach to record all necessary activity on the RDBMS that is required to faithfully reproduce the same activity on a test system, which the goal is capturing the RDBMS workload. Then captures could provide the replaying with all the necessary data to recreate the same workload on a test system so as to test and validate changes before these changes can be applied to a production system. The core idea is to capture all service calls of a client so that these calls can be replayed to another server.

In addition to debugging programs and testing systems, the concept of replaying the past also has been applied to reveal important media space events over time. Nunes et al. [13] created the TIMELINE visualization system that allows people to easily and rapidly explore a video history in detail. Features of the Timeline are that the system lets peoples do the following: 1) immediately see patterns of the activity within a video history via a technique called slit-scanning; 2) use minute, hour, day and week visualizations to present longitudinal overviews of the history at different time granularities; 3) explore patterns across different parts of the scene by moving the slit; 4) rapidly explore event details within a large video stream by scrubbing; 5) retrieve further details of the far past by selecting times of interest.

The need and benefits of a new framework and paradigm that incorporates the playing and replaying of the information is best appreciated through the Roslings Gapminder presentation software for interactive animated multi-dimensional visualization of development statistics [14, 15]. As the visualization in moving graphics is an intuitive method to understand relationships and it is an excellent way to exhibit patterns, the core idea behind this software is that to turn already existing development statistics into the meaningful knowledge by displaying time series as easily understandable moving graphics.

Experience from our earlier work [16, 17] suggested that "presentation, analysis and review of the information can be significantly simplified and enhanced through a new paradigm that combines the information visualization with a mechanism allowing the information to be managed, played and replayed in a dynamic and interactive manner on the basis of a formally constructed and meaningful domain (e.g. hospital domain) *information scenario*".

3   An Overview of the Proposed SOACH

In this research, a scenario is defined as *a structure description of multi-dimensional information clusters to express the sequence and/or linkage of real practices computerized in an information system.* The basic idea behind the *scenario* is that, in order to trace the changing history of certain information units, the specific information unit should be put into the context to reveal how it evolved and how it interacted with other information units in the application domain. Therefore, the default semantics of the scenario, which is used to represent the real daily medical activity in the hospital domain, is interpreted as *"who did what operated by whom in what time and where, under what condition and for what reason"*. Scenario can be either simple or complex. A simple scenario just describes one specific simple activity, such as, patient_take_test. But it can't give global descriptions of the hospital domain. Thus, the complex scenario is developed to represent the complex medical activity of the hospital domain. For example, a scenario about a patient therapy history is a complex scenario, which consists of several test-taking events or other treatment events. A complex scenario is composed of different existing scenarios (simple or complex) in order to show the dependencies and interactions in the application domain.

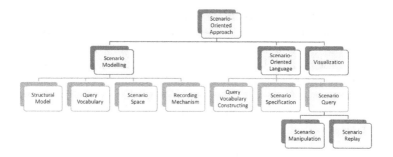

Fig. 1. The Composition of SOACH

Figure 1 illustrates the proposed SOACH for recording and replaying the healthcare information. In order to facilitate the process of replaying the healthcare information by following the SOACH, a *scenario model* together with a recording mechanism has been investigated and developed. This scenario model is mainly used to specify what kind of information is to be recorded and how these information units are linked. This model will support future play-back as the structural link on the conceptual level of information units are specified, hence a querying path (queries for replaying, etc.) can be decided at the conceptual level without concerning about logical or lower levels.

A *scenario-oriented* language also has been investigated and developed to support the SOACH. The scenario-oriented language consists of three main components: the *Query Vocabulary Construction* component, the *Scenario Specification* component and *Scenario-Oriented Query* component. The query vocabulary construction component will classify identifiers referred in information systems into different categories. The specification component provides the ability to specify scenarios by following the structure of the scenario. The query component provides a scenario-oriented query language that is used to manipulate scenarios. It also supports the concept of replaying information scenarios, by employing a REPLAY SCENARIO statement at the high-level and combing the information visualization technology, to help users to understand the domain information.

Detailed discussions about the *scenario model* can be found in [4, 6] and the *scenario-oriented language* was explicitly presented in [5].

4   An Architecture for Supporting the SOACH

This section illustrates the architecture for recording and replaying the healthcare information within the context of the scenario so as to support the SOACH. As shown in Figure 2, there are five main components in the architecture: 1) the user interface; 2) the specification component; 3) the query component; 4) the recording component; 5) information systems. It is worth noticing that the user interface overlaps with the specification component and the query component.

The *User Interface* component enables users to construct a new identifier to build the query vocabulary, create the scenario specification to describe the medical activity of concern. In addition, the User Interface provides users with functionalities to manage the life-cycle of the scenario, and furthermore, it enables users to replay the changing history of focused information units organized by the scenario. The *Scenario Replay Statement Input* module help users to construct their specific queries while the *Visualization of Replay Results* module displays replay results to make it human understandable.

The *Specification* component provides interfaces not only for constructing a new identifier, but also for specifying a new scenario to integrate related identifiers together. It also provides the service for translating the identifier construction statement and scenario specifications into SQL statements.

The *Recording* component provides the ability to implement the recording mechanism to store information clusters specified to be recorded into data repository by using the DBMS instance. *Domain Information Recording* and *Scenario Recording* are employed to record the needed information from two directions: The *Domain Information Recording* is used to record information sources of identifies referred in the hospital domain; The *Scenario Recording* is used to record the context of different elements that would constitute a real medical activity, which is expressed by the scenario.

Here, for a real user application software, replaying histories themselves are worth to be saved for mining hidden patterns, which can be further used for optimizing the system. In addition, system logs are also useful for finding errors and exceptions.

The *Query* component provides interfaces for specifying a manipulation statement, designating a replaying statement, and visualizing replaying results. More important, it provides services for translating the *Scenario-Oriented Query* language (the manipulation statement or the replaying statement) into SQL statements. In this architecture, the scenario-oriented query language is realized in the form of the XML document. Therefore a *Manipulation Parse Module* and a *Replay Parse Module* is developed to parse the corresponding XML document. After that, the parsed scenario-oriented query language acts as a knowledge base for generating corresponding SQL statements to manipulate and retrieve the related information stored in the database. The *Query Translation Processor* integrates the whole component into the system by encapsulating analysis and translation modules.

The *Information Systems* component retains the computerized daily medical activities executed in a computerized way in the hospital domain. Furthermore, it enables external systems to supply and receive information.

How to design and implement the SOPF by following the architecture is presented in the next section.

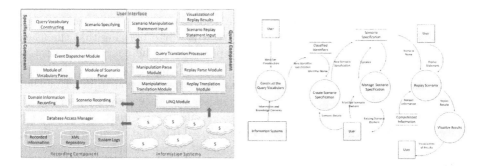

Fig. 2. The Architecture for Supporting the SOACH

Fig. 3. The Data Flow Diagram for the SOPF

5   The Platform: SOPF

The SOPF demonstrates the applicability of the SOACH for supporting the management of scenarios, by implementing the functionality to construct the query vocabulary, permitting the specification of the scenario, manipulating the scenario and supporting the replaying of scenarios. The SOPF utilizes available technologies, such as the database management system (DBMS) and the XML, as a base for implementing the *Scenario-Oriented Language*. The purpose of implementing such a platform is to manage the scenario in a computerized way so as to demonstrate the applicability of the SOACH. The SOPF could be regarded as a plug-in for existing information systems to provide the ability to replay the computerized information. Therefore, at a high level, the requirement of the SOPF can be stated as a need of software environment for providing the computer-based assistance in the specification, storage, manipulation, querying and replaying of the domain knowledge and/or information organized by the scenario so as to improve the management of the healthcare information within the context of the scenario.

The functional model of the SOPF is described in terms of data flow diagram (DFD) and describes what the system does. The DFD is used to present a description of the high-level functional relationship of the data that is computed by the SOPF. Figure 3 illustrates the DFD of the SOPF, showing main functional processes, data flows, the main data stored as well as external entities of the system. The processes illustrated in Figure 3 are listed as follows:

Construct The Query Vocabulary: In order to build the query vocabulary, the user actor specifies a new identifier, which will generate a relational table to monitor and store the related information, or be translated into a CHECK CONSTRAINT statement to ensure the validity of data in a database and to provide data integrity by limiting values that are accepted, which can be queried when replaying scenarios.

Table 1. Table of Data Flow for the DFD of Figure 3

FUNCTIONAL MODEL	INPUT	FROM	OUTPUT	TO	COMMENT
Construct the Query Vocabulary	•Identifier Construction •Information and knowledge Elements	User	Formatted Identifier Specification	Identifier Data Store	user creates a new identifier specification to monitor the related information
Create Scenario Specification	•New Scenario Specification •Identifier Name	User	Formatted New Scenario Specification	Scenario Specification Data Store	user creates a new scenario specification to manage the context information of different identifiers
Manage Scenario Specification	Changes	•User •Specification Data Store	Formatted Changes	•Scenario Specification Data Store •User	user modifies existing scenario specifications
Replay Scenario	•Replay Statement •Scenario Name •Needed Information	•User •Specification Data Store •Computerized Information	Replay Response	Visualize Results Process	user replays the predefined scenarios
Visualize Results	Replay Results	Replay Scenario Process	Formatted Replay Results	User	Displays the results to help users better understand the domain information

Create Scenario Specification: The user actor creates a new scenario specification to depict the context of related information and knowledge elements by referring different identifiers classified into different vocabularies. In addition, the simple scenario specification will be translated into a CREATE TABLE statement to create a relational table in a database so as to record the context information.

Manage Scenario Specification: The user actor may change the status of the pre-defined scenario, or modifies existing scenario specifications.

Replay Scenario: The user actor specifies a replay statement to review the changing history of certain information units, in other words, to retrieve scenario instances and the corresponding information.

Visualize Results: After executing the replay statement, replaying results will be visualized and be displayed on the screen to help users better understand the domain information.

Table 1 presents a detailed description for each process illustrated in Figure 3 in terms of the inputs, where they are coming from, and the outputs, where they are going to from the process.

6   A Case Study: MAP

The Microalbuminuria Protocol (MAP) is a CGP (Clinical Guidelines and Protocols) for the management and treatment of microalbuminuria in diabetes patients. There are several medical activities executed when the disease management of the MAP. These activities can be classified into: when patients are in the state of annual_urine_screening, they take the Dip-Stick Urine (DSU) test. When patients are in the state of other_infections_screening, they take the Urine Track Infection (UTI). Patients take the 24 Hour Creatine Clearance and Protein Loss (24CRCL_PL) test based on the result of the UTI. When patients are in the state of microalbuminuria screening, they take the Alubmin Creatine Ratio (ACR) test. When patients are in the state of confirmed microalbuminuria, two activities the checking Blood Pressure (BP) and the prescribing Angiotsin Converting Enzyme Inhibitors (ACE) will be executed for patients. When patients are in the state of Nephrology Referral (NPH), they will get a Referral Note.

After specifying the scenario of concern and retaining the needed information, users could express their query intent from several aspects on the computerized medical activity at high levels. When replaying the simple scenario, users could obtain the history information about one specific medical activity. While replaying the complex scenario, the history information about combined medical activities will be returned.

Query 1: List all taking ACR test events before 2009-01-01

Query 1 is an example of replaying the simple scenario. *Query 1* is used to review all test events executed when the patient took the ACR test before 2009-01-01. The phrase *before 2009-01-01* is employed to evaluate the temporal function provided in the REPLAY statement. The *BeforeOrAfter* function provides the ability to specify a time duration identified by a time stamp and a preposition 'before' or 'after'. Respecting to the *Query 1*, the employed *BeforeOrAfter* function tries to restrict all activities to be replayed with the time condition "happened before 2009-01-01". The screen-shot of replaying the *Query 1* is shown in Figure 4. The retrieved "taking ACT test" activities, which happened before 2009-01-01, are displayed on the screen one by one. Each retrieved activity is presented in a structural way and is labeled with a number to show the information for users. Such as the activity presented in the number *19*, the tag *From* and *To* indicate the execution time of this activity. The sentence *Dina Take ACRTest* respects to the information of "who did what". The tag *Operated_By* indicates the passive operation and the *Whom* presents the person who

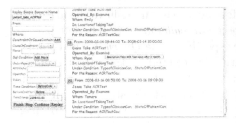

Fig. 4. Replaying the Query 1

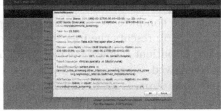

Fig. 5. Presenting the Detailed Information of the Retrieved Activity

executes the passive operation. The location information is indicated by the *In* tag. The tag *Under Condition* presents the constraint to indicate the activity was executed under what conditions. And the tag *For the Reason* indicates the information about why this activity happened. Furthermore, the *ToolTip* service is provided here to help users to view the detailed information for each returned identifier. As shown in Figure 4, when moving the mouse onto the *Examine* object (the gray object), the tooltip will be activated to show the detailed information of the *Examine*. Since the tooltip is activated only when a mouse pointer moves onto the identifier, the *childwindow* is utilized here to "freeze" the detailed information. More detailed information for the activity can be presented by clicking the *number* generated for each returned activity. Figure 5 shows the detailed information for the activity presented in the number *19*.

Query 2: List all activities executed when Julio was inspected for the microalbuminuria from 2008-01-01 to 2010-01-01

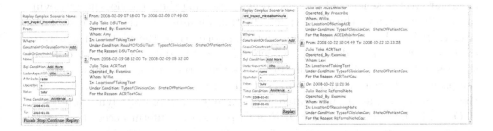

Fig. 6. Replaying the Query 2 While Starting the Replaying Process

Fig. 7. Replaying the Query 2 While Clicking the *Finish* Button

In the MAP, one of the most complex question is how to review the therapy history of a patient such as answering the question of "List all medical activities executed when Julio was inspected for the microalbuminuria from 2008-01-01 to 2010-01-01", which is mentioned at the beginning of this paper. Now, based on our assumption of the *global* scenario is composed by several medical activities executed when the patient was inspected for the disease, users have the ability to specify the complex scenario *patient inspect microalbuminuria*. The left part of the Figure 6 presents the user interface for specifying the *Query 2*. The complex scenario "patient_inspect_microalbuminuria" is selected as the target scenario to be replayed. Since users want to return the information from all aspects, the value of the *From* is set to null. In the *SqlCondition* part, the statement "name = 'Julio'" is described to return Julio's inspectional activities. Lastly, the specified interval of time is described in the *TimeCondition* part. After clicking the *Replay* button, the platform starts the execution of the query. In addition, in order to control the replaying process, three different functions, *stop*, *continue* and *finish*, are provided here. In the process of displaying generated sentences on the user interface, when users click the *stop* button, the displaying process will be paused, and the *continue* button enables the displaying process to continue. And if users want to display all results together, the *finish* button should be clicked. Figure 6 shows the screen-shot of replaying the *Query 2* while starting the replaying process. Figure 7 shows the screen-shot of the finished replaying process after clicking the *Finish* button.

7   Case Studying Findings and Discussion

According to evaluating the SOPF with the case study MAP, it can be noted here that, as a plug-in for multi hospital information systems, the SOPF exposes a *scenario* to its users for posting queries. This scenario is typically referred as the *context* of related information units, where the data resides at different sources. To answer queries using the pre-defined scenario, the platform needs reformulate a query posed over the scenario into queries over sources. In the SOPF, when constructing the query vocabulary, the identifier can be specified as a referential candidate to the schema of sources. When replaying the scenario, the retrieving process first retrieve the context information obtained by the target scenario. And then based on the retrieved context information, the platform generates queries over referred identifiers, which refer to the data residing at different sources. Intuitively, the identifier describes the structure of the data source or the path how to refer to data sources (to describe where the real data is), while the scenario provides an integrated and "virtual" view of underlying sources.

Overall, the benefit of the SOPF is to provide a uniform access to a set of heterogeneous data sources, freeing the user from the knowledge about where the data is, how they are stored, and how they can be accessed. That is to say, the SOPF enables users to focus on specifying *what* they want, rather than thinking about *how* to obtain answers. As a result, it frees users from tedious tasks of finding relevant data sources, interacting with each source in isolation using a particular interface, and combing the data from multi sources.

In our previous research, a representation method of visualizing replaying results and displaying results in a more user-friendly and graphic manner has been investigated and developed. Three main panels are designed for supporting the representation method: *a puzzle panel*, which is the main area for displaying recorded information units; *an index panel*, where each operation is visualized as a shape and the detailed information about the operation can also be retrieved by interacting with the shape; *a fish-eye mechanism* was also provided to ensure the minimal space between shapes that users are interested in; *a control panel*, which not only provides buttons for replaying a solving process, but also offers a slider with a drag-able square so as to enhance replaying experiences. For further discussion on visualization of retrieved scenarios, please refer to [17].

8 Conclusions

This paper presented an architecture and a platform to support the recording and replaying of the healthcare information. The developed SOPF, which is a platform for managing the scenario, can be regarded as a plug-in for existing information systems. This will help users to review the information from multiple applications by using one platform. Unfortunately, the method of incorporating the SOPF into the existing information system is not fully investigated and developed in this research. The biggest problem involved in this integrating is that how to bridge the gap between the design of the existing information system and the requirement of the SOPF. In detailed, it means how to make the SOPF has the ability to monitor, record and retrieve the information from the data repository which has been pre-designed and executed for the existing information system. For simplicity, this method can be regarded as a problem which is relevant to "schema mapping". How to integrating the SOPF with existing information systems will be left for future research.

Acknowledgments. This project is sponsored by the National Natural Science Foundation of China (Project No. 61300090), the Fundamental Research Funds for the Central Universities (Project No.ZYGX2013J080), and the Scientific Research Foundation for the Returned Overseas Chinese Scholars, State Education Ministry.

References

1. Rosson, M.B., Carroll, J.M.: Scenario-based design. In: Human- Computer Interaction: Development Process, pp. 146–161. CRC Press (2009)
2. Alspaugh, T.A., Anton, A.I.: Scenario support for effective requirements. Information and Software Technology 50, 198–220 (2008)
3. Hsu, S.H., Chang, J.W.: Developing a scenario database for product innovation. In: Kurosu, M. (ed.) HCD 2009. LNCS, vol. 5619, pp. 585–593. Springer, Heidelberg (2009)
4. Ding, Y., Wu, B., Zhou, E., Wu, J.: The scenario-oriented method for recording and playing-back healthcare information. In: Cruz-Cunha, M.M., Varajão, J., Powell, P., Martinho, R. (eds.) CENTERIS 2011, Part III. CCIS, vol. 221, pp. 175–184. Springer, Heidelberg (2011)

5. Ding, Y., Wu, B.: Making Use of Scenario for Supporting the Replay of Information in Computerized Information System. In: Proceedings of The IADIS International Conference Information Systems 2012, Berlin, German, pp. 368–371 (2012)

6. Ding, Y., Wu, B., Wu, J., Zhou, E.: The Scenario-Oriented Method for Recording and Replaying the Complex Information. In: Proceedings of 11th International Conference on Information Technology and Telecommunication, Cork, Ireland, pp. 61–68 (2012)

7. Bullon, S.: Longman dictionary of contemporary english, 4th edn. Pearson ESL (2006)

8. Guo, Z., Wang, X., Tang, J., Liu, X., Xu, Z., Wu, M., Kaashoek, M.F., Zhang, Z.: R2: an application-level kernel for record and replay. In: Proceedings of the 8th USENIX Conference on Operating Systems Design and Implementation, OSDI 2008, pp. 193–208. USENIX Association, Berkeley (2008)

9. VMWare. Understanding full virtualization, paravirtualization, and hardware assist. Tech. rep., VMWare Inc. (2007)

10. Joukov, N., Wong, T., Zadok, E.: Accurate and efficient replaying of file system traces. In: Proceedings of the 4th Conference on USENIX Conference on File and Storage Technologies, pp. 25–38. USENIX Association, Berkeley (2005)

11. Galanis, L., Buranawatanachoke, S., Colle, R., Dageville, B., Dias, K., Klein, J., Papadomanolakis, S., Tan, L.L., Venkataramani, V., Wang, Y., Wood, G.: Oracle database replay. In: Proceedings of the 2008 ACM SIGMOD International Conference on Management of Data, SIGMOD 2008, pp. 1159–1170. ACM, New York (2008)

12. Colle, R., Galanis, L., Buranawatanachoke, S., Papadomanolakis, S., Wang, Y.: Oracle database replay. Proceedings of the VLDB Endowment 2, 1542–1545 (2009)

13. Nunes, M., Greenberg, S., Carpendale, S., Gutwin, C.: What did i miss? visualizing the past through video traces. In: Bannon, L., Wagner, I., Gutwin, C., Harper, R., Schmidt, K. (eds.) Proceedings of the 2007 Tenth European Conference on Computer-Supported Cooperative Work, pp. 1–20. Springer, London (2007)

14. Rosling, H.: Debunking third-world myths with the best states you've ever seen (2009), http://www.ted.com/index.php/talks/view/id/92

15. Rosling, H., Zhang, Z.: Health advocacy with gapminder animated statistics. Journal of Epidemiology and Global Health 1, 11–14 (2011)

16. Wu, B., Mansour, E., Dube, K.: Complex Information Management Using a Framework Supported by ECA Rules in XML. In: Paschke, A., Biletskiy, Y. (eds.) RuleML 2007. LNCS, vol. 4824, pp. 224–231. Springer, Heidelberg (2007)

17. Zhou, E., Wu, B., Wu, J., Ding, Y.: An architecture and a prototype for querying and visualising recorded context information. In: Beigl, M., Christiansen, H., Roth-Berghofer, T.R., Kofod-Petersen, A., Coventry, K.R., Schmidtke, H.R. (eds.) CONTEXT 2011. LNCS, vol. 6967, pp. 321–334. Springer, Heidelberg (2011)

Design and Development of a 3-Lead ECG System Based on the ISO/IEEE 11073-10406 Standards

Zhuqing Q. Xiong[1,2], Honghui H. Fan[3], Weizhong Z. Wang[1],
Gaosheng S. Xie[1], and Bangyu Y. Hwang[1]

[1] Institute of Biomedical and Health Engineering,
Shenzhen Institutes of Advanced Technology, Guangdong, China
[2] College of Information Engineering, Nanchang University of Aeronautics, Jiangxi, China
[3] School of Computer Engineering Jiangsu University of Technology, Jiangsu, China

Abstract. Improving the quality of life with the least expense has been conducted by incorporating advanced technology, especially for Personal Health Devices (PHDs), into the medical service market. To guarantee the compatible extensibility of the relative health system, standards which manage and send information from the users of PHDs have been defined recently by the Continua Alliance, IEEE Standards Association, and the IEEE-EMBS affiliated 11073 Personal Health Data Working Group. ECG device is a typically one and is widely used in the monitoring and diagnosing of heart disease. Part 10406 is a device specialization of basic ECG, 1- to 3-lead ECG, and approved by IEEE 11073 Standards Committee until September 2011 [1]. We designed a 3-lead ECG system, which might be the first ECG device based on the 11073-10406 and android platform. Such a device could increase the interconnectivity of the ECG system.

1 Introduction

High mortality and disability rate in heart disease have brought about serious harm to human health, prevention and treatment of heart disease have become a hot issue of the medical community. Moreover, they have also become an important content for individual and family's health. Since ECG signal is regular and easy to be monitored, ECG monitoring has played an important role in the medical monitoring system of heart disease [2].

The development of mobile Internet has led to the boom of mobile medical technology, which plays an important role in electronic medical technology. In addition, with the popularity of Android phone, the importance of smart phone or tablet in health monitoring system as the terminals is more and more obvious [3]. People can use smart phone to gather and save medical data in time. But in China, few cases are there that android phone is used as terminal equipment for ECG monitoring system. Furthermore, medical devices from different vendors can hardly be compatible with each other because of their different protocol standards, which greatly restricts the development of Personal Health Devices (PHDs). In order to solve this problem, the IEEE-EMBS affiliated 11073 Personal Health Data Working Group and developed

Y. Zhang et al. (Eds.): HIS 2014, LNCS 8423, pp. 141–147, 2014.

IEEE 11073 Standards, which support different medical equipments from some major manufacturers to work together. Major objectives of IEEE 11073 PHD: to provide real-time Plug and Play function for medical instruments; to provide efficient exchange between physiological parameters of the patient and the outside world; to ensure the physiological parameters can be recorded, acquired and processed in the absence of a large number of software and hardware [4]. The IEEE 11073-10406 PHD is especially designed for typical ECG devices.

To meet the requirements of medical service market, we designed a software system for ECG terminal based on android phone and the IEEE 11073-10406. This paper is aimed primarily at software processing of ECG signal transmission, rather than the hardware part. In our system, we display ECG waveform and calculate the heart rate. Android phone or tablet is connected with the ECG acquisition hardware via USB (Universal Serial Bus). The whole system is cost-effective, which allows people to have a multi-faceted collection of ECG data with ease and greatly improves the compatibility and usability. This paper mainly focuses on designing and developing the ISO/IEEE 11073-10406 Standards on the android platform.

2   System Model

In this study, the 3-lead system for smart-phone on android platform is designed and developed. The system manages individual's heart condition by gathering and monitoring ECG signal in real time. Our system consists of three sections, the modular of ECG signal gathering (agent), the modular of USB transmission, and Android phone or tablet for collecting ECG data and displaying ECG waveform which acts as manager of IEEE 11073-10406 Standards. Data transmission of this 3-lead system conforms to IEEE 11073-10406 Standards. The system is shown in Fig. 1.

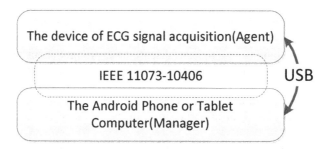

Fig. 1. System architecture

For its lower cost and higher transmission rate, USB is used as wired transmission to exchange data between medical devices for ECG signal acquisition and android phone. In this 3-lead system, both the ECG signal acquisition and android phone support IEEE 11073 standard protocol. The modular of ECG signal acquisition, which the Stm32F103 and ADS1294 are used in, collects the measured data from different non-standard ECG devices and exchanges these values with android phone or android tablet according to the IEEE 11073-10406 Standards. The Stm32F103 and ADS1294 is responsible for collecting data and calculating the heart rate through a series of algorithms such as low-pass filtering, high-pass filtering, derivative, moving window integral and thresholding. Android software shows ECG waveform and heart rate in real time when it is connected with a USB port.

3   System Design and Implementation

3.1   The Whole Android System

The main function of android phone is to draw ECG waveform and display heart rate. As shown in Fig. 2, the entire android software mainly consists of three portions, the portion of USB transmission for identifying the peripheral and establishing connection, the portion of IEEE 11073-10406 Standards for exchanging measured values between agent and manager, and the portion of waveform and heart rate displaying.

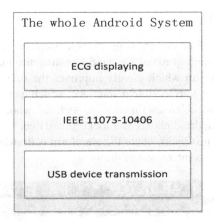

Fig. 2. Android software architecture

Android phone identifies and configures USB peripherals in main UI thread and the specific process is described later. If peripherals are connected with smart phone successfully, the program would start a broadcast to send a notification. When BroadcastReceiver class receives the notification, it informs other programs or threads to be ready to communicate with the module of ECG signal acquisition according to ISO/IEEE 11073-10406 PHD standard protocol. Fig. 3 shows this process. IEEEThread is responsible for writing code of interchanging messages between agent and smartphone-based manager with IEEE 11073-10406 standard protocol. DataReceiverThread is responsible for receiving ECG data from IEEEThread and noticing WareformThread to draw ECG waveform. WareformThread is primarily responsible for drawing dynamic electrocardiogram waveforms.

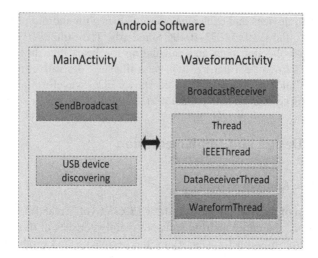

Fig. 3. Software components of android program

3.2   Drawing ECG Waveform

SurfaceView is employed as the drawing control, because we can execute another thread for drawing dynamic graphics to avoid blocking the main thread, and it has double buffering mechanism which greatly improves the drawing efficiency. SurfaceView should work with SurfaceHolder interface, which can be obtained by calling getHolder. If we apply lockCanvas() method to lock the whole painting area, splash screen might appear on android phone. But lockCanvas(Rect rect) method could solve this problem, because it just locks where the wareform is drawing, without modifying the other area. Fig. 4 shows the results of drawing.

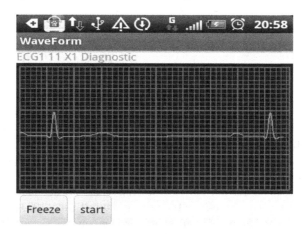

Fig. 4. ECG waveform on smartphone

3.3   IEEE 111073 Standard Protocol

ISO/IEEE 11073 PHD, a new medical standard, is designed for some typical PHD devices. It defines the communication protocol between medical equipments and manager. This standard is divided into three main components: Domain Information Model (DIM), Service Model(SM) and Communication Model (CM). Moreover, it composes of the 11073-20601 Optimized Exchange Protocol and other 11073-104zz specializations. The IEEE 11073-10406 Standards are especially developed for the basic electrocardiogram (1- to 3- lead ECG) devices. It describes the service layer of application and the issues of data exchanging protocol for typical ECG devices. The communication between the two devices is based on the Agent/Manager concept of ISO namespace in IEEE 11073 Standards. In this 3-lead ECG system, the module of ECG signal acquisition acts as Agent, and the smartphone application acts as Manager that collects the measured ECG data and manages individual's heart condition. The manager is designed on Android platform and employs USB interface to communicate with the agent. The Agent connects and corresponds with the Manager based on IEEE 11073-20601 and IEEE 11073-10406 standard protocol. ECG system that we designed follows IEEE 11073-10406 PHD standard, making possible the interoperability with any ECG equipment of any other manufacturers.

3.4   The Android USB Communication

Android supports USB peripherals via two modes: USB accessory mode and USB host mode. In USB accessory mode, the peripherals connected with the android phone act as the USB hosts and power the bus, while the USB accessories must adhere to Android accessory communication protocol. In USB host mode, the Android devices play the role of host and are bus-powered. And Android phones must follow Android host protocol.

USB host mode is adopted in this study. The smartphone or tablet with android platform acts as the host of USB communication. A mobile phone and a tablet are equipped with powerful CPU and large RAM, thus they are faster in processing ECG signal compared with ECG acquisition device. Android phone and tablet for measurement should support USB OTG(On-The-Go). The basic ECG signal acquisition hardware acts as the USB slave. As USB host mode requires Android 3.1 (API level 12) or higher platform, what we have adopted is android 4.1 platform. USB API supported by Google can be directly applied by USB application developers on android 3.1 or higher platform. These USB classes, such as UsbManager, UsbDevice, UsbInterface, UsbEndpoint, UsbDeviceConnection, UsbRequest and so on, are in the package of android.hardware.usb. In our software, we use an intent filter to be notified when the peripheral is connected. Along with the intent filter, we specify the product and vendor ID of USB devices. When the ECG signal acquisition hardware that matches with the intent filter is connected with Android phone, it would communicate with Android phone successfully.

4   The Experimental Results

An electrocardiogram simulator is used in our system as the ECG source; a Lenovo Tablet A1000-T and HTC S510b is also employed as Android devices for testing. Android tablet can effectively receive and display signals from the ECG acquisition device based on the STM32 via USB correspondence. The system can display all the waveform from simulator in real time. Besides, we also calculate and show the heart rate. After repeated modifications and tests, the system proves its reliability and stability. Fig. 5 shows the testing environment and results.

5   Conclution

Smart phone and tablet are widely used nowadays, and USB port is one of their standard peripherals. People can monitor ECG signal with ease at any time via an ECG acquisition device. From the testing results, we can see that the system is user-friendly, low-cost and fairly reliable. The new medical technique of managing and interchanging ECG data between the ECG signal acquisition and smartphone-based manager based on IEEE 11073-10406 standard protocol guarantees the capability and extensibility of the ECG system. With it, the elderly and patients can monitor their heart condition with this system anytime, anywhere.

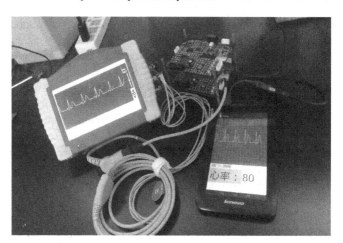

Fig. 5. The experiment result

Acknowledgements. The authors gratefully acknowledge the financial support from China National Natural Science Fund of China (61302124), Natural Science Fund of Jiangsu Province (BK20130235), Natural Science Foundation of the Higher Education Institutions of Jiangsu Province (13KJB520006), Program of six talent tops of Jiangsu Province (DZXX-031).

References

1. ISO/IEEE11073-10406 Health informatics. Personal Health Devices communication. Device Specialization - Basic ECG (1-3 lead)
2. Harmah, D.J., Kathirvelu, D.: An ubiquitous miniaturized android based ECG monitoring system. In: 2013 Internation Conference on Emerging Trends in Computing, Communication and Nanotechnology (ICE-CCN), pp. 117–120 (2013)
3. Filipović, N., Stojanović, R., Debevc, M., Devedžić, G.: On line ECG Processing and Visualization Using Android SmartPhone. In: 2013 2nd Mediterranean Conference on Embedded Computing (MECO), pp. 93–96 (June 2013)
4. IEEE Std 11073-20601^{TM}, Health informatics – Personal health device communication – Part 20601: Optimized exchange protocol
5. Gakare, P.K., Patel, A.M., Vaghela, J.R., Awale, R.N.: Real Time Feature Extraction of ECG Signal on Android Platform. In: 2012 International Conference on Communication, Information & Computing Technology (ICCICT), pp. 1–5 (2012)
6. Reisner, A.T., Clifford, G.D., Mark, R.G.: The Physiological Basis of the Electrocardiogram. In: Clifford, G.D., Azuaje, F., McSharry, P.E. (eds.) Advanced Methods for ECG Analysis. Artech House, Boston (2006)
7. Lim, J.-H., Park, C., Park, S.-J.: Home Healthcare Settop-box for Senior Chronic Care using ISO/IEEE 11073 PHD Standard. In: Proc. of 32nd IEEE EMBS, August 31 (2010)
8. Cano-Garcia, J.M., Gonzalez-Parada, E., Alarcon-Collants, V., CasilariPerez: A PDA-based Portable Wirelss ECG Monitor for Medical Personal Area Network. In: IEEE MELECON, Benalmadena (Malaga), Sain, May 16-19 (2006)

Data Integration in a Clinical Environment Using the Global-as-Local-View-Extension Technique

Georgi Straube, Ilvio Bruder, Dortje Löper, and Andreas Heuer

Database Research Group, Dept. of Comp. Science, University of Rostock, Germany
metis@informatik.uni-rostock.de

Abstract. Medical data is stored across institutions in heterogeneous systems with differences in both, data structures and their semantics. Often, additional information from other data sources is required, e.g. for decision making. The extension of all the data combined from different sources represents the global data or global knowledge. Thus, granting participants access to this global knowledge is crucial for a successful clinical treatment. Accessing this information through the local system is called global-as-local-view-extension. This paper presents an approach for realizing this by using the entity-attribute-value model in accordance with a special schema mapping technique as well as inverses of schema mappings between local and global repositories.

1 Introduction

Hospitals, physicians, care givers, and other healthcare participants work with data about patients. These data comprise patients' personal data, treatment data, medication data, vital signs, etc. They manage their data in their own systems according to their own needs. This means, they use different software with different interfaces, different database systems, different database models and different data models. What happens, if a patient is referred from a general practitioner to a specialist? The data from one system, e.g. from a general practitioner, with its used models have to be transformed to data for the specialist's system with the data models there. Unfortunately, this transformation is often arranged using paper documents which are printed or handwritten in the source system and then manually transferred to the target system. Furthermore, data in the different systems are redundant but not implicitly consistent. If data about one patient, located in different systems, has to be merged, it can be a difficult task to identify the data sets corresponding to this one patient. In fact, a global data set is needed for identifying data sets from different, i.e. local, data systems. An even better solution could be that everyone is obligated to use a global system with standardized data. However, this is not very practicable because every physician or facility already has their own established systems and it would be a non-trivial and expensive task to transform the system and the stored data. Therefore, a solution is needed which addresses both problems: providing a global

Y. Zhang et al. (Eds.): HIS 2014, LNCS 8423, pp. 148–159, 2014.

view of integrated local data besides a data usage on local systems. This paper presents a solution based on the global-as-local-view-extension technique [5]. After a more detailed problem description in section 2, the database techniques for information integration are discussed. Section 4 then presents the global-as-local-view-extension technique based on a specialized schema mapping and its inverse mapping. Thereafter, some experiments and examples are described.

2   Problem Description

In the medical environment, there is a strong demand for exchanging data. Each data source has different software systems, different data schemas, and different interfaces. This issue is well-known under the term heterogeneity. Many problems arise if we try to integrate heterogeneous systems. The conceptional idea is having a global view over all data from the different sources. In fact, there are many problems integrating the software and hardware interfaces. This paper focusses on describing the integration of the heterogeneous data models. Such data models could be a relational model from a database management system, an XML Document Type Definition from an XML database, or any other data model. Comparing the relational with the XML data model already reveals some major differences. On the one hand, the relational database model is based on tables, i.e. relations, and sets of rows, i.e. tuples. On the other hand, XML describes the information structure using hierarchically ordered information elements.

The scenario for the integration technique described in this article is a medical environment. This environment contains a hospital using SAP i.s.h.med[1] with the patient's master data and vital signs, a specialist for radiation therapy using a Conquest DICOM server[2], and a general practitioner storing his own medical care data using an HL7 Clinical Document Architecture XML format. One concrete problem arises with the data integration of DICOM images and data collected by a specialist into a hospital management software based on SAP, and the subsequent transferring of all data to the general practitioner.

Figure 1 shows these three data sources. The upper part of the figure describes a scenario using a point-to-point communication between every participating system. The major disadvantage is the definition of a mapping between each of the participating systems, especially if a new system joins the network. For n participating systems, $n * (n - 1)/2$ schema mappings have to be defined. The bottom part of the figure illustrates the same scenario, but introduces an integration layer which communicates with the different sources. Thus, the heterogeneous models of the sources are integrated into a global model. This global model has to be flexible and robust regarding the information in the source schemas. In our approach, we use an extended entity-attribute-value model (EAV model) for the integration.

Furthermore, we envision that the participants gain access to the global data through their own local systems. In our approach presented herein, we have

---

[1] SAP i.s.h.med is a hospital information system from Siemens based on SAP for Healthcare.

[2] http://ingenium.home.xs4all.nl/dicom.html

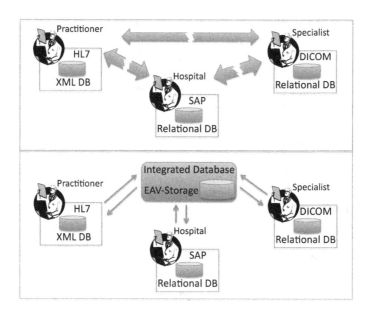

Fig. 1. Integration problem in a medical environment. Top: Data exchange without integration, Bottom: Data Exchange using integration.

chosen the global-as-local-view-extension technique. Therefore, after mapping a local data model to the global schema, the inverse mapping is needed to integrate the global data.

3   Database Techniques for Data Integration

Concerning data integration, Haas has identified four steps towards a successful integration [7]:

1. **Understanding:** This step comprises all means of analyzing the given data sources concerning their structural and semantic characteristics.
2. **Standardization:** Based on the analysis, a target schema is developed. This also includes decisions regarding granularity (e.g. full name vs. first name and last name) and naming conventions of the data to be stored as well as regulations for the cleansing processes.
3. **Specification:** Once the integration schema is defined, the mappings from the data sources to the target schema need to be specified. This step also comprehends technical decisions for the integration, e.g. which techniques and technologies are used along with the designated execution engine.
4. **Execution:** This task carries out the actual integration of the data from the data sources to the target schema. Depending on the approach chosen, the integrated data will either be materialized in the target system or it is only integrated virtually. A hybrid approach is also possible.

This paper mainly offers a contribution for the second and third task.

A schema mapping describes how the entities from a source schema (also named local schema) are mapped to the corresponding entities in a target schema (also named global schema). Formally, a source schema S of a database and a target schema T of another database are sets of relation symbols [17]: $S = (S_1, ..., S_n)$ and $T = (T_1, ..., T_m)$ where $S_1, ..., S_n, T_1, ..., T_m$ represent relation symbols. Their instances I (source instance) and J (target instance) respectively, represent a set of relations (and one relation comprises a set of corresponding tuples) based on the relation symbol definitions. A mapping $M = (S, T, \Sigma)$ syntactically describes a set of rules Σ in a logical formalism that maps the relation symbols in S to the relational symbols in T. Semantically, this mapping can be specified as $M = (S, T, W)$ where W is a set of those pairs (I, J) that comply with all the rules in Σ. Then J as the target instance can be seen as a solution for I (the source instance).

Depending on the approach, different kinds of mappings can be defined [10]: Mapping rules that specify one target relation as a view over one or more source relations are called global-as-view (GaV) mappings. In contrast to that, rules that define one source relation as a view over several target relations are named local-as-view (LaV) mappings. Those two concepts can be combined to global-local-as-view (GLaV) techniques, also named query correspondence assertions [11]. Basically, GLaV rules represent mappings that specify a view on target relations as a view on source relations. The global schema remains the access point for querying the integrated information. Therefore, an institution has to communicate with two systems: their own local one and the global one. To overcome this drawback, Flach et al. focus on extending each local schema by adding new structural elements (e.g. database relations or XML elements) from other source schemas [5]. That way, local systems can include information from other sources systems as well. Within this approach, the global schema is only used as an intermediary one for schema mapping. It does not serve for querying purposes. Instead, each local system can be queried for all integrated data directly. In order to use this global-as-local-view-extension (GaLVE), mappings between schemas need to be inverted. Approaches for inverting schema mappings can be found in the designated literature (e.g. [3]).

Concerning clinical environments, the networks are still highly heterogeneous and lack flexible interfaces. Standardizations and an incremental approach along with generic models are predicted to be the basis for future IT systems [9].

The field of healthcare integration offers diverse research directions for different technical ways of integrating information. Some examples are XML-based approaches [8], approaches based on message exchange [14,2], and agent-based approaches [6,15].

All of these approaches have one thing in common: They integrate towards one global target system which then contains all the information (materialized or virtually). Queries for the integrated information need to be issued towards that global system. In contrast to that, the GaLVE technique mentioned above offers direct access to the integrated information through the local system.

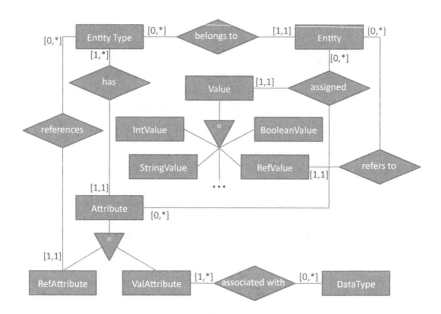

Fig. 2. The extended entity-attribute-value model as an entity-relationship diagram

As a representation of the global schema, we chose the entity-attribute-value (EAV) model. It offers a generic approach for storing information in a flexible and compact way. The main difference to a conventional data model is that the structure is also represented as data (within entity and attribute objects). The EAV model can be extended by classes and relationships to an EAV/CR model [13]. Figure 2 shows a relational representation of the entity types, entities, attributes and values. Values can be of different types which is why they are subclassed. Attributes either have a single value or can be a complex structure again consisting of another entity.

We already used the EAV approach for a concept of integrating healthcare data [12] for a home environment. This approach offers flexibility regarding the current structure and future structural changes as well as a compact storage capacity along with simple restoring capabilities.

4   Integration Technique for a Clinical Environment

The integration technique described in this article requires not only a mapping of local data sources to a global (intermediate) schema but also an inverse mapping. Initially, schema mappings and the notion of inverse mappings have been studied as candidates for a formalism underlying the integration technique. The following drawbacks have been identified:

– The concept of schema mappings is mainly suited for describing mappings between two relational database schemas. Other data models are not supported to the same extent.

- The definition of inverse mappings requires every attribute of the local schema to be also present in the global schema. As a result, there will be many null values in the global schema because attributes that are only present in one (or few) local data source(s) will be null for instances from other local sources.
- Fagin [3] introduced a necessary condition (named unique solutions property) for deciding whether a schema mapping is invertible. However, it is sufficient for only a special sub-case of schema mappings (local-as-view mappings). Hence, it is not always possible to decide whether a schema mapping is invertible or not.
- The definition of inverse schema mappings proposed by Fagin is quite restrictive. As a result, there are simple schema mappings which are not invertible in the sense of this definition. Other less restrictive definitions exist ([4], [1]), however, they are more suitable for recovering materialized data than for the formulation of precise inverse mappings.

The null value problem as well as the lack of support for data models other than the relational data model, motivated the use of the entity-attribute-value (EAV) model as an intermediary layer for the integration of different data sources. Initially, we tried to formulate the mapping to the EAV model using schema mappings and inverse schema mappings. However, the underlying formalism of schema mappings is not expressive enough to capture the semantics of this mapping. This problem occurs because the mapping to the EAV model requires a mapping of data structures to data. On the other hand, schema mappings describe correspondences between data structures only. As a further consequence of this, the necessary condition for invertibility cannot be fulfilled.

Therefore, the use of schema mappings has no longer been pursued. Instead, we now map the data sources, i.e. their respective data models, to the EAV model (see figure 3 for an overview of this mapping). An advantage of this approach is that mappings don't have to be created for each individual schema of a given data model. The integration is then performed in the EAV model. Afterwards, the integrated data is mapped back to a schema in a specific data model.

The extended EAV model consists of entity types with attributes. There is a distinction between value-based attributes which have one or more primitive data types, such as string, and reference attributes describing relationships between entity types. Both types of attributes have a cardinality feature. Reference attributes are bidirectional and are therefore assigned inverse cardinalities.

The EAV model supports the concept of identifying attributes. If the source data model supports this notion as well, then the information which attributes uniquely identify an entity in a given data model will be preserved. An example is the relational data model which has the primary key concept. In the case of reference attributes, referencing and referenced attributes can be annotated if the data model provides this information.

Regarding the mapping of relational databases, a relation schema is represented as an entity type. All attributes of the schema become value-based attributes of the entity type with a minimal cardinality of 0, if null values are

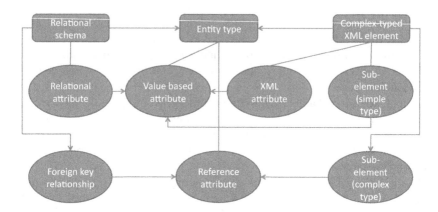

Fig. 3. Mapping of relational and XML data sources to the EAV model

allowed for the relational source attribute, and 1 otherwise[3]. As an example, consider the schema `DICOMPatients` of the DICOM database. The attributes `PatientNam` and `PatientBir` with types `varchar(64)` and `char(8)` of this schema are mapped to value-based attributes of the data type `string` with cardinality 0:1. Foreign key relationships are covered as reference attributes. For instance, the attribute `PatientID` of the schema `DICOMStudies` is a foreign key referencing the primary key `PatientID` of the schema `DICOMPatients`. It will be mapped to a reference attribute belonging to the entity type `DICOMStudies` and referencing the entity type `DICOMPatients`. Since the value of the foreign key attribute `PatientID` may be null, the cardinality of this reference attribute is 0:1 because a foreign key relationship links a tuple from the referencing relation to at most one tuple from the referenced relation. Conversely, a tuple from the referenced relation can be linked to none or multiple tuples from the referencing relation via the foreign key relationship. Hence, the inverse cardinality of the reference attribute is 0:n where n denotes an unlimited maximal cardinality.

The mapping of XML data sources involves the actual XML document and an associated XML schema file. An XML element e with a complex type[4] is mapped to an entity type with simple-typed XML attributes of the element and simple-typed subelements becoming value-based attributes of the entity type. The nesting of subelements with a complex type is captured as a reference attribute.

An excerpt from an XML schema file, part of the HL7 CDA specification, is presented in listing 1.1. It contains the definition of a complex type `POCD_MT000040.Patient` which is referenced in a subelement declaration in another part of the schema file. This declaration as well as the definitions of other

---

[3] For the remainder of this article, cardinalities are denoted as min:max.

[4] An XML element with a complex type may feature attributes and/or nested subelements beside the actual content. A simple-typed XML element must not contain neither attributes nor subelements.

referenced types, such as II, CE or EntityClass, are omitted for this example. All referenced types are complex types. Thus, all XML attributes and subelements appearing in the definition of POCD_MT000040.Patient are being mapped to entity types. The links between POCD_MT000040.Patient and these entity types are reflected by reference attributes. For instance, the nesting of element birthplace would be mapped to a reference attribute with a minimal cardinality of 0 and a maximal cardinality of 1.

The cardinality of entity type attributes, which result from the mapping of subelements, corresponds to the value of the XML schema attribute minOccurs/maxOccurs. If these XML schema attributes are missing, a value of 1 is assumed, as defined by the XML schema specification. In the case of XML attributes mapped to entity type attributes, the maximal cardinality is always 1 because XML attributes can only occur at most once per element. The minimal cardinality depends on whether the XML attribute has been declared as being required (use="required", use="fixed") or optional (use="optional").

```
1  <xs:complexType name="POCD_MT000040.Patient">
2    <xs:sequence>
3      <xs:element name="id" type="II" minOccurs="0"/>
4      <xs:element name="name" type="PN" minOccurs="0"
            maxOccurs="unbounded"/>
5      <xs:element name="birthTime" type="TS" minOccurs="0"/>
6      <xs:element name="maritalStatusCode" type="CE" minOccurs="0"/>
7      <xs:element name="religiousAffiliationCode" type="CE" minOccurs="0"/>
8      <xs:element name="birthplace" type="POCD_MT000040.Birthplace"
            minOccurs="0"/>
9    </xs:sequence><xs:attribute name="nullFlavor" type="NullFlavor"
            use="optional"/>
10   <xs:attribute name="classCode" type="EntityClass" use="optional"
            fixed="PSN"/>
11   <xs:attribute name="determinerCode" type="EntityDeterminer"
            use="optional" fixed="INSTANCE"/>
12  </xs:complexType>
```

Listing 1.1. Excerpt from exemplary HL7 CDA XML schema

After mapping the local data sources to the EAV model, the integration process can be carried out. The process is based on the integration method developed by Spaccapietra et al. which makes use of assertions [16] specifying correspondences between designated objects. Assertions between entity types can be defined on the foundation of assertions between their value-based attributes. Apart from that, assertions can be specified between paths which result from the linking of reference attributes. This allows for avoiding redundant references in the integrated schema. The integration process is guided by five rules:

1. Entity types and paths in source schemas for which there is no assertion defined are transferred into the integrated schema without change.
2. The second rule describes the integration of entity types which are asserted to be equivalent. It determines how the attributes of the integrated entity type are created depending on the correspondences between the source attributes. Details may be found in [16]. If there is no correspondence for a source attribute, the attribute is inherited by the integrated entity type.

3. If there are equivalent paths of length 1, i.e. paths consisting of a single reference attribute, they will be merged into one path in the integrated schema.

4. If there is an assertion expressing the equivalence of a path of length 1 and a longer path, it suffices to transfer the longer path to the integrated schema: The connection expressed by the path of length 1 is already covered by the longer path. On the other hand, two equivalent paths composed of two or more reference attributes must both be transferred to the integrated schema. Otherwise, information loss might occur.

5. The last rule specifies how an equivalence assertion between an entity type e and a value-based attribute a is handled. An assertion of this type expresses structural heterogeneity. This structural heterogeneity is removed by transforming the value-based attribute into a reference attribute. The newly created reference attribute refers to the entity type e' to which the source entity type e has been mapped during the integration process.

After the integration process is completed, a new schema with integrated entity types and entity types that have been transferred from the source schemas without change is created. The flexibility of the EAV model implies that its semantical expressiveness is weak, i.e. it conveys little information about the semantics of the contained data. Thus, in most cases it is impractical to query the global schema directly. For that reason, the data is mapped back from the EAV model to one of the source data models. For the relational data model, this inverse mapping is defined as follows:

- An entity type e is mapped to a relation schema r_1. All value-based attributes with a cardinality of 0:1 or 1:1 are represented as relational attributes of this schema. Value-based attributes with other cardinalities must be incorporated into another relation schema r_2 which is then linked to r_1 via a third schema r_3 and corresponding foreign key relationships.
- A value-based entity type attribute with more than one data type must be splitted into several relational attributes, one for each data type.
- A reference attribute is expressed via foreign key relationships. If the reference attribute has a cardinality of 0:1 or 1:1, it suffices to introduce a foreign key between the referencing relation and the referenced relation. Otherwise, an intermediary relation must be introduced which will reflect the reference attribute through foreign keys pointing to the corresponding relations.

In the case of XML, an entity type is mapped to an XML element. If an entity type attribute is value-based and has a cardinality of 0:1 or 1:1, it can be transferred to an XML attribute of the XML element. The cardinality is reflected through the specification of either use="required" (1:1) or use="optional" (0:1). Value-based attributes with different cardinalities can be captured through subelements because in contrast to XML attributes a subelement of the same name can occur more than once per element. Reference attributes are captured using the key referencing construct provided by XML schema.

5 Experiments

In this section, the integration process described in the previous section will be demonstrated. Table 1 shows an example of how the content of relation DICOMPatients looks like for one single patient. Similarly, listing 1.2 contains an excerpt from a HL7 CDA document, referring to data of the same patient.

Both data sets are identified as equivalent by the patient ID. Entity types of both source schemas can be integrated according to the rules presented in Section 4. As a result, a new integrated schema will be created.

Table 1. Patient data in DICOM

DICOMPatients			
PatientID	PatientNam	PatientBir	PatientSex
0002	John Doe	12.01.1950	M

```
1  <patientRole>
2    <id extension="12345" root="2.16.840.1.113883.19.5"/>
3    <patient>
4      <name><given>John</given> <family>Doe</family></name>
5      <administrativeGenderCode code="M"
           codeSystem="2.16.840.1.11383.5.1"/>
6      <birthTime value="19500112"/>
7    </patient>
8    ...
9  </patientRole>
```

Listing 1.2. Patient data in HL7 CDA

The transformation of a relational data source to XML will be demonstrated with an example of the database of the Conquest DICOM server. Considering again the relation schema DICOMPatients having the attributes PatientID: varchar(64), PatientNam: varchar(64), PatientBir: char(8), PatientSex: varchar(16), AccessTime: int, qTimeStamp: int, qFlags: int and qSpare: varchar(64), listing 1.3 contains the mapping of DICOMPatients to the complex XML type DICOMPatients_Type. The corresponding XML element DICOMPatients is declared locally, nested within the declaration of the root element conquest. Also, all other XML elements, which result from the mapping of each relation schema of the database conquest, are declared in there. The information that the attribute PatientID is a uniquely identifying one is reflected through the use of the XML Schema key concept (see line 7 of listing 1.3). In turn, this property originates from PatientID being the primary key of the source relation DICOMPatients.

An example for an XQuery expression in listing 1.4 returns as a result date, time and processing device for all images. A nested XQuery expression is presented in listing 1.5. It retrieves all studies for a given patient providing information about the study's date, description and physician in charge.

```
1  <xs:complexType name="DICOMPatients_Type">
2    <xs:attribute name="PatientSex" use="optional" type="xs:string"/>
3    <xs:attribute name="PatientBir" use="optional" type="xs:string"/>
4      ...
5    <xs:attribute name="PatientNam" use="optional" type="xs:string"/>
6    <xs:attribute name="PatientID" use="required" type="xs:string"/>
7    <xs:key name="DICOMPatients_Key">
8     <xs:selector xpath="/conquest/DICOMPatients"/>
9     <xs:field xpath="PatientID"/>
10   </xs:key>
11 </xs:complexType>
```

Listing 1.3. The relation schema DICOMPatients as a complex XML type

```
1  for $image in /conquest/DICOMImages
2  return
3    <image>
4     <date>{$image/string(@ImageDate)}</date>
5     <time>{$image/string(@ImageTime)}</time>
6     <device_name>{$image/string(@DeviceName)}</device_name>
7    </image>
```

Listing 1.4. A simple XQuery example

```
1  for $patient in /conquest/DICOMPatients
2  return
3    <patientStudies>
4     <patient name="{$patient/string(@PatientNam)}">
5      for $patient_study in /conquest/DICOMStudies[@PatientID =
           $patient/string(@PatientID)]
6      return
7       <study date="{$patient_study/string(@StudyDate)}"
             physician="{$patient_study/string(@ReferPhysi)}">
8        {$patient_study/string(@StudyDescr)} </study>
9     </patient>
10   </patientStudies>
```

Listing 1.5. A nested XQuery example

6   Conclusions

This paper describes an approach to provide a user with access to a globally integrated information repository through a local system. This is mainly based on mappings from the source data schemas to the globally integrated data schema and, more importantly, their inverse mappings. This technique is called GaLVE (global-as-local-view-extension). We showed the applicability in a clinical environment with relational and XML data sources. The concrete environment for the experiments contained SAP i.s.h.med with the patient's master data and vital signs, a Conquest DICOM server, and an HL7 Clinical Document Architecture XML format.

Nevertheless, some open issues still remain. This article does not discuss the concrete type of integration. It is possible for the integration to copy the data (also known as materialized integration) or to distribute the queries to the respective source (also known as virtual integration). Especially for the second type, it is necessary to specify an adequate query transformation process, which has to be done in future work.

References

1. Arenas, M., Pérez, J., Riveros, C.: The recovery of a schema mapping: bringing exchanged data back. ACM Transactions on Database Systems 34(4), 22 (2009)
2. Bortis, G.: Experiences with Mirth: An Open Source Health Care Integration Engine. In: 30th Int. Conf. on Software Engineering, pp. 649–652 (2008)
3. Fagin, R.: Inverting schema mappings. ACM Transactions on Database Systems (TODS) 32(4), 25 (2007)
4. Fagin, R., Kolaitis, P.G., Popa, L., Tan, W.-C.: Quasi-inverses of schema mappings. ACM Transactions on Database Systems 33(2), 11 (2008)
5. Flach, G., Heuer, A., Langer, U., Meyer, H.: Transparent queries in federated database systems. In: Workshop on Federated Databases: Inst. Report, No. ITI-96-01, pp. 45–49. Univ. of Magdeburg (1996) (in German)
6. Fraile, J.A., Bajo, J., Corchado, J.M.: AMADE: Developing a Multi-Agent Architecture for Home Care Environments. In: Iberagents 2008: Proceedings of the 7th Ibero-American Workshop in Multi-Agent Systems, Lisboa, Portugal, pp. 43–54 (2008)
7. Haas, L.: Beauty and the beast: The theory and practice of information integration. In: Schwentick, T., Suciu, D. (eds.) ICDT 2007. LNCS, vol. 4353, pp. 28–43. Springer, Heidelberg (2006)
8. Hägglund, M., Scandurra, I., Moström, D., Koch, S.: Integration Architecture of a Mobile Virtual Health Record for Shared Home Care. In: 19th MIE Conf. Studies in Health Technology and Informatics, vol. 116, pp. 340–345 (2005)
9. Lenz, R., Beyer, M., Kuhn, K.A.: Semantic integration in healthcare networks. International Journal of Medical Informatics 76(2-3), 201–207 (2007)
10. Lenzerini, M.: Data integration: A theoretical perspective. In: 21st ACM Symposium on Principles of Database Systems, PODS 2002, pp. 233–246 (2002)
11. Leser, U.: Combining heterogeneous data sources through query correspondence assertions. In: 1st Workshop on Web Information and Data Management, in Conjunction with CIKM 1998, pp. 29–32 (1998)
12. Löper, D., Klettke, M., Bruder, I., Heuer, A.: Enabling flexible integration of healthcare information using the entity-attribute-value storage model. Health Information Science and Systems 1(1), 9 (2013)
13. Nadkarni, P.M., Marenco, L., Chen, R., Skoufos, E., Shepherd, G., Miller, P.: Organization of Heterogeneous Scientific Data Using the EAV/CR Representation. Journal of the American Medical Informatics Association 6(6), 478–493 (1999)
14. Neumann, C.P., Lenz, R.: $\alpha-$ flow: A document-based approach to inter-institutional process support in healthcare. In: Rinderle-Ma, S., Sadiq, S., Leymann, F. (eds.) BPM 2009. Lecture Notes in Business Information Processing, vol. 43, pp. 569–580. Springer, Heidelberg (2010)
15. Schweiger, A., Sunyaev, A., Leimeister, J.M., Krcmar, H.: Toward seamless healthcare with software agents. In: Communications of the Association for Information Systems, pp. 692–709 (2007)
16. Spaccapietra, S., Parent, C., Dupont, Y.: Model independent assertions for integration of heterogeneous schemas. The VLDB Journal 1(1), 81–126 (1992)
17. ten Cate, B., Kolaitis, P.G.: Structural characterizations of schema-mapping languages. Commun. ACM 53(1), 101–110 (2010)

Fall Detection with the Optimal Feature Vectors
Based on Support Vector Machine

Jing Zhang[1], Yongfeng Wang[2], Yingnan Ma[3], Xing Gao[3], Huiqi Li[1],
and Guoru Zhao[1,*]

[1] Shenzhen Key Laboratory for Low-cost Healthcare and Shenzhen Institutes of Advanced
Technology, Chinese Academy of Sciences, Shenzhen 518055, China
[2] School of Mechanical Engineering, Hebei University of Technology, Tianjin 300130, China
[3] Beijing Research Center of Urban System Engineering, Beijing, China

Abstract. Falls have caused extensive interest of the researchers for it becomes
the second largest accidental injury to death in the world. And there are lots of
approaches to fall detection at present. However, on account for the complexity
of this problem, a preferable effective method for fall detection hasn't been
present so far. This paper adopts a relatively high-predicted and stable SVM
classifier to predict falls. 10 healthy young subjects participated in this study
based on the Xsens MVN Biomech system. With the extraction of feature
vectors, as well as the exploration of the best position, it found that the waist
would be the best to measure body's motion, and the simple accelerometer can
offer the preferable features for the classifier to determinate the falls well.
Meanwhile it can get a high accuracy up to 96% by setting an optimal C and g
with five-fold cross-validation testing.

Keywords: Fall detection, Support Vector Machine, feature extraction.

1 Introduction

As the second external cause of unintentional injury, falls have become a major public
health problem, especially in the elderly. It leads to 20-30% of mild to severe injuries,
and are underlying cause of 10-15% of all emergency department visits [1,2]. The
resulting falls detection for elderly has attracted more and more people to research it
for its potential applications. Among the existing methods, the wearable sensing with
accelerometers and gyroscopes seem to be more convenient and acceptable than the
other two main technologies: video-based sensing and ambient sensing [3,11]. Based
on the thresholds relevant to the acceleration or other kinematic parameters in
different position, it could detect falls with acceptable accuracy around over 85%,
which have some discount with its sensitivities or specificities [4,5,6]. Meanwhile
there are another algorithm based on SVM distinguishing falls from other general
activities, it can get the results but not to set a threshold which depends on statistical
learning theory [7,8,9].

---

* Corresponding author.

Y. Zhang et al. (Eds.): HIS 2014, LNCS 8423, pp. 160–166, 2014.
© Springer International Publishing Switzerland 2014

SVM is one of the most practical machine learning techniques on the basis of statistical learning theory, which is permitted by Vapnik [12], with the structural risk minimization of statistical learning theory. In this study, an algorithm based on SVM is presented on account of its advantages in the small samples, non-liner and high dimensional problems. The purpose was to find the best position for the sensor and extract the optimal feature vectors [13,14] to classify the falls and ADLs by optimized the C and g.

2   Methods

In this paper, an algorithm with SVM was applied to the fall detection. With Xsens system, the collected data was pre-processed and set up a new database for SVM to classify the ADLs and the falls on the platform of MATLAB.

2.1   Measurements

For the sake of safety, the arranged experiments were performed by healthy youths instead of the elders. The simulated-falls and others activities of daily living (ADLs) trails were recorded from 10 healthy young subjects (3 female and 7 male students) based on the Xsens MVN Biomech system, which were ranged in age from 23 to 33 years. With the Xsens system, the kinematic data of the subjects could be obtained for it is integrated a 3D accelerometer, a 3D gyroscope and a 3D magnetometer, which included the component acceleration, angular velocity and magnetic field of each axis. In addition, each activity was self calibrated with the detection system before they were recorded. In the experiment, there were 4 multiple MTx sensor modules set in the follow positions: chest, right waist, right thigh, right shank, which is shown in figure 1.

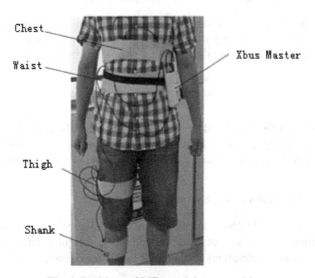

Fig. 1. Positions of MTx modules on a subject

For the activities, the participants were asked to perform the specified actions: falls and ADLs, while the ADLs included jogging, running, walk-run, go-upstairs, go-downstairs and stand-sit-stand, and other 4 kinds of falls were forward fall, left-fall, right-fall, backward fall. Meanwhile, all simulated falls were performed on a protective mat for the sake of safety.

2.2   SVM

SVM classifies the data by mapping the vector from low-dimensional space to high-dimensional space with kernel function. Given a liner separable dataset Φ: (xi,yi), i=1,…,n, $x_i \in R_d$ is the input variables, and $y_i \in \{+1,-1\}$ is the class-label, then a separating hyperplane set can be described in any inner product space as follows:

$$\begin{cases} \omega^T \cdot x_i + b \geq 1, \ y_i = 1 \\ \omega^T \cdot x_i + b < -1, y_i = -1 \end{cases} \tag{1}$$

The distance between the 2 hyperplanes can be calculated with geometry which is 2/‖ω‖. As the distance should be maximized, it is transferred into a quadratic programming problem. Considering the non-liner problem in general, the constrained condition could be soften with penalty parameter C and slack variable ξ_i (C>0 and ξ_i ≥0), the quadratic optimization can be written as follow:

$$\begin{cases} \max \sum_{i=1}^{n} \alpha_i - \frac{1}{2} \sum_{i=1}^{n} \sum_{j=1}^{n} \alpha_i \alpha_j y_i y_j (x_i \cdot x_j) \\ s.t. \ \sum_{j=1}^{l} y_i \alpha_i = 0, 0 \leq \alpha_i \leq C, i = 1,2,\cdots,l \end{cases} \tag{2}$$

In fact, a SVM need introduce a kernel function to overcome the curse dimensionality, as well. Among the several common kernel functions, the RBR is selected for its good application in many areas, which is shown in (3):

$$K(x_i, x_j) = \exp(-\frac{\| x_i - x_j \|^2}{2\sigma^2}) \tag{3}$$

By means of MATLAB embedded the LibSVM, it can help to classify the ADL and the falls effectively. In the classification system, five-fold cross-validation testing was used to search for the best C and g to improve the accuracy of classification.

2.3   Feature Translation and Extraction

With the help of Xsens MVN Biomech system, the 3D accelerations (a) and the 3D angular velocities (ω) can be obtained. Instead of the original data, the correlation coefficients (cc's) of accelerations and angular velocities of each axis were taken into account to act as the feature vectors for classification [10], which included the correlation coefficients between every axis of the accelerations and the angular velocities, and the correlation coefficients between the component of each axis and the sum of the accelerations and the angular velocities separately. Then 12 feature vectors could be obtained for the classifier at last. Furthermore, it needs to find out the optimal combination in order to acquire the relatively high accuracy with these SVs. As the features were corrective and the dimension was not so high, it was feasible to adopt the exhaustive method extract the final feature vectors.

In addition, as there were 4 sensors used to measure the different motions in different position, the correlation coefficients between each two sensors also could be considered as the feature vectors, which produced 6 feature vectors in this way.

3   Results

3.1   The Inner-Axis Correlation Coefficients of One Sensor

The rebuilding dataset by the way of the inner-axis correlation coefficients of one sensor is listed in Table 1.

Table 1. The basic feature vectors of activities

	x- and y- axes	y- and z- axes	z- and x- axes
set 1	$cc\ (a_x,a_y)$	$cc\ (a_y,a_z)$	$cc\ (a_z,a_x)$
set 2	$cc\ (a_x,a)$	$cc\ (a_y,a)$	$cc\ (a_z,a)$
set 3	$cc\ (\omega_x,\omega_y)$	$cc\ (\omega_y,\omega_z)$	$cc\ (\omega_z,\omega_x)$
set 4	$cc\ (\omega_x,\omega)$	$cc\ (\omega_y,\omega)$	$cc\ (\omega_z,\omega)$

Based on the whole feature vectors, the best measuring position should be firmed. With the calculated result, it found that classified accuracies were similar with less than 2% disparity in the three positions of chest, waist and thigh, while the result of the shank is 10% less than other three positions.

As it had the highest performance of ROC, the waist was selected as the best measuring position for detect the body kinematic information.

Combined the 12 features with every set regularly, the dataset was divided into two groups, while the first 130 samples were set for training and the rest of them were set for testing. And the results are shown in table 2.

It's obvious that the data derived from the gyroscope has little effect on the train and test from the group 3, 4 and 6. Comparing the group 1 and 2, the accuracy classified with the correlation coefficients of each axis is better than that between every axis and the sum. Though the whole features used as the vectors have the highest testing accuracy relatively, the training accuracy is not as good as the group 1. On the other hand, the slight benefit of the testing accuracy is obtained at the cost of another gyroscope.

Table 2. The results of the 1st classification

	Features	Training accuracy	Testing accuracy
1	Set1	93.08%	96.15%
2	Set2	83.78%	90%
3	Set3	53.85%	77.69%
4	Set4	70.77%	67.69%
5	Set1&2	90.77%	95.38%
6	Set3&4	62.31%	69.23%
7	Set1&3	90.77%	96.15%
8	Set2&4	91.54%	92.69%
9	Set1&2&3&4	92.31%	96.92%

3.2   The Correlation Coefficients of Different Sensors

In addition, there was another trial with the correlation coefficients between every two sensors. And the classified results are shown in the table 3.

Table 3. The results of the 2nd classification

	Combinations	Training accuracy	Testing accuracy
1	Waist &Thigh	94.62%	93.85%
2	Waist &Chest	87.69%	90.77%
3	Thigh &Chest	96.15%	94.62%

With the three set of results, it is confirmed that the correlation coefficients of x/y/z- acceleration between the thigh sensor and the chest sensor has the best accuracy. While it has no obvious performance with other feature vectors, the results aren't listed here.

4   Discussion and Conclusion

To determinate the falls and the ADLs, the correlation coefficients between the different parameters were adopted as the feature vectors of SVM. Generally, the more feature vectors there are, to a certain extent, the classified accuracy will be higher. On the other hand, a plethora of feature vectors may generate data redundancy and it would increase the complexity of calculation in a higher dimension. Though the dimension in this study is a little low, it proved that the more feature vectors didn't highlight the dramatic superiority with the finite features. In addition, it need obtain these features at the cost of another sensor. In the second analysis with the parameters in the different positions, the sensor combination of the thigh and the chest showed the best accuracy of the training and testing respectively. But it also has no more advantage than the result from one sensor in the first group analysis. Considering the testing cost and its performance, one accelerometer with the correlation coefficients between each two sensors can achieve a high precision accuracy to classify the falls and ADLs.

In this study, there are still some shortcomings. In spite of its good performance with small samples, the samples of activities are not enough to approach to the true situation with the learning capacity. And all of the activities are performed in a laboratory environment rather than in the real world, which leads to some distortion in the simulated actions of the subjects relative to the real falls of the elders.

For the further study, fall detection should extend to the fall pre-impact and fall protection. The fall detection based on SVM is off-line analysis in this study, which can't content the timeliness of fall protection in spite of its high accuracy. In the future, it needs more work to realize fall detection on-line with SVM, so that it can provide an affective and real-time basis for the protective study of fall to analyze.

Acknowledgments. This study has been financed partially by the National Natural Science Foundation of China (Grant Nos. 51105359 and 61072031) and the National Basic Research (973) Program of China (Grant No. 2010CB732606), and was also supported by the Guangdong Innovation Research Team Fund for Low-cost Healthcare Technologies, the International Science and Technology Cooperation Program of Guangdong Province (Grant No. 2012B050200004) and Beijing financial fund for Elderly health and safety services and key technology development (Grant No. PXM2013-178215-000001).

References

1. World Health Organization.Falls,
   http://www.who.int/mediacentre/factsheets/fs344/en/index.html
2. Thierauf, A., Preuss, J., Lignitz, E.: Retrospective analysis of fatal falls. Forensic Science International, 92–96 (2010)
3. Nouy, N., Fleury, A.: Fall detection-principles and methods. In: The 29th IEEE EMBS, Lyon, pp. 1663–1666 (2007)
4. Guoru, Z., Zhanyong, M., Ding, L., Kamen, I.: Exploration and implementation of a pre-impact fall recognition method based on an inertial body sensor network. J. Sensor, 15338–15355 (2012)
5. Woon-Sung, B., Dong-Min, K., Faisal, B., Jae-Young, P.: Real life application fall detection system based on wireless body area net work. In: The 10th IEEE CCNC-eHealth, pp.62 – 67 (2013)
6. Maarit, K., Antti, K., Ilkka, W., Timo, J.: Determination of simple thresholds for accelerometry-based parameters for fall detection. In: The 29th IEEE EMBS, Lyon, pp. 1367–1370 (2007)
7. Shin-Hong, L., Wen-Chang, C.: Fall detection with the Support Vector Machine during scripted and continuous unscripted activities. J. Sensor,12301–12316 (2012)
8. Shaoming, S., Tao, Y.: A wearable pre-impact fall detection using feature selection and Support Vector Machine. In: The ICSP Proceedings of IEEE, pp. 1686–1689 (2010)

9. Guangyi, S., Cheung-Shing, C., Wen- Jung, L., Kwok-Sui, L., Yuexian, Z., Yufeng, J.: Mobile human airbag system for fall protection using MEMS sensors and embedded SVM classifier. IEEE Sensor Journal, 495 – 503 (2009)

10. Dirk, W., Bert-Jan, B., Chris, B., Hermie, H., Peter, V.: Automatic identification of inertial sensor placement on human body segments during walking. Journal of Neuro Engineering and Rehabilitation (2013)

11. Jerene, J., Tam, N., Donald, L., Z.S., Bishara, J., Dentino, B.R.: A Fall Detection Study on the Sensors Placement Location and a Rule-Based Multi-Thresholds Algorithm Using Both Accelerometer and Gyroscopes. In: IEEE International Conference on Fuzzy Systems, Taipei, pp. 666–671 (2011)

12. Chuxiong, M., Yu, W., Yonghong, Z., Jian, Q., Ming, Z., Xiaodong, W.: A SVM classifier combined with PCA for ultrasonic crack size classification. In: CCECE /CCGEI of IEEE, Niagara Falls, pp. 1627–1630 (2008)

13. Xiangui, K., Matthew, S., Anjie, P. K.J., Ray, L.: Robust Median Filtering Forensics Using an Autoregressive Model. In: TIFS of IEEE, pp. 1456–1468 (2013)

14. Joshua, A., Damon, W., Gerry, D., Philip, M., Kelvin, B., George, G.: Genetic-Based Type II Feature Extraction for Periocular Biometric Recognition: Less is More. In: International Conference on Pattern Recognition, p. 20.

Pre-impact and Impact Detection of Falls
Using Built-In Tri-accelerometer of Smartphone

Liyu Mao[1], Ding Liang[1], Yunkun Ning[1], Yingnan Ma[2], Xing Gao[2], and Guoru Zhao[1,*]

[1] Shenzhen Key Laboratory for Low-Cost Healthcare
and Shenzhen Institute s of Advanced Technology,
Chinese Academy of Sciences, Shenzhen 518055, China
[2] Beijing Research Center of Urban System Engineering, Beijing, China

Abstract. Falls in elderlies are a major health and economic problem. Research on falls in elderly people has the great social significance under the population aging. Previous smartphone-based fall detection systems have not both fall detection and fall prevention, and the feasibility has not been fully examined. In this paper, we propose a smartphone-based fall detection system using a threshold-based algorithm to distinguish between Activities of Daily Living (ADL) and falls in real time. The smartphone with built-in tri-accelerometer is used for detecting early-warning of fall based on pre-impact phase and post-fall based on impact phase. Eight healthy Asian adult subjects who wear phone at waist were arranged to perform three kinds of daily living activities and three kinds of fall activities. By comparative analysis of threshold levels for acceleration, in order to get the best sensitivity and specificity, acceleration thresholds were determined for early pre-impact alarm (4.5-5m/s^2) and post-fall detection (21-28 m/s^2) under experimental conditions.

Keywords: smartphone, tri-accelerometer, fall detection, fall prevention.

1 Introduction

In aging society, elderlies increase dramatically. Falls affect over one third of elderlies in the world, and it is a major cause of injuries even death in elderlies [1]. Falls in elderly people have become a major health problem around the world, not only for the disabling fractures and psychological illness, but also for its' high social and economic costs. One of the most critical challenges faced by healthcare for the elderly is the realization of early fall recognition and alarm to prevent falls and keep elderlies doing activities of daily life safely [2].

Current work on automatic fall detection methods can be classified into three main categories in terms of the sensors they use: video-based methods [3], acoustic-based methods [4] and wearable sensor-based methods [5]. A majority of fall detection systems require some specific hardware or software design [6, 7]. This increases cost and limits its usage to the wealthiest people of society only. Many systems also

---

* Corresponding author.

Y. Zhang et al. (Eds.): HIS 2014, LNCS 8423, pp. 167–174, 2014.
© Springer International Publishing Switzerland 2014

have significant installation and training times, which causes the average person to tend to reject the system.

Currently, Smartphones have built-in motion sensors and global positioning system (GPS) navigation. These features may enable them to be appropriate tools to detect and report fall information to a remote party over the smartphone network. Researchers have already developed some smartphone-based fall detection systems [8,9,10,11,12].These systems make use of the embedded sensors (accelerometer, gyroscope and magnetometer) to detect a fall, but use different algorithms. The principle of functioning is very similar: a fall is detected if the embedded sensors reach a given threshold or the system reaches determine conditions of a specific algorithm; if there are no movements for a certain amount of time, the system automatically sends an alarm (phone call, text message, email etc.) to a set of contacts. These systems can detect a fall only after it has already occurred but cannot be used to prevent them from happening in the first place. In [13] used the built-in accelerometer and gyroscope of the smartphone to identify abnormal gaits in users for fall prevention and can alert the user about their abnormal walking pattern.

However, these studies have not both fall detection and fall prevention, and the feasibility has not been fully examined. This is the main contributions of this paper and the differences between this work and other existing studies. In this paper, we propose a smartphone-based fall detection system which is responsible for fall detection and fall prevention by built-in tri-accelerometer of smartphone. Fall prevention is to alert the users about the possibility of falling. Fall detection can detect a fall after it has already occurred and the system sends an alarm to caregivers/doctors for immediate help. In addition, we conducted an experiment to verify the feasibility of this system. According to our experimental investigation, the sensitivity and specificity of the impact detection were 100% when the threshold is set to 21-28 m/s^2 and the optimal sensitivity and specificity of the pre-impact recognition are about 98.61% when the threshold is set to 4.5-5m/s^2. Fall detection using a smartphone is a feasible and highly attractive technology for older adults, especially those living alone. It does not require the user to wear any physical sensors on the body, is highly secure, and is inexpensive because it requires only a smartphone.

2   Methods

2.1   Algorithm

Previous research has shown that the root-sum-of-square of the 3D accelerometer signals (Acc) (1) can be used to distinguish falls from ADL (Activities of Daily Living). Sensors provided us three channels of Acc component signals: Acc_x, Acc_y, Acc_z. The threshold of the impact always used for fall detection [14,15,16]. As shown in Figure 1[17], during a fall, the acceleration decreases sharply to a minimum as the person falls(pre-impact phase); the impact of landing causes a sharp increase in acceleration to a maximum value(impact phase). The acceleration profiles of everyday activities would unlikely reach these levels and could therefore be used as thresholds for detection. There were two thresholds in Acc that could be used to classify falls from ADLs, one for impact detection; while another for pre-impact detection.

$$Acc = \sqrt{Acc\_x^2 + Acc\_y^2 + Acc\_z^2} \qquad (1)$$

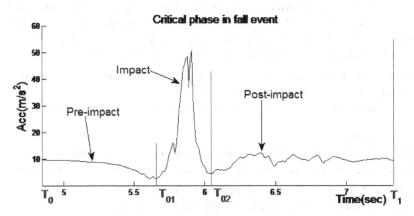

Fig. 1. Each phases of a fall event

2.2 System Design

The fall detection system is responsible for pre-impact recognition/alarm (i.e., prediction/alarm of a fall event before it happens) and post-fall detection (i.e., detection of a fall event after it already happened). The smartphone with built-in tri-accelerometer was utilized to collect the signal which represents the body movement. Then the median filter with n=3 is applied to the raw data to attenuate the noise [18]. At the same time, the smartphone compare with two thresholds for impact detection and pre-impact detection. Pre-impact recognition/alarm attempts to identify high-risk gait patterns and alert the user to save them from an imminent fall through vibration and voice prompt. When the smartphone identify a post-fall, a Pop-Up appears on the screen of the smartphone with options: 1) alarm, 2) reset. If the option of alarm is selected or the elderly person is unconscious at the end of a predefined time interval, it collects the geographic coordinates via the Global Positioning System (GPS) (i.e., if you are outdoors) or the cell-tower positioning (i.e., if you are indoors). Then an SMS with the time and the suspected fall location is automatically sent. The smartphone would also make an audible signal to attract the attention of any nearby persons. If there was no serious problem the user could reset the phone and make a phone call/send a text to the remote party indicating all was well [8].

2.3 Experiments

It is impossible to let elderlies perform fall activities. Eight healthy young male adult subjects (age: (23±3.45) years, weight: (60±7.68) kg) participated in this study. Subjects gave informed consent to participate in this procedure, which was approved by the CAS Ethics Board. [17]Head and waist are relevant sites for accelerometer detection of falls, using simple thresholds and posture detection [19]. So the smartphone in this system is worn on the waist.

Activities of Daily Living (ADL)

Subjects were asked to perform ADL in the laboratory. Each subject performed each ADL three times; every activity was performed from standing position and end with standing position. Only ADL that may trigger a fall detecting algorithm hold true meaning. And the ADL should come from people's daily life. With these considerations into account, we chose the following activities as testing ADL:

--Sitting down and standing up from a chair, the height of the chair was 50cm;
--Walking 5m, turn around, and walking back;
--Lying down and getting up from a bed, the height of the bed was 50cm.

Fall Experiments

Subjects performed fall activities on large crash mats (Fig. 1) after ADL were all completed. Each fall type was performed three times. Two types of fall were selected:

--Lateral fall (include left side and right side fall);
--Back-forward fall (include backward fall and forward fall).

Specificity and Sensitivity

The sensitivity and specificity of fall detection were calculated using the following definitions:

$$\text{Specificity} = \frac{\text{No.of true negatives}}{\text{No.of true negatives} + \text{No.of false positives}} \quad (2)$$

$$\text{Sensitivity} = \frac{\text{No.of true positives}}{\text{No.of true positives} + \text{No.of false negatives}} \quad (3)$$

Where true positive is a fall correctly identified as a fall. False positive is an everyday activity incorrectly identified as a fall. True negative is an everyday activity correctly excluded as not a fall. False negative is a fall incorrectly excluded as not a fall [8].

3   Results

As shown in Figure 2, the system can identify all fall events by detecting the impact phase and the threshold is 25m/s^2. As shown in table 1, the sensitivity and specificity were 100% when the threshold is set to 21-28 m/s^2. False positives will occur when the threshold below 21m/s^2. The system will occur undetected when the threshold above 28m/s^2.

As shown in Figure 3, the system can detect early-warning of fall based on pre-impact phase by setting the threshold to 5m/s^2. As shown in table 2, optimal sensitivity and specificity are about 98.61% when the threshold is set to 4.5-5m/s^2.

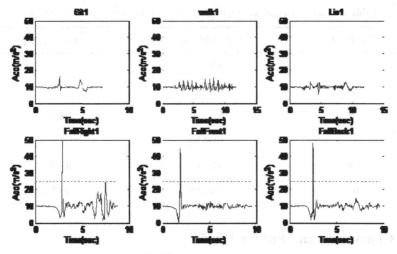

Fig. 2. Fall detection based on impact

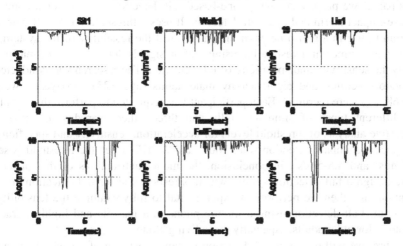

Fig. 3. Early-warning of fall based on pre-impact phase

Table 1. Accuracy evaluation with different threshold (Impact phase)

Threshold	Sensitivity	Specificity
18	100.00%	88.89%
20	100.00%	98.61%
21	100.00%	100.00%
28	100.00%	100.00%
29	97.22%	100.00%
32	95.83%	100.00%

Table 2. Accuracy evaluation with different threshold (Pre-impact phase)

Threshold	Sensitivity	Specificity
3	83.33%	100.00%
4	90.28%	98.61%
4.5	98.61%	98.61%
5	98.61%	97.22%
5.5	98.61%	87.50%
6	100.00%	80.56%

4   Conclusion and Future Work

In this paper, we propose a smartphone-based fall detection system which combines early pre-impact alarm and post-fall detection. It uses a threshold-based fall-detection algorithm to use in a real-time environment. To test the feasibility of the system, we design an experimental investigation using motion signals detected by the smartphone to study the sensitivity and specificity of fall detection. The research was conducted in a laboratory setting, and eight healthy male adults (age: (23 ± 3.45) years, weight: (60 ± 7.68) kg) were recruited. Each participant was requested to perform three trials of three different types of simulated falls and three other everyday activities. By comparative analysis of threshold levels for acceleration, sensitivity and specificity of pre-impact and impact detection were 100% and 98.61% when the threshold is set to 21-28 m/s^2 and 4.5-5m/s^2. In conclusion, the main contributions of this paper are that we design a fall detection system which is responsible for fall detection and fall prevention, and then we perform an experimental to fully examine the feasibility of this system. Fall detection using a mobile phone is a feasible and highly attractive technology for older adults, especially those living alone.

In future, we will design a fall detection system consisting of a smartphone and a remote server. The remote server aims to perform user management and provide useful information for family, healthcare providers and doctors. It can get analysis and statistical information of falls, the elderly profile and physical condition, etc. Besides, we can charge to user rely on useful information and user management.

Acknowledgements. This study has been financed partially by the National Natural Science Foundation of China (Grant Nos. 51105359 and 61072031) and the National Basic Research (973) Program of China (Grant No. 2010CB732606), and was also supported by the Guangdong Innovation Research Team Fund for Low-cost Healthcare Technologies, the International Science and Technology Cooperation Program of Guangdong Province (Grant No. 2012B050200004) and Beijing financial fund for Elderly health and safety services and key technology development (Grant No. PXM2013-178215-000001).

References

1. Bourke, A.K., O'Brien, J.V., Lyons, G.M.: Evaluation of a threshold-based tri-axial accelerometer fall detection algorithm. Gait Posture 26(2), 194–199 (2007)
2. Thierauf, A., Preu, J., Lignitz, E., Madea, B.: Retrospective analysis of fatal falls. J. Forensic Sci. Int. 198(1-3), 92–96 (2010)
3. Alemdar, H., Yavuz, G.R., Özen, M.O., Kara, Y.E., İncel, Ö.D., Akarun, L., Ersoy, C.: A Robust Multimodal Fall Detection Method for Ambient Assisted Living Applications. In: Proc. of IEEE Signal Processing and Communications Applications Conference, SIU 2010, Turkey (2010)
4. Zigel, Y., Litvak, D., Gannot, I.: A Method for Automatic Fall Detection of Elderly People Using Floor Vibrations and Sound Proof of Concept on Human Mimicking Doll Falls. Proc. of Transactions on Biomedical Eng. 56(12), 2858–2867 (2009)
5. Luo, S., Hu, Q.: A Dynamic Motion Pattern Analysis Approach to Fall Detection. In: Proc. of IEEE International Workshop on Biomedical Circuits and Systems, pp. 1–5 (2004)
6. Bouten, C.V.C., Koekkoek, K.T.M., Verduin, M., Kodde, R., Janssen, J.D.: A Triaxial Accelerometer and Portable Data Processing Unit for the Assessment of Daily Physical Activity. Proc. of Transactions on Biomedical Engineering 44(3) (1997)
7. Biddargaddi, N., Sarela, A., Klingbeil, L., Karunanithi, M.: Detecting Walking Activity in Cardiac Rehabilitation by Using Accelerometer. In: Proc. of International Conference on Intelligent Sensors, Sensor Networks and Information, pp. 555–560 (2007)
8. Lee, R.Y.W., Carlisle, A.J.: Detection of falls using accelerometers and mobile phone technology. Age and Ageing, 1–7 (2011)
9. Yavuz, G., Kocak, M., Ergun, G., Alemdar, H.O., Yalcin, H., Incel, O.D., Ersoy, C.: A Smartphone Based Fall Detector with Online Location Support. In: Proceedings of PhoneSense, pp. 31–35 (2010)
10. Dai, J., Bai, X., Yang, Z., Shen, Z., Xuan, D.: PerFallD: A pervasive fall detection system using mobile phones. In: Proceedings of the 8th IEEE International Conference on Pervasive Computing and Communications Workshops (PERCOM Workshops), pp. 292–297 (2010)
11. Sposaro, F., Tyson, G.: iFall: an Android application for fall monitoring and response. Journal of Eng. Med. Biol. Soc., 6119–6122 (2009)
12. Jiangpeng, D., Xiaole, B., Zhimin, Y., Zhaohui, S., Dong, X.: Mobile phone-based pervasive fall detection. Journal of Personal Ubiquitous Computing 14(7), 633–643 (2010)
13. Majumder, A.J.A., Rahman, F., Zerin, I., et al.: iPrevention: towards a novel real-time smartphone-based fall prevention system. In: Proceedings of the 28th Annual ACM Symposium on Applied Computing, pp. 513–518. ACM (2013)
14. Kangas, M., Vikman, I., Wiklander, J., Lindgren, P., Nyberg, L., Jämsä, T.: Sensitivity and specificity of fall detection in people aged 40 years and over. Gait & Posture 29(4), 571–574 (2009)
15. Kangas, M., Konttila, A., Lindgren, P., Winblad, I., Jämsä, T.: Comparison of low-complexity fall detection algorithms for body attached accelerometers. Gait & Posture 28(2), 285–291 (2008)

16. Bourke, A.K., van de Ven, P., Gamble, M., O'Connor, R., Murphy, K., Bogan, E., McQuade, E., Finucane, P., ÓLaighin, G., Nelson, J.: Evaluation of waist-mounted tri-axial accelerometer based fall-detection algorithms during scripted and continuous unscripted activities. Journal of Biomechanics 43(15), 3051–3057 (2010)

17. Liang, D., Zhao, G., Guo, Y., Wang, L.: Pre-impact & impact detection of falls using wireless body sensor network. In: 2012 IEEE-EMBS International Conference on Biomedical and Health Informatics (BHI), pp. 763–766 (2012)

18. He, Y., Li, Y., Bao, S.D.: Fall Detection by built-in tri-accelerometer of smartphone. In: 2012 IEEE-EMBS International Conference on Biomedical and Health Informatics (BHI), pp. 184–187. IEEE (2012)

19. Kangas, M., Konttila, A., Winblad, I., Jamsa, T.: Determination of simple thresholds for accelerometry-based parameters for fall detection. In: 29th Annual International Conference of the IEEE Engineering in Medicine and Biology Society, EMBS 2007, pp. 1367–1370 (2007)

Portable Assessment of Emotional Status and Support System

Pei-Ching Yang[1], Chia-Chi Chang[1], Yen-Lin Chen[1], Jung-Hsien Chiang[1,*],
and Galen Chin-Lun Hung[2,*]

[1] Department of Computer Science and Information Engineering,
National Cheng Kung University, Tainan, Taiwan
{yang.peiching,chia_chi_chang,aegis30263,
jchiang}@iir.csie.ncku.edu.tw
[2] Department of Addiction Science, Taipei City Psychiatric Center,
Taipei City Hospital, Taipei, Taiwan
galenhung@tpech.gov.tw

Abstract. In this paper, we propose a system that can capture and assess users' emotional status and provide support. The system includes a user profile database, an expert knowledge rule base, an education material database, and a portable emotion-sensing module. A user answers standardized questionnaires and visual analogue scales regarding to different emotions including depression, anxiety and stress, while recording daily activities and contextual factors leading to mood change through the portable emotion-sensing module in real time. The portable emotion-sensing module stores these variables in the cloud-based user profile database via Wi-Fi. The expert knowledge rule base in the cloud server receives values and distributing patterns of the variables to determine the corresponding mood symptoms and their severity. The educational material database, based on mindfulness-based cognitive therapy, returns guidance and encouragements to the portable emotion sensing module through the internet to provide the user with real-time support.

In the focus group testing, we invited twenty medical professionals and ten graduate school students to evaluate the system. Preliminary results showed that participants found the system helpful in achieving better awareness of their ever-changing emotional states, and that mindfulness-based audio guidance indeed helped them reduce stress and negative emotions. Subsequent pilot studies on patients with mild to moderate depression will help elucidate the clinical feasibility and efficacy of the proposed system.

Keywords: emotional status, moderate depression, portable emotion sensing module.

1   Introduction

The 2004 World Health Organization's report indicated that five of the ten leading causes of disability were psychiatric conditions. Psychiatric and neurologic conditions

---

* Corresponding author.

Y. Zhang et al. (Eds.): HIS 2014, LNCS 8423, pp. 175–183, 2014.

account for 28% of all years lived with disability, but only 1.4% of all deaths and 1.1% of years of life lost [1]. Thus, psychiatric disorders, while traditionally not regarded as a major epidemiological problem, are shown by consideration of disability years to have a huge impact on populations. Current predictions indicate that by 2030 depression will be the leading cause of disease burden globally [1, 2]. Major depression, along with its frequent comorbidity with chronic illness, is associated with lost productivity and excess mortality.

Given that depression is one of the most common and debilitating psychiatric disorders and is the leading cause of suicide. It is important not just to treat the clinically identifiable episodes, but also to recognize prolonged negative emotion and intervene early in order to achieve secondary prevention and avoid relapse of depression. A public health strategy capable of reaching the general, non-clinical population is, therefore, warranted.

It seems that everyone has a smartphone these days and a smartphone serves not only as a communication tool but also has powerful functions as a portable computer. Therefore, many medical personnel are devoted to develop mobile application to monitor and intervene various health conditions, depression alike.

Utilizing mobile programs to facilitate the access of psychological and behavioral interventions can promote popularity and participation of users [3]. For example, a lot of research point out that computer-based programs of cognitive behavior therapy can improve the symptom of depression [4, 5]. Furthermore, mobile applications have the advantage of real-time feedback [6]. The patients have more flexibility to interact with the app and to receive support at their convenience. Interacting with the app, they are able to preserve personal privacy and avoid the stigma of seeking help for mental illnesses [7]. To have a cordial talk with patients is critical in mobile application interaction [8].

Smartphone and mobile applications represent a unique opportunity to explore new modalities of monitoring, treatment, and research of mental health conditions [9]. However, available mobile applications for mood tracking and management are far from comprehensive, and users can neither receive professional guidance nor learn any self-help skills from those applications.

To address the unmet demand from the clinical aspect, we aim at developing a mobile app capable of monitoring, analyzing and responding to patients emotional states. We first review the research regarding human emotion tracking via a mobile system. We then describe our smartphone-based system. Finally, we briefly present the results of our focus-group study.

2   Related Work

In human daily emotion, there exist some underlying constructs including emotional tone (positive, negative or neutral) and degree of arousal (calmness or anxiety). A personal emotion model can be correlated with different cognitive and behavioral patterns to generate relevant predictions and feedbacks.

Currently, one of the common methods for assessing human emotion is standardized questionnaire to assess the degree of depression and stress. The questionnaire most commonly used in the mental health field is the Patient Health Questionnaire 9

(PHQ-9) and Perceived Stress Scale (PSS), respectively. Another way of assessing emotion is providing a visual analogue scale (VAS) for the users to rate their subjective emotional state.

The free app DS 憂鬱情緒檢測 by EzMoBo is a mobile application to fill in an online questionnaire for tracking depression. The app Sad Scale by Deep Pocket Series LLC sets up several questionnaires including a general depression scale, a depression scale for children, a post-partum depression scale, and a geriatric depression scale. The results for each questionnaire can be stored for physicians' use and can also be emailed, including emailing the results via a graph.

These preliminary results show the effective emotion self-tracking would be desirable. Self-tracking regularly is an effective way to monitor and understand one's own mood status, with the next reasonable step being providing users with real-time analysis of current emotional state and related support and guidance. However, available mobile apps lack the corresponding features.

3   Material and Method

In this research, we propose and implement a portable system for emotional status examination and support. The system can collect 3 emotional parameters (depression, anxiety, and stress) and their physical (somatic perceptions, daily activity level), psychological (thoughts), and environmental (location, accompanying persons, tasks in hand) correlates. The system provides feedback according the results of the cloud system computing and analyzing, based on pre-determined rules set by standardized questionnaires or expert opinions. The system also provides instant messaging for background mental health professionals to provide participants with real-time support and guidance.

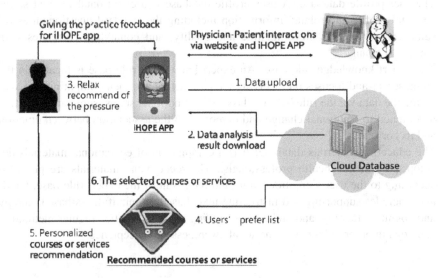

Fig. 1. System architecture

The development process consists of five stages: (1) deciding on the specifications, (2) selecting the platform, (3) creating the design, (4) testing the prototype, and (5) collecting the feedback of the focus group users and modifying the app.

3.1   System Architecture

The portable assessment of psychological status and support system consists: iHOPE mobile application, the user profile database, the expert's knowledge rule base and the education material database. The system architecture is as in Fig.1.

Firstly, we implement the iHOPE mobile application to provide the users to track their daily emotions and their correlates. Tracked variables include:

- Level of depression, anxiety and stress assessed by VAS
- Level of depression and stress assessed by PHQ-9 and PSS, respectively
- Daily activity level measured by g-sensor built in the smartphone
- Factors affecting mood change including time, place, persons, tasks, somatic feelings, thoughts and sleep quality

These data first store in mobile local database until detecting the Wi-Fi network and then all the data is uploaded via the Wi-Fi network to the cloud server that stores data into the relation database.

Secondly, the experts' knowledge database provide the users' state classification to provide different feedback contents and education materials.

Finally, background mental health professionals use the web service to reply to the users' question and problems, and provide instant support and guidance.

1. The user profile database: A user profile database is a cloud database that stores personal profile and related information including the standard questionnaires results, activity record, sleeping time and quality, and contextual correlates with emotional change.
2. The expert knowledge rule base: An expert knowledge rule base is located in the cloud server and focuses on receiving the parameters and then computing and analyzing the data via the rule base to classify the emotional status, summarize the factors related to emotional change and demonstrate the association between emotion and its correlates.
3. The education materials database: It is a compilation of educational materials developed by mental health professionals.. The recommend materials are provided according to the user's emotion status and the result of the expert rule base. Guidance includes supporting and instructing texts based on mindfulness-based therapy and cognitive therapy, and audio clips guiding users to practice regular meditation and yoga in order to increase emotional awareness and acceptance.

Example 1: if GHQ-9 scores 20 or above, the current emotional state is categorized as severely depressive, and the user receives the following suggestion:" It seems that you have severe depression, you will need immediate medical attention and proper pharmacotherapy may be warranted."

Example 2: if a user indicates 3 or more times that when his mood gets worse, the accompanying person is mother, he receives the following feedback: " It seems that when your mood turns worse, your mother is usually aside. Would you wonder why?"

Example 3: if there is an inverse association of mood state and daily activity for 3 days, the user receives the following suggestion:" it seems that your mood gets worse when you're physically inactive, would you like to try some exercise?"

3.2   Case Study

We performed an evaluation of iHOPE. We invited twenty medical professionals and ten graduate school students to try out the system on a daily basis for two weeks, and they are asked to fill out the questionnaire for feedback after two weeks of practice. The participants all used the smartphone in a regular basis in their daily lives.

Firstly, the participants download and install the iHOPE application and then input the basic information into the application. Secondly, the participants write down their emotion into the application and answers standardized questionnaires and visual analogue scales regarding to different emotions including depression, anxiety and stress, while recording daily activities and contextual factors leading to mood change through the portable emotion-sensing module in real time. Thirdly, the application shows the result of every record. iHOPE push to send real-time notifications to log the patients' emotion scales 4 times a day regularly and to log the patients' sleeping time and quality on 7:30 am.

Of the 20 participants offered to use the app, 12 evaluated them and considered the system easy to use and indicated that they found the user interface to be user-friendly and interesting. They found this app helpful in visualizing their ever-changing emotions and contributing factors. The guided meditations are practiced in various degrees, and an introductory course is demanded. Two respondents suggested: "Application could be developed for iOS version." One respondent indicated: "It would be preferable if some rewards are built in to encourage continuous use of the app."

Here appears to be technical limitations to use the mobile app, primarily because when pedometer is turned on, it consumes additional power and the smartphone needs to be charged more than once a day.

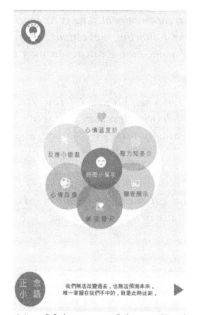

(a).   Main menu of the application

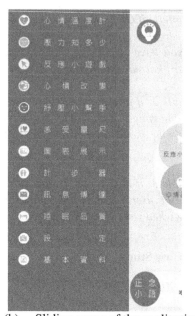

(b).   Sliding menu of the application

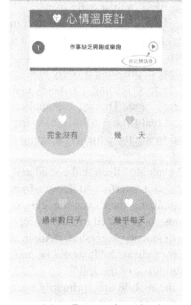

(c).   Depression check

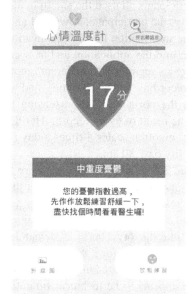

(d).   Depression score

Fig. 2. The iHOPE application interface for Chinese-language

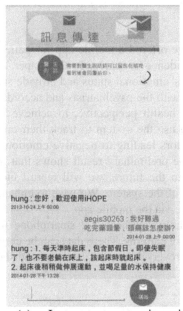

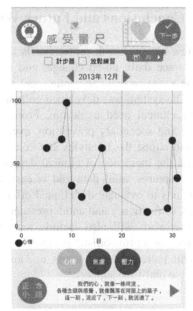

(a). Instant text messaging with physician

(b). Mood charts of depression score

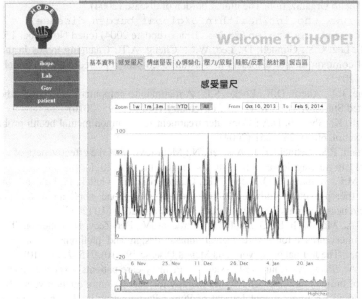

(c). The history of the emotion scales

Fig. 3. The iHOPE real-time information service

4   Conclusions and Future Work

Very few mental health professionals to date have offered a mobile app for patients and to trace daily mood change, and related evidence is scarce. In this paper, we propose a system that can capture and assess users' emotional status and provide support. The system was developed collaboratively with the psychiatrists and according to their clinical need to design. From a public health perspective, to achieve the primary and secondary prevention, everyone can use the system to track their emotions and adjust the lifestyles and contextual factors leading to negative emotion to decrease the incidence of clinical depression. The preliminary result shows that the system captures valid data and is easy to use. In the future, we will recruit more participants to evaluate the clinical effectiveness of the system. We wish to enhance patients' self-efficacy and antidepressant adherence via the mobile app.

Future work will also include recognizing daily routines (e.g. smartphone use behaviors) as a probabilistic combination of activity patterns. These data can be correlated with patients' mood, stress, and anxiety and reversely predict current mood state to provide real-time support.

References

1. World Health Organization. The global burden of disease (2004),
   http://www.who.int/healthinfo/global_burden_disease/
   2004_report_update/en/index.html (update 2004) (cited November 15, 2012)
2. Fu, T.S., Lee, C.S., Gunnell, D., Lee, W.C., Cheng, A.T.: Changing trends in the prevalence of common mental disorders in Taiwan: a 20-year repeated cross-sectional survey. Lancet. (2012)
3. Cartreine, J.A., Ahern, D.K., Locke, S.E.: A roadmap to computer-based psychotherapy in the United States. Harvard Review of Psychiatry 18(2), 80–95 (2010)
4. Cavanagh, K., Shapiro, D.A.: Computer treatment for common mental health problems. J. Clin. Psychol. 60(3), 239–251 (2004)
5. Foroushani, P.S., Schneider, J., Assareh, N.: Meta-review of the effectiveness of computerised CBT in treating depression. BMC Psychiatry 11, 131 (2011)
6. Morris, M.E., Kathawala, Q., Leen, T.K., Gorenstein, E.E., Guilak, F., Labhard, M., et al.: Mobile therapy: case study evaluations of a cell phone application for emotional self-awareness. Journal of Medical Internet Research 12(2), e10 (2010)
7. Depp, C.A., Mausbach, B., Granholm, E., Cardenas, V., Ben-Zeev, D., Patterson, T.L., et al.: Mobile interventions for severe mental illness: design and preliminary data from three approaches. The Journal of Nervous and Mental Disease 198(10), 715–721 (2010)
8. Beattie, A., Shaw, A., Kaur, S., Kessler, D.: Primary-care patients' expectations and experiences of online cognitive behavioural therapy for depression: a qualitative study. Health expectations: An International Journal of Public Participation in Health Care and Health Policy 12(1), 45–59 (2009)
9. Torous, J., Friedman, R., Keshvan, M.: Smartphone Ownership and Interest in Mobile Applications to Monitor Symptoms of Mental Health Conditions. JMIR mhealth and uhealth 2, 1 (2014)

10. Zhong, E., et al.: User demographics prediction based on mobile data. In: Pervasive and Mobile Computing (2013)
11. Chittaranjan, G., Blom, J., Gatica-Perez, D.: Mining large-scale smartphone data for personality studies. In: Personal and Ubiquitous Computing (2011)
12. LiKamWa, R., et al.: MoodScope: Building a Mood Sensor from Smartphone Usage Patterns (2013)
13. Whittaker, R., et al.: A multimedia mobile phone based programme to prevent depression in adolescents (2011)
14. Whittaker, R., et al.: MEMO—A Mobile Phone Depression Prevention Intervention for Adolescents: Development Process and Postprogram Findings on Acceptability from a Randomized Controlled Trial. Journal of Medical Internet Research (2012)
15. Burns, et al., Harnessing Context Sensing to Develop a Mobile Intervention for Depression. Journal of Medical Internet Research 13(3) (2011)
16. Tan, G., T.K.D., Farmer, L., Sutherland, R.J., Gevirtz, R.: Heart Rate Variability (HRV) and Posttraumatic Stress Disorder (PTSD): A Pilot Study (2011)
17. Kuehl, L.K., Deuter, C., Richter, S.: Mental stress induced changes in high-frequency HRV can be explained by vagal withdrawal (2011)
18. Morris, M.E., et al.: Mobile Therapy: Case Study Evaluations of a Cell Phone Application for Emotional Self-Awareness. Journal of Medical Internet Research The Leading Peer-Reviewed eHealth Journal (2010)

Mining Order-Preserving Submatrices
Based on Frequent Sequential Pattern Mining

Yun Xue[*], Yuting Li, Weijun Deng, Jiejin Li, Jianxiong Tang,
Zhengling Liao, and Tiechen Li

School of Physics and Telecommunication Engineering,
South China Normal University, Guangzhou, China, 510006
xueyun@scnu.edu.cn, Yuting_Li2011@163.com,
{junupwards,ltch2013}@gmail.com, 602520319@qq.com,
tomjx@sina.cn, lzl1991@yahoo.com

Abstract. Order-Preserving Submatrices (OPSMs) have been widely accepted as a pattern-based biclustering and used in gene expression data analysis. The OPSM problem aims at finding the groups of genes that exhibit similar rises and falls under some certain conditions. However, most methods are heuristic algorithms which are unable to reveal OPSMs entirely. In this paper, we proposed an exact method to discover all OPSMs based on frequent sequential pattern mining. Firstly, an algorithm is adjusted to disclose all common subsequences (ACS) between every two sequences. Then an improved data structure for prefix tree was used to store and traverse all common subsequences, and Apriori Principle was employed to mine the frequent sequential pattern efficiently. Finally, the experiments were implemented on a real data set and GO analysis was applied to identify whether the patterns discovered were biological significant. The results demonstrate the effectiveness and the efficiency of this method.

Keywords: OPSM, biclustering, all common subsequences, Apriori Principle, frequent sequence, the prefix tree.

1 Introduction

DNA microarrays are a breakthrough in experimental molecular biology. The resulting expression data can be viewed as an $M \times N$ matrix with M genes (rows) and N conditions (columns), in which each entry gives the expression level of a given gene under a given condition.

To analyze genetic data, clustering is introduced to group either genes or conditions. According to [1], clusters can be uncovered by either hierarchical or partitioned clustering techniques. However, standard clustering methods are limited to derive the local model as they deal separately with either the rows or the columns of the dataset. As a result, traditional methods such as k-means [18] and hierarchical clustering [19] do not perform well for high-dimensional gene expression data.

Y. Zhang et al. (Eds.): HIS 2014, LNCS 8423, pp. 184–193, 2014.
© Springer International Publishing Switzerland 2014

Because genes tend to be co-expressed or co-regulated only under a few conditions and there are still possibilities that some gene may share some common experimental conditions. Consequently, the idea to perform simultaneous row-column clustering was introduced by Hartigan [22], and first applied on gene expression data by Cheng and Church [2]. These simultaneous clusters, designated as biclusters, can be found by a greedy iterative search method based on mean squared residue proposed by Cheng and Church. Since then, various biclustering methods were introduced to mine the biclusters where the genes exhibit highly correlated activities for given conditions[3][4][5][6][7][8].

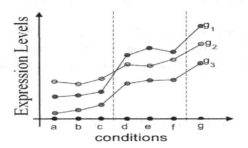

Fig. 1. The Order-Preserving Matrix

Due to the high level of noise in typical microarray data, it is usually more meaningful to compare the relative order of expression levels rather than their exact values. Genes that exhibit simultaneous rises and falls of their expression values across different time points or experiments reveal interesting patterns and knowledge. However, the classical distance-based biclustering algorithm is difficult to handle the problem of missing values ,therefore, the OPSM model, a pattern-based subspace clustering method, was originally launched by BenDor et al. in 2003[9]. The OPSM, which is manifested in Fig. 1, is a kind of coherent evolution bicluster where genes exhibit simultaneous rises and falls of the expression values across different time points or experiments. In other words, the OPSM problem focus on the relative order of the expression levels of each gene rather than the exact values [10], so the OPSM problem is competent to find the hidden patterns in noisy data [11].Whereas the OPSM problem itself is an NP-hard problem, and there are some drawbacks of the pioneer OPSM algorithm [9].Firstly, this algorithm was based on a given probability model. Secondly, the greedy heuristic mining did not guarantee that all OPSMs could be found. Finally, only one OPSM could be found at a time which was very sensitive to parameters and initialization. So after that, several improved methods have been raised to cope with the OPSM problem [12][13].

By sorting elements in the row sequences and replacing them with their corresponding column labels, the data matrix can be transformed into a sequence database, and OPSM mining is reduced to a special case of the sequential pattern mining problem. A sequential pattern uniquely specifies an OPSM with all the supporting row sequences, and the number of supporting row sequences is the support count of the pattern. A common subsequence whose support count is beyond a minimum support threshold, min_sup, is called a frequent sequential pattern.

Therefore, the problem of mining significant OPSM is equivalent to find the complete set of frequent sequential patterns. A new approach based on all common subsequences is proposed in the paper. Firstly, we acquire all common subsequences of every two rows by findACS [14][15]. Then, an exact method based on Apriori principle and frequent sequences patterns mining have been suggested in this paper to mine all salient OPSMs. Thus, the complete set of OPSMs will be obtained, including some biological significant OPSMs which many conventional OPSM mining methods ignore.

The rest of the paper is organized as follows. Section 2 describes the OPSM problem and the model. The algorithm to mine the OPSMs is introduced in section 3. The experiment result and the performance evaluation are given in Section 4. Section 5 concludes the paper.

2   The OPSM Problem and the Model

Microarray data is an $M \times N$ matrix D whose element d_{ij} represents the expression level of the ith gene under the condition j. The goal of the paper is to uncover the OPSMs in D. An example of D is shown in Fig. 2.

	conditions				
	1	2	3	4	5
1	4392	284	4108		228
2	401	281	120	275	298
genes 3	318	280	37	277	215
4	401	292	109	580	238
5	2857	285		271	226

	Column Labels				
1	5	2	3	1	
2	3	4	2	5	1
genes 3	3	5	4	2	1
4	3	5	2	1	4
5	5	4	2	1	

Fig. 2. A microarray data matrix D   **Fig. 3.** An example of transformed matrix C

2.1   The OPSM Problem

The Order-preserving submatrices B(OPSMs) have been employed to discover significant tendency of gene expression levels across a subset of conditions as a subspace cluster model. If the raw expression data of each row is sorted in an ascending order and its values are replaced by their corresponding column labels, the OPSM problem is able to be converted into the frequent sequential mining problem. After this operation of data preprocessing, the column transformed matrix C is formed which is illustrated in Fig. 3. Matrix C is an $M \times N$ matrix whose elements $C_{i_0 j_0}$ are the label of the column from the original matrix. Each row of the matrix C is a sequence indicating a one-by-N pattern of gene's whose expression values are in an ascending order. Therefore, a k-subsequence of each row represents a one-by-K pattern with similar tendency.

A frequent sequential pattern (FSP) is a common subsequence with support beyond a minimum support threshold δ. Such a frequent sequential pattern suggests the expression levels of co-regulated genes change (rise or fall) synchronously under certain conditions, which reveals OPSM information.

Based on such perspective, the searching of OPSMs $\{B_k = (I_k, J_k), k = 1, ... N\}$ can be transformed into finding common subsequences of length $\|J_k\|$ shared by $\|I_k\|$ ordered row sequences, where $\|I_k\|$ and $\|J_k\|$ are the number of involved genes and conditions. A significant OPSM should satisfy the minimum support threshold δ since a small scale OPSM may be random produced.

2.2   FindACS

An existing algorithm for counting all common subsequences (ACS) is adopted, which is called FindACS [14]. FindACS calculates similarity based on the number of all the common sequences between the two sequences, which could unearth all common subsequences between two sequences. This guarantees all the OPSMs could be found under the given condition $\delta = 2$. The original pseudo code of FindACS is given in Fig. 4.

By this algorithm (FindACS), all common subsequences of every two rows are obtained, but it raises exponential computation complexity as well as space complexity in the process of patterns storing, database traversing and support counting.

2.3   The Prefix-Tree

While most existing algorithms for OPSM model which are starting from a short sequence pattern to obtain all the frequent sequential patterns by the column extension, the paper find all the ACS which have different length and meet the support of no less than 2 instead to get all the frequent sequential patterns satisfying the support threshold. However, due to the large size of the ACS collection, it is hard to store and traverse all the candidates. In order to reduce the time and space complexity, a modified prefix tree is adopted to store and search all the ACS we acquired above.

The prefix-tree model is constructed in this sub-section, which is capable to reveal the k-frequent sequential pattern just by traversing the k-candidate prefix-tree instead of jointing.

The prefix tree model is an approach based on common subsequences searching which are subsequences of two sequences. Subsequence is defined as a sequence that can be derived from another sequence by deleting some characters without changing the order of the remaining characters. On the contrary, the supersequence is defined as a sequence that contains a series of sequences. That is say, if A is the subsequence of B, then B is one of supersequences of A. If a common sequence has length of K, it would be called as common k-subsequence. A frequent subsequence is a subsequence that meets the minimum support threshold (δ) and the column threshold(ξ).

The prefix tree records each frequent item in the database C. Nodes of the tree are sorted by certain order, such as by the dictionary order or by the support order. Each node in the tree maintains a triple (item, count, and branch), item denotes the last item of a sequence, count is the support of sequence and branch is a branch of the tree pointing to its child. Each branch (from the root node to a leaf node) represents a candidate sequence.

Find ACS-find the set of all common subsequences
          Of two sequences.

Data: Sequence α

Output: A list, $L_{\alpha\beta}$, of all common subsequences of α and β

1.   Init: $S=\varepsilon$, ind(S)=0, $L=\varepsilon$
2.   **for** (i=0; i<$|\alpha|$; i++) **do**
3.   x= $\alpha[i]$
4.   **if** $\beta[j] = x$ **then**
5. $S' = \varnothing$
6.   **for** every $Z \in L$ **do**
7.   **if** j> ind(Z) **then**
8. $S' = S' \cup Z$
9.   end
10.   **end**
11. $S = yx, \forall y \in S'$
12.   Ind(S)=j
13. $L = L \cup S$
14.   **end**
15.   **end**
16. $L_{\alpha\beta}=U_{x\in L}X$

Fig. 4. Pseudo-code of findACS [15]

3   Frequent Sequence Mining

In this part, the algorithm based on common ACS and Apriori Principle is described. At the beginning, the flowchart of the algorithm is illustrated in Fig. 5.

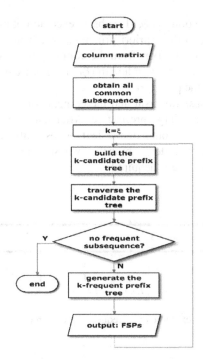

Fig. 5. Flowchart of FSPs discovery

Firstly, the ξ-candidate prefix tree would be generated by the candidate ξ-subsequences matrix. Fig. 6 illustrates the 2-candidate prefix tree for $\xi=2$. The leave nodes of the prefix tree record the labels of the rows of a common subsequence (a branch). For example, {1, 4} is the subsequence of row 4 and row 5.

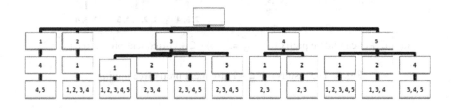

Fig. 6. An example of 2-candidate prefix tree

After that, the ξ-frequent prefix tree is constructed just by deleting the infrequent subsequences that dissatisfy the support. Fig. 7 is the ξ-frequent prefix tree.

Next specific steps are detailed to construct the $(\xi+1)$-candidate prefix tree. Firstly traverse the ξ – frequent tree, if the first ξ prefixes of the common $(\xi+1)$ subsequence are the same as a branch in the ξ-frequent tree then inserting the $(\xi+1)^{th}$ element of the common $(\xi+1)$-subsequences into the $(\xi+2)^{th}$ layer of the ξ-frequent prefix tree. Simultaneously, the leave nodes of the ξ-frequent prefix tree would be revised. If the first ξ prefixes of the common (ξ+1) subsequence do not match any paths of the ξ -frequent tree, according to the Apriori principle, which means the common subsequence consisting of the ξ prefixes from the common (ξ+1) subsequence is not frequent, the common subsequence with length (ξ+1) is not frequent either and it should not be added as a path to the prefix tree.

This reduces meaningless traversal and the comparison between sequences, which is very time-consuming in a large prefix tree. After that, we get the (ξ+1)-candidate tree. Then compare the row count of the leaf nodes with the support threshold to prune infrequent branches and delete branches whose length is less than the support. Finally, the (ξ+1)-frequent tree is acquired.

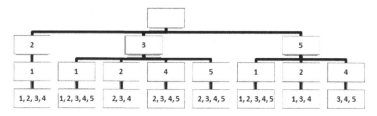

Fig. 7. An example of 2-frequence prefix tree with "δ=3"

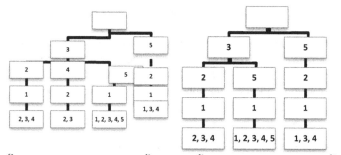

(a) (ξ+1)-candidate prefix tree (ξ=2) (b) (ξ+1)-frequent prefix tree (ξ=2)

Fig. 8. The results of (ξ+1)-frequent prefix tree mining

4   Experiments Results

The algorithm was implemented on the platform Matlab R2011b with i3 380 CPU and 4G memory, and the operating system is Windows Server 2007. The real datasets is Yeast Galactose data of (Ideker et al[21][16][17])which is a 205 by 80 real microarray data set obtained from a study of gene response to the knockout of various genes in the Galactose utilization (GAL) pathway of the baker's yeast, columns corresponding to the knockout conditions and rows corresponding to genes that exhibit responses to the knockouts.

4.1   Results

To evaluate the quality of the OPSMs that have been found by this approach, we applied the algorithm to the 205-by-80 microarray data set [16][17] with our measurements to study the quality of the OPSMs in data and the result is shown in Fig. 9.In this experiment, the threshold number of rows δ was 20, the threshold number of columns ξ was 7. The results are summarized in Fig. 9 and one example of overlapping is also shown in Fig. 10.

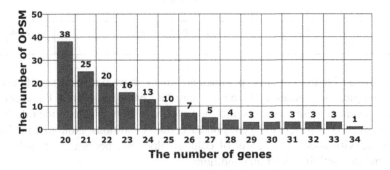

Fig. 9. Results for 205-by-80 microarray data set

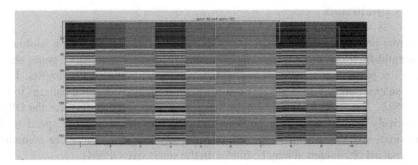

Fig. 10. One example of overlapping from found OPSMs

Totally 154 clusters are found with many clusters containing overlapping. 64 percent of clusters had 23 genes or fewer, and 85 percent of clusters had 30 genes or fewer. From Fig. 10, we can clearly see that there is considerable overlap between two clusters, where their ID is 48 and 183 respectively. The first cluster (its ID is 48) has 25 rows and 7 columns, and the second cluster (ID is 183) has 24 rows and 6 columns. Both have 16 rows (genes) and 4 columns (conditions) in common.

4.2   Go Analysis

To assess the biological relevance of the biclusters, the Gene Ontology (GO) is analyzed and the p-values are obtained from the hypergeometric distribution. For this, we used the functions from the three GO categories, biological process, molecular function and cell component at level higher than3. Table1 shows p-values computed using the GOToolbox and the utilities from the 205-by-80 microarray data set [16][17].

Table 1. Biological relevance of the biclusters

Bicluster ID	Genes	Conditions	GO-Category	GO-Level	P-Value
07	176(YBR028C)	8	protein amino acid phosphorylation	9,7,8	0.0221942
10	62(YAR010C)	8	transposition, RNA-mediated	4	0.0215646

The generated biclusters whose p-values are small show statistical significance as well as biological significance in one or more GO categories. Table1 presents the expression levels of these biclusters and shows the algorithm is able to identify highly correlated expression patterns of genes under certain conditions. Note that the highly correlated activity under this subset of columns does not necessarily translate into highly correlated activity under all conditions.

5   Conclusion

The order-preserving submatrices (OPSMs) have been accepted as a biologically meaningful bicluster model. OPSMs consisting of a small number of genes sharing expression patterns over many conditions are very interesting to biologists. In this paper, an exact algorithm is put forward based on frequent sequential patterns to mine the OPSMs. The experiment results show that this approach can discover the OPSMs exhaustively. Future work will be done to accelerate the computing speed to find some small size OPSMs which have comparatively less rows and more columns as some unusual phenomenon may be hidden in the small size OPSMs.

Acknowledgements. The authors thank gratefully for the colleagues who have been concerned with the work and have provided much more powerfully technical supports. The work is supported by Guangdong Science and Technology Department under Grant No.2009B090300336,No.2012B091100349; Guangdong Economy & Trade Committee under Grant No. GDEID2010IS034; Guangzhou Yuexiu District science and Technology Bureau under Grant No 2012-GX-004; National Natural Science Foundation of China (Grant No:71102146, No.3100958) ; Science and Technology Bureau of Guangzhou under Grant No. 2011J4300046.

References

1. Treshansky, A., McGraw, R.: An overview of clustering algorithms. In: SPIE (2001)
2. Cheng, Y., Church, G.: Biclustering of expression data. Ismb. 93–103 (2000)
3. Getz, G., Levine, E., Domany, E.: Coupled two-way clustering analysis of gene microarray data. Proc. Natl. Acad. Sci. U.S.A. 97, 12079–12084 (2000)
4. Gu, J., Liu, J.S.: Bayesian biclustering of gene expression data. BMC Genomics 9(suppl. 1), S4 (2008)
5. Lazzeroni, L., Owen, A.: Plaid models for gene expression data. Stat. Sin. (2002)
6. Tanay, A., Sharan, R., Shamir, R.: Discovering statistically significant biclusters in gene expression data. Bioinformatics. 18(suppl. 1), S136–S144 (2002).
7. Yang, J., Wang, H., Wang, W., Yu, P.: Enhanced biclustering on expression data. In: Third IEEE Sympesium Bioinforma. Bioengineering, BIBE 2003 (2003)
8. Yu, P.: δ-clusters: capturing subspace correlation in a large data set. In: Proceedings 18th International Conference on Data Engineering, pp. 517–528. IEEE Comput. Soc. (2002)
9. Ben-Dor, A., Chor, B., Karp, R., Yakhini, Z.: Discovering local structure in gene expression data: the order-preserving submatrix problem. J. Comput. Biol. 10, 373–384 (2003)
10. Madeira, S.C., Oliveira, A.L.: Biclustering algorithms for biological data analysis: a survey, http://www.ncbi.nlm.nih.gov/pubmed/17048406
11. Zhang, M., Wang, W., Liu, J.: Mining approximate order preserving clusters in the presence of noise. In: Data Eng., ICDE 2008 (2008)
12. Gao, B., Griffith, O., Ester, M.: On the Deep Order-Preserving Submatrix Problem: A Best Effort Approach. Trans. 24, 309–325 (2012)
13. Liu, J., Wang, W.: OP-cluster: clustering by tendency in high dimensional space. In: Third IEEE International Conference on Data Mining, pp. 187–194. IEEE Comput. Soc. (2003)
14. Wang, H.: All Common Subsequences.pdf. IJCAI (2007)
15. Wang, H., Lin, Z.: A Novel Algorithm for Counting All Common Subsequences. In: 2007 IEEE International Conference on Granular Computing (GRC 2007), pp. 502–502. IEEE (2007)
16. Yeung, K.Y., Medvedovic, M., Bumgarner, R.E.: Clustering gene-expression data with repeated measurements (2003),
http://www.ncbi.nlm.nih.gov/pubmed/16901101
17. Medvedovic, M., Yeung, K.Y., Bumgarner, R.E.: Bayesian mixture model based clustering of replicated microarray data (2004),
http://www.ncbi.nlm.nih.gov/pubmed/14871871
18. Macqueen, J.: Some Methods for Classifiation and Analysis of Multivariate Observations (1967)
19. Kaufman, L., Rousseeuw, P.J.: Finding Groups in Data: An Introduction to Cluster Analysis. Google (2009)
20. Gao, B., Griffith, O., Ester, M.: On the Deep Order-Preserving Submatrix Problem: A Best Effort Approach. Trans. 24, 309–325 (2012)
21. Ideker, T., Thorsson, V., Ranish, J.A., Christmas, R., Buhler, J., Eng, J.K., Bumgarner, R., Goodlett, D.R., Aebersold, R., Hood, L.: Integrated genomic and proteomic analyses of a systematically perturbed metabolic network. Science 292, 929–934 (2001)
22. Hartigan, J.: Direct Clustering of a Data Matrix. J. Am. Statistical Assoc. 67(337), 123–129 (1972)

Unsupervised Segmentation of Blood Vessels from Colour Retinal Fundus Images

Xiao-Xia Yin[1], Brian W.-H. Ng[2], Jing He[1], Yanchun Zhang[1], and Derek Abbott[2]

[1] Centre for Applied Informatics, College of Engineering and Science, Victoria University, Melbourne, VIC 8001, Australia
[2] Centre for Biomedical Engineering and School of Electrical & Electronic Engineering, The University of Adelaide, SA 5005, Australia

Abstract. This paper represents an algorithm based on curvature evaluation and Entropy Filtering techniques with texture mapping for guideline. The method is used for the detection of blood vessels from colour retinal fundus images. In order to evaluate vessel-like patterns, segmentation is performed with respect to a precise model. We evaluate the curvature of blood vessels via carrying out eigenvalue analysis of Hessian matrix. This method allows to extract the fine retinal image ridge but introduces the effect of central light reflexes. We apply entropy filtering techniques to calculate the segmentations in relation to central reflex vessels. For efficient differentiation of vessels from analogous background patterns, we use spectral clustering to partition the image texture. It is an alternative of traditional intensity thresholding operation and allows more automatic processing of retinal vessel images. The detection algorithm that derives directly from this modeling is based on five steps: 1) image preprocessing; 2) curvature evaluation; 3) entropy filtering; 4) texture mapping; 5) morphology operation with application of vessel connectivity constraints.

Keywords: retinal vasculature, spectral clustering, fundus image, Sobel edge detection, central light reflex, entropy filtering, morphological operation.

1 Introduction

The vessel segments from different image texture are linearly combined to produce final segmentation for a retinal image. In this paper, we propose a comprehensive method for segmenting the retinal vasculature in fundus camera images. Different from the state-of-the-art methods, we explore graph partitioning to pre-group together the vessels using morphology based spectral clustering technique. This aims to obtain a color map of the fundus images according to texture feature of vasculature instead of complex threshold processing for the evaluation of multi-scale image. We use eigenvalue analysis of the Henssian matrix to obtain curvature of vessel images in order to find the retinal image ridge. For the texture based region where small vessels are dominant, we apply a Sobel edge

Y. Zhang et al. (Eds.): HIS 2014, LNCS 8423, pp. 194–203, 2014.

detector and a morphological closing operation on the enhanced image to calculate an initial mask of vessels and then remove the noise from background. For the texture based region where consists of main large vessels, we extract vessel segments via a single threshold operation on the curvature based enhanced image. This reduces the computational complexity and avoids multi-threshold operation. In order to eliminate the effect of central light reflex, we apply entropy filtering technique to calculate the segment in relation to central reflex vessels. The vessel segments from different image texture are linearly combined to produce final segmentation for a retinal image. On DRIVE, visual inspection on the segmentation results shows that the proposed method produces accurate segmentation in comparison with manual segmentation from an expert. Meanwhile, we demonstrate an efficient method for vessel width measurements obtained using the segmentations produced by the proposed method. The result is accurate and close to the measurements provided by the expert. The advantages of the proposed method include its efficiency with its simplicity and scalability to deal with high resolution retinal images.

The paper is organized as follows. Section 2 summarizes the methodology we use to for the analysis of retinal vessel images. Section 3 represents the method that is designed for retinal width measurement. Section 4 reports and discusses our experimental results. Section 5 concludes the paper.

2   Methodology

2.1   Image Source

We obtained human retinal images from publicly available databases. The source of fundus images used to test the segmentation was the DRIVE (Digital Retinal Image for Vessel Extraction) database [1]. The image to be analysed is 565×584 pixels in size, and was captured in digital form using a Canon CR5 nonmydriatic 3CCD at $45°$ field of view as part of a screening programme in the Netherlands. The image set contains representative images that are large, showing visible pathologies and have vessels exhibiting prominent central light reflexes. One set of gold standard segmented binary image showing blood vessels was made available. In our case, colour images were ere converted to grayscale by extracting the green channel information and treating this as containing gray levels, because the green channel exhibits the best contrast for vessel detection [2]. For convenience, the fundus image is truncated to the dimension of 512×512 pixels. To improve the local contrast of the retinal image, a morphological top-hat transform as preprocessing is suggested [3]. The top-hat transformation of an retinal image is described via the equation: $\mathbf{I}_T = \mathbf{I} - (I \circ \mathbf{S})$. The symbols of S is a defined structure element (SE) and $(\circ)$ denotes the opening operator. About the details of mathematic morphological algorithm, pls refer to [3].

2.2   Morphology Based Spectral Clustering for Vessel Texture

The eye fundus photographs present inadequate contrast, lighting variations, noise influence and anatomic variability affecting both the retinal background texture and the blood vessels structure. Spectral Clustering methods are promising approaches to perceptual retinal vessel segmentation that take into account global image properties as well as local spatial relationships. The method is represented as [4,5,6], which integrates complex wavelet transforms with spectral clustering for a measure of spatial variation in texture though the morphological algorithm of watersheds. It consists of four major stages. First, a dual-tree complex wavelet transform in the decimated domain is carried out to reduce the computational complexity. Next, a median filter is used to filter the texture subband magnitude before the application of the gradient operator. The filter is separable-, scale-, and orientation-adaptive, aiming to make a nonlinear edge-pre-serving smoothing and remove artificial noise from retinal images. Afterwards, an over segmented image based on the gradient image and watershed transform is created. The gradient image is computed as the combination of the the gradient and modulated intensity gradient. The implementation of watershed relies on the morphological H-minima transform, as the latter controls watershed over segmentation. In the fourth stage, the over-segmented image is the input for the image region similarity graph (RSG) construction. It is an undirected weighted graph where the set of nodes corresponds to the atomic region. For each pair of regions, the set of links repents relationships and the link weights represent similarity measurers between the regions. Finally, spectral clustering is applied on the RSG to group together those pieces which have come from the same perceptual region. It affords a weighted mean cut criterion for possible fragment combinations.

2.3   Eigenvalue Analysis of Hessian Matrix

To analyze the local behavior of the preprocessed image $I_T(x)$, Taylor expansion in the neighborhood of a point x_0 is computed up to the second order. The equation is represented as follows:

$$I_T(x_0 + \delta x_0) \approx I_T(x_0) + \delta x_0^T \nabla_0 + \delta x_0^T \mathcal{H}_0 \mathcal{H}_0 \delta x_0, \tag{1}$$

where δx_0 and $\mathcal{H}_0$ are the gradient vector and Hessian matrix of the image computed in x_0. In this framework, differentiation operators of I_x is as a convolution with derivatives of Gaussian:

$$\frac{\partial}{\partial x} I_T(x) = I_T(x) \times \frac{\partial}{\partial x} G(x) \tag{2}$$

where the D-dimensional Gaussian is defined as:

$$G(x) = \frac{1}{(2\pi\sigma^2)}^{D/2} e^{-\frac{\|x\|^2}{2\sigma^2}}. \tag{3}$$

The third term in Eq. 1 gives the second order directional derivative

$$\delta x_0^T \mathcal{H}_0 \delta x_0 = (\frac{\partial}{\partial \delta x_0})(\frac{\partial}{\partial \delta x_0}) I_T(x_0) \tag{4}$$

The idea behind eigenvalue analysis of the Hessian is to extract the principal directions in which the local second order structure of the image can be decomposed [7]. In this case, the direction of smallest curvature along the vessel can be computed directly.

2.4   Entropy Filtering Technique

Entropy filtering is a technique to filter an image via selecting of an optimum threshold value [8]. The optimum threshold value is determined according to the pixel intensity from the histogram of the image that exhibits the maximum entropy over the entire image. In order to represent spatial structural information of an image, a co-occurrence matrix is generated from the image with top-hat preprocessing. It is a mapping of the pixel to pixel greyscale transitions in the image between the neighboring pixel to the right and the pixel below each pixel in the image.

The co-occurrence matrix is a $P \times Q$ dimensional matrix $C = [c_{ij}]_{P \times Q}$. The c_{ij} is defined as follows:

$$c_{ij} = \sum_{l=1}^{P} \sum_{l=1}^{Q} \delta, \tag{5}$$

where $\delta = 1$, if

$$\begin{cases} I_T(l, k) = i \text{ and } I_k(l, k+1) = j, \\ I_T(l, k) = i \text{ and } I_k(l+1, k) = j \end{cases}$$

and otherwise, $\delta = 1$.

The probability of co-occurrence satisfies the equation, $p_{ij} = \frac{c_{ij}}{\sum_i \sum_j c_{ij}}$. The candidate threshold $0 \leq s \leq L - 1$ divides the co-occurrence matrix into four regions representing within object (P_A), within background (P_C), object to background (P_B), and background to object class transitions (P_D). The second-order entropy of the object $(H_A^{(2)}(s))$ and background $(H_C^{(2)}(s))$ are defined as:

$$\begin{cases} H_A^{(2)}(s) = -\frac{1}{2} \sum_{i=0}^{s} \sum_{j=0}^{s} (P_{ij}/P_A)^A \log_2(P_{ij}/P_A) \\ H_C^{(2)}(s) = -\frac{1}{2} \sum_{i=s+1}^{L-1} \sum_{j=s+1}^{L-1} (P_{ij}/P_C) \log_2(P_{ij}/P_C) \end{cases}$$

Finally, the total second-order entropy of the object and the background are calculated, and the optimal thresholds are found by maximizing the entropies as a function of threshold.

2.5   Width Measurement

We design a vessel width measurement method to identify a pair of edge points representing the width of a vessel at a specific center point. The first step is to apply a morphological thinning algorithm [9,10,11] on the resultant segmentation for centreline computation. Thinning iteratively removes exterior pixels from the detected vessels, finally resulting in a new binary image containing connected lines of 'on' pixels running along the vessel centers. Thereafter, we apply the skeletonisation operation on the vessel segmented binary image to detect the vessel centerlines. Skeletonisation is a binary morphological operation which removes pixels on the boundaries of objects without destroying the connectivity in an eight-connected scheme. The pixels remaining make up the image skeleton without affecting the general shape of the pattern [12]. Therefore, the one pixel thin vessel centerline is obtained with a recognizable pattern of the vessel. The pixels that consist of vessel centerline are viewed as a series of specific center points for width measurements.

All edge points are detected on the vessel centerline image using a 3 × 3 window. This is realised based on the following steps. First, we conduct convolution operation between the window and vessel centerline image. We consider only three windowed centreline pixels that consist of three unique positions along its horizontal or vertical orientation or both. This avoids vessel crossing to be detected with two adjacent branchings on the vessel centerline image. We linearly extrapolate and rotate the centreline pixels with window as such that each of the resultant profile enables to contain widest segmented pixels and pixels from additional background region. The principle is to approximate the tangent of centreline at any point of it via the connected neighbor pixels in the local region. The connected pixels consist of three unique coordinates along a horizontal or vertical direction. The resultant profiles perpendicularly cross through tangents and go through the pixel with central coordinate. For only one unique x position, we directly find its perpendicular line. Such a resultant profile overlaps with vessel segment and its background, and the distance between the central coordinate pixel and the pixels from vessel segment is calculated. The edges of the extracted segments are located with the largest distance from the central coordinate point.

3   Experimental Results

We implemented our proposed method by MATLAB version R2013a. As mentioned earlier, the green channel is processed for the DRIVE database. In fact, vessels clearly stand out from background in green channel for images of DRIVE database. The algorithm described in Section 2 is followed. First, top-hat based morphology preprocessing is applied on the selected channel shown in Fig. 1(a) aiming for contrast enhancement. Accordingly, morphology based spectral clustering is carried out in order to partition the fundus region. We obtain colorful mapping of the vessel texture, demonstrated in Fig. 1(b). These different regions are regrouped into two parts. One is from the largest texture region which includes most of the blood vessels with small size and low contrast (red region). The other is to group together the remaining small regions as these regions mainly consist of major vessels from the retinal image. Afterwards, eigenvalue analysis of Hessian matrix is conducted for an enhanced image. This is illustrated in Fig. 1(c). To extract the blood vessels from background, the Sobel edge detector is applied. As illustrated in Fig. 1(d), we then utilise morphological closing

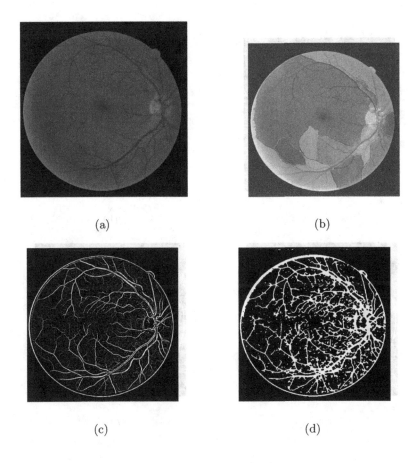

(a)   (b)

(c)   (d)

Fig. 1. Application of vessel segmenation to a DRIVE database image. (a) Illustration of an original image selected from green chanel. (b) Colorful mapping of the vessel texture via morphology based spectral clustering. (c) Illustration of the vessel segmentation via eigenvalue analysis of Hessian matrix. (d) The combination of the Sobel edge detector and morphological closing to achive the primitive segmentation with background pixels.

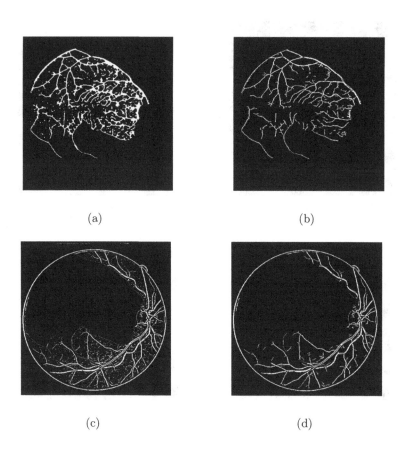

(a)

(b)

(c)

(d)

Fig. 2. Analysis of vessel segmenation according to Fig. 1. (a) Illustration of the red labeled texure related region from Fig. 1(d). (b) The extraction of vessel segmentation of (a) from background pixels. (c) Illustration of the remaining regions of Fig. 1(d) with the region representated by (a) excluded. (d) The extraction of vessel segmentation of (c) from background pixels.

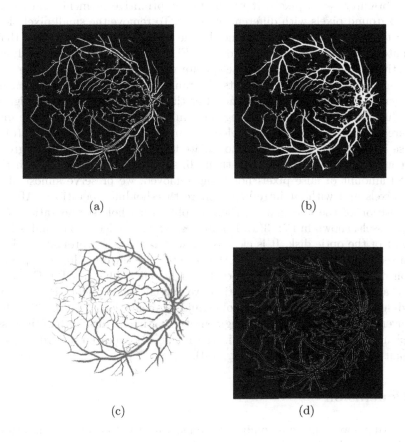

Fig. 3. Analysis of vessel segmenation according to Fig. 2. (a) The combination of segments from Fig. 2(c) and (d). (b) Illustration of the application of entropy filtering to eliminate the effect of central light reflex. (c) Overlays of the detected vessel segmentations (yellow) to the gold stand segmentation (green), with the overlapping region labeled by blue color. (d) Illustration of the vessel edge in the image according to the resultant segmentation with application of our width measurement method.

to the edge profiles to assist to identify thick vessels by filling in any 'holes' in the silhouette of the vessels created during the processing procedure. A set of linear structuring elements (SE) are selected at 12 different directions with angular resolution of 15°. Due to background intensity variation from nonuniform illumination, the intensity values of some background pixels is comparable to that of brighter vessel pixels. It results in the primitive segmentation containing background pixels with different intensity. To remove the small pixel blocks, we use texture mapping as guideline. In the red labeled related region that is dominated by the small vessels, shown in Fig. 2(a), we continually analyse its connectivity constraints of the vessels, before and after thresholding the intensity image. The vessel region consists of a range of connected pixels that should be larger than 16 and 18, before and after thresholding, respectively. Fig. 2(b) is an illustration of the resultant segment. In the remaining parts of the image that are associated with color labeled texture regions, shown in Fig. 2(c), we analyse its connectivity only once to isolate the vessel pixels from background, with connected components larger than 16, shown in Fig. 2(d). Though there is small amount of false pixels not being removed, we preserve almost all the vessel pixels and without introducing more thresholding operations. After the superposition of the two images, then we obtain a whole segmentation of the retinal vessels, shown in Fig. 3(a). It removes the circle edge of the fundus image and part of the optic disk. It is clear to show that there is a pronounced bright region seen running through one of the vessels. The entropy filtering operation is applied to eliminate the effect of central light reflex, illustrated in Fig. 3(b).

To evaluate the retinal segmentation, we overlay the segmentation generated according to our method with the gold stand segmentation. The Fig. 3(c) shows good overlapping between the two segmentations. Finally, the width of the vessels are calculated and the vessel edge in the image is delineated according to the resultant segmentation shown in Fig. 3(d).

4   Conclusion

In this paper, we explore a combined model, which is to evaluate curvature of retinal vessels via eigenvalue analysis of hessian matrix with entropy filtering technique to remove central light reflexes. The spectral clustering for texture mapping used as guideline to separate the retinal texture aiming to reduce the amount of connectivity constraints and manual methods of intensity thresholding analysis. The algorithm described here fully automates the analysis of retinal vessel widths. It allows the fast calculation of diameters all along the length of each vessel rather than at specific points of interest, thereby producing more fine-grained results that would be possible manually or using interactive, computer-assisted software. The algorithm described here is general enough to offer a practical alternative to manual measurements for a wide range of studies.

References

1. Staal, J., Abramoff, M., Niemeijer, M., Viergever, M., van Ginneken, B.: Ridge-based vessel segmentation in color images of the retina. IEEE Transactions on Medical Imaging 23(4), 501–509 (2004)
2. Hoover, A., Kouznetsova, V., Goldbaum, M.: Locating blood vessels in retinal images by piecewise threshold probing of a matched filter response. IEEE Transactions on Medical Imaging 19(3), 203–210 (2000)
3. Miri, M., Mahloojifar, A.: Retinal image analysis using curvelet transform and multistructure elements morphology by reconstruction. IEEE Transactions on Medical Imaging 58(5), 1183–1192 (2011)
4. Zana, F., Klein, J.-C.: Segmentation of vessel-like patterns using mathematical morphology and curvature evaluation. IEEE Transactions on Image Processing 10(7), 1010–1019 (2001)
5. O'Callaghan, R., Bull, D.: Combined morphological-spectral unsupervised image segmentation. IEEE Transactions on Medical Imaging 14(1), 49–62 (2005)
6. Yin, X.X., Ng, B.W.-H., Yang, Q., Pitman, A., Ramamohanarao, K., Abbott, D.: Anatomical landmark localization in breast dynamic contrast-enhanced MR imaging. Medical & Biological Engineering & Computing 50(1), 91–101 (2012)
7. Frangi, A.F., Niessen, W.J., Vincken, K.L., Viergever, M.A.: Multiscale vessel enhancement filtering. In: Wells, W.M., Colchester, A.C.F., Delp, S.L. (eds.) MICCAI 1998. LNCS, vol. 1496, pp. 130–137. Springer, Heidelberg (1998)
8. Chanwimaluang, T., Fan, G.: An efficient blood vessel detection algorithm for retinal images using local entropy thresholding. In: Proceedings of the 2003 International Symposium on Circuits and Systems, ISCAS 2003, vol. 5, pp. V21–V24 (2003)
9. Patton, N., Aslam, T.M., MacGillivray, T., Deary, I.J., Dhillon, B., Eikelboom, R.H., Yogesan, K., Constable, I.J.: Retinal image analysis: concepts, applications and potential. Progress in Retinal and Eye Research 25(1), 99–127 (2006)
10. Mendonça, A.M., Campilho, A.: Segmentation of retinal blood vessels by combining the detection of centerlines and morphological reconstruction. IEEE Transactions on Medical Imaging 25(9), 1200–1213 (2006)
11. Bankhead, P., Scholfield, C.N., McGeown, J.G., Curtis, T.M.: Fast retinal vessel detection and measurement using wavelets and edge location refinement. PLoS ONE 7(3), art. no. e32435 (2012)
12. Louisa, L., Lee, S.-W., Suen, C.: Thinning methodologies—a comprehensive survey. IEEE Transactions on Pattern Analysis and Machine Intelligence 14(9), 869–885 (1992)

Mobile Graphic-Based Communication: Investigating Reminder Notifications to Support Tuberculosis Treatment in Africa

Haji Ali Haji, Hussein Suleman, and Ulrike Rivett

University of Cape Town, 7701 Rondebosch, South Africa
hajiali10@hotmail.com, hussein@cs.uct.ac.za,
ulrike.rivett@uct.ac.za
http://www.uct.ac.za

Abstract. Visual communication is a method of communication using visual elements, which is suggested to be more effective than text or voice, and has the additional advantage that it, can also be used by who are unable to read. In this paper, the findings of a user requirements study, which was conducted at MnaziMmoja Hospital in Zanzibar, are presented. In a cross-sectional study, twenty nine people including TB patients and TB Health care workers were interviewed. The findings show that participants agreed that the use of mobile graphic-based communications could support TB patients in their treatment. The contribution of this work is the process to investigate and develop a new mobile graphic-based application for push notification services that are literacy-level and language agnostic.

Keywords: visual communication, mobile graphic-based, tuberculosis.

1 Introduction

The rapid adoption of mobile technology in developing countries has provided new avenue to reach and improve the level of care for the under-served, at-risk populations with infectious diseases such as Human Immunodeficiency Virus (HIV) or Tuberculosis (TB).

According to the World Health Organization (WHO) [1], almost nine million infections of TB occurred in 2011, and more than one million people die every year from this disease. Sub-Saharan Africa carries the greatest proportion of new cases, with over 260 cases per 100 000 people in 2011 [1]. The majority of patients fail to take their medication at the appropriate time. As a result, the recovery rates increase, resistant strains develop and medication success is reduced.

The standard approach to treating TB is by Direct Observed Therapy Short-course (DOTs), an intervention where the patient is observed by another person taking medication in order to ensure adherence. A full recovery from TB is only possible if patients strictly follow the prescribed medication regime for a minimum period of six months. Patients are required to take between three and five tablets daily for seven days per week [1,2].

Y. Zhang et al. (Eds.): HIS 2014, LNCS 8423, pp. 204–211, 2014.
© Springer International Publishing Switzerland 2014

The DOTs generally requires healthcare workers to remind and observe patients a time of taking their daily TB medication. This process necessitates adequate human labour that is a challenge in developing countries [2]. The technology-assisted DOTs seek to reach more patients at a lower cost through automated reminders via mobile phones. The process needs a few human labour and cost less.

Mobile phones have become very popular and affordable. The number of mobile phones reached almost six billion in the world by the end of 2012. Of that, more than 86% of the 660 million new mobile cellular subscribers were from developing countries [3]. Additionally, most mobile phones today have advanced applications. Multimedia Message Services (MMS) are a standard telephone message system, allowing the sending and receiving of multimedia objects (image, audio and video) [4].

In recent years, the use of cell phones for medical care has increased rapidly. Short Message Service (SMS) and telephone calls are the most common mobile interventions currently used in medical reminder applications. Various studies indicate how SMS text messages [5,6] and telephone calls [7,8] encourage patients to follow their treatment as scheduled. There is potential for mobile technology to help people to reduce missed medications and appointments [9,10].

Different mobile reminder methods; including SMS text message and telephone call have been proposed, as approaches have limited use by some people. Compared to voice call the text message has potential, but only for literate people. Voices call reminder system faced by language barrier. It also requires good network connection during implementation, as shown in the research conducted by Chen et al [11].

The aim of this paper is to present the findings obtained during the user requirements study. Several reminder notifications were suggested by participants and these will be used in the development of the mobile graphic-based application. Based on the findings, people can better understand pictures better than text [12]. Picture languages enable people who speak different languages from different countries to understand one another.

2   Related Works

2.1   Mobile Healthcare Systems

Mobile health, or mHealth, refers to the use of mobile devices, such as phones, to support the practice of medicine and public health. It is a rapidly-growing field with potential for frequent use of mobile phones for healthcare services [13].

The growing field of mHealth in low-income regions has seen an increasing number of projects targeting patients, such as those with TB. The advantages of mobile reminder systems are indicated in the research of Okuboyeyo et al [14] and Lester et al [15]. In their studies found that mobile phone reminder applications are more effective at reducing missed medication than manual reminder systems, or no reminders at all, among a wide range of patients. The two mobile interventions that have been recently used for reminders: SMS text messages and telephone calls.

2.2   SMS Text Messages

Studies carried out by Akhter et al [16] and Barclay [17] focused on text message reminders system that encourage patients to take their medication regularly. The studies reported that mobile reminders were most helpful to reduce the number of missed medications, compared to the manual reminder systems. SMSs can be sent a few minutes before the medication time to remind patients to take their tablets at the right time.

Text messaging can also be used to remind patients of clinic appointment times. SMSs could be forwarded to a patient's phone 24 hours prior to the appointment day and also a few minutes before the appointment time [18]. This can help patients to attend the clinic more regularly for medical consultations. However, the problem of the language barrier is a major challenge, as addressed in the study of Prasad and Anand [18].

Moreover, text messaging systems are used as a "store and forward" communication technique. It is more preferable in the areas where network connections are unstable [19]. The "store and forward" helps to store the messages if the recipient's cell phone is not available and forward it as soon as the phone becomes reachable [20]. The concept of "store and forward" will be considered in this study.

Although text messages have potential in helping patients to take their medication and keep appointment times more effectively, the problems of language and literacy barriers are still challenges facing that intervention, especially in the rural areas of developing nations [13],[18].

2.3   Telephone Calls

Research conducted by Parikh et al [21] and Hanauer et al [22] indicated how telephone call reminder methods encouraged patients to follow their medication regimes. Parikh et al [21] investigated the effectiveness of telephone reminders to out-patients. Their study showed positive results for those patients who were receiving the calls.

However, telephone call communication is real-time. The approach requires good network coverage and high management costs [20], and this is challenging in the majority of developing nations. Chen et al [11] indicated that during their study the majority of reminder calls were not delivered, due to the unavailability of the recipients' phones.

In this study several multimedia picture-based applications will be developed. The approach is to push graphic reminders that are literacy-level and language-agnostic. Unlike text or voice, images do not lead to language and literacy barriers. Therefore, it is hoped that the use of pictures in mobile reminder systems will be helpful to encourage the patients to aware to their treatment regimes.

Images have become a more powerful way of communication than writing [12]. Use of images in medical diagnosis has been rapidly increasing with positive resources [23, 24].

Pictures and other visualizations are the only media that connect people from different areas in the world, who speak different languages, regardless of their age or literacy levels [25,26,27].

3   Materials and Methods

Participatory action research (PAR) is used as the core research method. PAR consists of two aspects:

- **Action:** Research should be more than just finding out; research should also involve an action component that seeks to engender positive change.

- **Participation:** Research is a participatory process that requires the equal and collaborative involvement of the 'community of research interest' [28].

This method is useful as the development process for the study is expected to be cyclic. The strategy is to involve the target users as co-researchers; the PAR accommodates user-centred design [29].

Data for this study was collected through a survey. This enables the researcher to collect first-hand information on users' preferences and identify the required solution.

In-depth interviews were conducted to understand the key issues. Both TB health workers and TB patients were interviewed semi-structured. Face-to-face interviews were carried out in group and individually.

The user requirements study was conducted in Zanzibar from July to August 2013, in the department of infectious disease at MnaziMmoja Hospital.

4   Results and Discussion

4.1   Outline of User Requirements

A user requirements study aimed to identify the challenges that face TB health workers and patients during treatment. It also aimed to identify the reminder notifications to use in the application. Furthermore, the study aimed to find out the number of people who were infected with TB and rate of transmission and how those who infected are treated.

Twenty nine people participated in the data collections process including TB patients, TB health workers, TB coordinator, TB pharmacist, TB data manager and TB patient's supporter. The interview sessions were conducted in groups and individually. Interviewed patients were both inpatients and home-based care patients.

Table 1. Outline of interview sessions

Session No.	Type	No. of Participants	Participants Status
1	Group	5	4 Health workers and 1 TB coordinator
2	Group	5	Health workers
3	Individual	1	Pharmacist
4	Individual	1	Data manager
5	Group	2	Patients
6	Individual	1	Patient
7	Group	3	Patients
8	Individual	1	Patient's supporter
9	Group	4	Patients
10	Individual	1	Patient
11	Group	2	Patients
12	Group	3	Health workers

A total of twelve sessions were conducted, including: seven groups and five individual sessions, as shown in Table 1 below. Each session lasted for 30 to 45 minutes. The researcher was assisted by the health worker in each patient's interview session. This was to ensure that the conversations were done in a safe environment for the researcher and patients.

4.2   Participants' Demographic Information

Figure 1 below shows the gender of participants who participated in the user requirement study, where 17 of participants (59%) were females compared to 12 (41%) of whom were males. Participants were categorised into six different statuses. There were twelve health providers, thirteen patients, one coordinator, one data manager, one pharmacist and one patient's supporter, as shown in Figure 1 below.

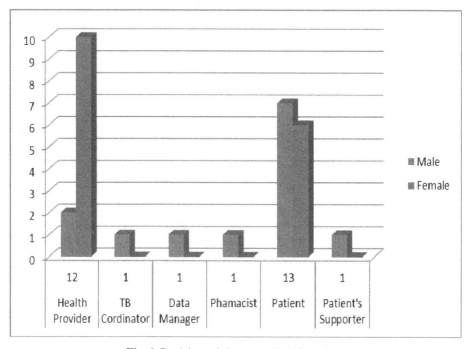

Fig. 1. Participants' demographic information

It was found that all interviewed participants had mobile phones. This shows that the majority of target users have mobile phones that could support them for accessing the proposed mobile application. Furthermore, participants were asked about their awareness regarding the use of mobile phones for health care service ("Do you think the mobile phone can support you in your treatment?") It was found that all participants (100%) agreed the use of phones for healthcare services. Furthermore, interviewed patients were illiterate and semi-literate. They were excited as the idea of the use of pictures as reminders.

4.3   Collected Reminder Notifications

The researcher was able to identify the challenges that face the TB health workers and patients during their treatment. Such challenges include poor infrastructure, unsafe working environments, insufficient working instruments and lack of financial support. It was also found that patients did not frequently attend the clinic for consultations due to several reasons, such as unaffordable transport cost and little knowledge of the TB disease. All patients believed that the use of mobile phones could help them to follow the medication procedures as prescribed.

Participants proposed various types of reminder notifications that may be used in the tuberculosis treatment, as indicated in Table 2 below. This assisted the researcher to develop the graphic-reminder notifications using professional graphic design software. The graphic-reminder will be used to remind the patient of the medication or appointment process. The concept of this system is to push graphic-reminder notifications so that TB patients can receive medication or appointment reminders at specific times as suggested by a health care professional. The intention is to develop an application that will accessible to any type of mobile phone that supports multimedia. The first experiment is about a cross platform application that could be insured on different smartphones.

Table 2. Collected reminder notifications

S/N	Reminder item
1	Please take your medication
2	Please visit the hospital for consultation
3	You are required to send your sputum smear for checking
4	You are required to collect your medication at the hospital for upcoming days
5	Different consultation and reminders regarding disease care: do this, don't do that
6	If you see "this" sign please visit clinic or see a doctor as soon as possible
7	Meal suggestions. That is: You are advised to get vegetables from time to time, take a glass of milk, etc

The study also confirmed, as found in the literature review, that patients failed to follow the medication procedures as recommended by health workers. This hampers the effective treatment of the patients for the prescribed period. All participants supported the idea that the proposed mobile picture-based communication can help them to follow the medication regimes.

5   Conclusion

Currently, the use of mobile graphic-based communication to support TB treatment and other infectious diseases such as HIV is a new area, particularly in Africa. The preliminary findings show that people support the use of a mobile picture-based application.

Picture communication will enable every person to easily understand the meaning, unlike text. It is expected that the findings of the study will help TB patients to follow the treatment regimes. The next phase of the study is to develop the collected text-based reminder notifications into graphic-reminder. After that the mobile graphics-based application will be developed and evaluated.

Acknowledgement. I would like to express my gratitude to the Hasso Platner Institut (HPI) for funding me in my study. I would also like to express my thanks to Mr. Khamis Abubakar and Ms. Rahma Ali for their support during data collection. And all people who participated in the interview.

References

1. WHO. Global Tuberculosis Report 2012 (2002),
   `http://www.who.int/tb/publications/global_report/en/`
2. Gordon, A.L., Nigro, C.C.M., Poling, P.C.: UC Berkeley: Technology Assisted DOTs (2008), `http://groups.ischool.berkeley.edu/`
   `Technology%20Assisted%20DOTS`
3. ITU Statistical, International Telecommunication Limited: Key statistical highlights (2012), `http://www.itu.int/ITU-D/ict/`
   `2011%20Statistical%20highlights_June_2012`
4. ITU. Making mobile phones and services accessible for persons with disabilities, A joint report of ITU – The International Telecommunication Union and G3ICT – The global initiative for inclusive ICTs (2012), `http://www.itu.int/ITU-D/sis/PwDs/`
   `Documents/Mobile_Report.pdf`
5. Pop-Eleches, C., Thirumurthy, H., Habyarimana, J., Graff Zivin, J., Goldstein, M., de Walque, D., Bangsberg, D.: Mobile Phone Technologies Improve Adherence to Antiretroviral Treatment in Resource-Limited Settings: A Randomized Controlled Trial of Text Message Reminders. Aids 25, 825–834 (2011)
6. Mohammed, S., Siddiqi, O., Ali, O., Habib, A., Haqqi, F., Kausar, M., Khan, A.J.: User engagement with and attitudes towards an interactive SMS reminder system for patients with tuberculosis. Journal of Telemedicine and Telecare 18(7), 404–408 (2012)
7. Piette, J.D., Weinberger, M., McPhee, S.J.: The effect of automated calls with telephone nurse follow-up on patient-centered outcomes of diabetes care: A randomized, controlled trial. Medical Care 38(2), 218–230 (2000)
8. Kunawararak, P., Pongpanich, S., Chantawong, S., Pokaew, P., Traisathit, P., Srithanaviboonchai, K., Plipat, T.: Tuberculosis treatment with mobile-phone medication reminders in northern Thailand. Southeast Asian Journal of Tropical Medicineand Public Health 42(6), 1444 (2011)
9. Roux, P., Kouanfack, C., Cohen, J., Marcellin, F., Boyer, S., Delaporte, E., Spire, B.: Adherence to antiretroviral treatment in HIV-positive patients in the Cameroon context: promoting the use of medication reminder methods. JAIDS Journal of Acquired Immune Deficiency Syndromes 43, S40-S43 (2011)
10. Mosen, D.M., Feldstein, A.C., Perrin, N., Rosales, A.G., Smith, D.H., Liles, E.G., Glasgow, R.E.: Automated telephone calls improved completion of fecal occult blood testing. Medical Care 48(7), 604–610 (2010)
11. Chen, Z.W., Fang, L.Z., Chen, L.Y., Dai, H.L.: Comparison of an SMS text messaging and phone reminder to improve attendance at a health promotion center: A randomized controlled trial. Journal of Zhejiang University Science B 9(1), 34–38 (2008)
12. Marsh, E.E., White, M.D.: Taxonomy of relationships between images and text. Journal of Documentation 59(6), 647–672 (2003)

13. Kaplan, W.A.: Can the ubiquitous power of mobile phones be used to improve health outcomes in developing countries? Globalization and Health 2, 9 (2006), doi:10.1186/1744-8603-2-9
14. Okuboyejo, S., Ikhu-Omoregbe, N.A., Mbarika, V.: A Framework for the Design of a Mobile-Based Alert System for Outpatient Adherence in Nigeria. African Journal of Computing & ICT 5(5), 151–158 (2012)
15. Lester, R.T., Ritvo, P., Mills, E.J., Kariri, A., Karanja, S., Chung, M.H., Plummer, F.A.: Effects of a mobile phone short message service on antiretroviral treatment adherence in Kenya (WelTel Kenya1): A randomised trial. The Lancet. 376(9755), 1838–1845 (2010)
16. Akhter, K., Dockray, S., Simmons, D.: Exploring factors influencing non-attendance at the diabetes clinic and service improvement strategies from patients' perspectives. Practical Diabetes 29(3), 113–116 (2012)
17. Barclay, E.: Text messages could hasten tuberculosis drug compliance. The Lancet. 373(9657), 15–16 (2009)
18. Prasad, S., Anand, R.: Use of mobile telephone short message service as a reminder: the effect on patient attendance. International Dental Journal 62(1), 21–26 (2012)
19. Perron, N.J., Dao, M.D., Righini, N.C., Humair, J.P., Broers, B., Narring, F., Gaspoz, J.M.: Text-messaging versus telephone reminders to reduce missed appointments in an academic primary care clinic: A randomized controlled trial. BMC Health Services Research 13(1), 1–7 (2013)
20. Sidney, K., Antony, J., Rodrigues, R., Arumugam, K., Krishnamurthy, S., D'souza, G., Shet, A.: Supporting patient adherence to antiretroviral using mobile phone reminders: Patient responses from South India. AIDS Care 24(5), 612–617 (2012)
21. Parikh, A., Gupta, K., Wilson, A.C., Fields, K., Cosgrove, N.M., Kostis, J.B.: The effectiveness of outpatient appointment reminder systems in reducing no-show rates. The American Journal of Medicine 123(6), 542–548 (2010)
22. Hanauer, D.A., Wentzell, K., Laffel, N., Laffel, L.M.: Computerized Automated Reminder Diabetes System (CARDS): E-mail and SMS cell phone text messaging reminders to support diabetes management. Diabetes Technology & Therapeutics 11(2), 99–106 (2009)
23. Waran, V., Bahuri, N.F.A., Narayanan, V., Ganesan, D., Kadir, K.A.A.: Video clip transfer of radiological images using a mobile telephone in emergency neurosurgical consultations (3G Multi-Media Messaging Service). British Journal of Neurosurgery 26(2), 199–201 (2012)
24. Ohtsuka, M., Uchida, E., Nakajima, T., Yamaguchi, H., Takano, H., Komuro, I.: Transferring images via the wireless messaging network using camera phones shortens the time required to diagnose acute coronary syndrome. Circulation Journal: Official Journal of the Japanese Circulation Society 71(9), 1499 (2007)
25. Sipe, L.R.: Revisiting the Relationships Between Text and Pictures. Children's Literature in Education 43(1), 4–21 (2012)
26. Smith, K.L., Moriarty, S., Kenney, K., Barbatsis, G. (eds.): Handbook of visual communication: Theory, Methods, and Media. Routledge (2013)
27. Hyodo, K., Chihara, K., Yasumuro, Y., Imura, M., Manabe, Y., Masuda, Y., Naganawa, M.: Doctor-to-Patient communication by 2.5 G mobile phone; preliminary study. International Congress Series, vol. 1281, pp. 196–199. Elsevier (2005)
28. Walter, M.: Participatory action research. Reason 71 (1998)
29. Avison, D.E., Lau, F., Myers, M.D., Nielsen, P.A.: Action research. Communications of the ACM 42(1), 94–97 (1999)

Multiscale Geometric Active Contour Model and Boundary Extraction in Kidney MR Images

Ling Li[*], Jia Gu, Tiexiang Wen, Wenjian Qin, Hua Xiao, Jiaping Yu

1. Shenzhen Institutes of Advanced Technology, Chinese Academy of Science
Shenzhen Key Lab for Low-Cost Healthcare
Ling.li@siat.ac.cn

Abstract. Active contour methods (ACM) are model-based approaches for image segmentation and were developed in the late 1980s. ACM can be divided into two classes: parametric active contour model and geometric active contour model. Geometric method is intrinsic model. Because of its completeness in mathematics, geometric active contour model overcomes many difficulties of the parametric active contour model. However, in medical images with heavy structural noise, the evolution of the geometric active contour will be seriously affected. To handle this problem, this paper proposed a multiscale geometric active contour model, based on the multiscale analysis method—bidimensional empirical mode decomposition. In the human kidney MR images, the proposed multiscale geometric active contour model successfully extracts the complex kidney contour.

Keywords: active contour method, bidimensional empirical mode decomposition, MR images segmentation, multisacle active contour method.

1 Introduction

SINCE active contour models (ACM) firstly introduced by kass et al [1], which are based on the theory of surface evolution and geometric flows, have been widely studied and successfully used in image segmentation field with promising implementation results. As usual, ACM can be divided into two classes: parametric active contour models (PACM) [1] and geometric active contour models (GACM), GACM is proposed by Caselles et al [2] and Malladi et al [3]. The first ones have been studied for many years which will not appear in this paper; While the second ones which based on curve evolution theory and level set method have been a hot topic in medical image segmentation field in recently years due to its capability of processing images with intensity inhomogeneity which often occurs in Magnetic Resonance (MR) images, Computed Tomography (CT) images, X-ray images and Ultrasound (US) images. In this paper we mainly discuss the GACM [4][5].

GACM are proposed based upon curve evolution theory and level set method, following is the main idea: expressing contours as the zero level set of an implicit function

---

[*] Corresponding author.

Y. Zhang et al. (Eds.): HIS 2014, LNCS 8423, pp. 212–219, 2014.
© Springer International Publishing Switzerland 2014

defined in a higher dimension, usually refer as the level set function, and to evolve the level set function according to a partial differential equation (PDE) [6]. This approach shows several advantages over the conventional PACM. Firstly, the contours represented by the level set function may break or merge naturally during the evolution, and the topological changes are thus automatically handled. Secondly the level set function always remains a function on a fixed grid, which allows efficient numerical schemes [6] to solve.

The existing GACM can be categorized into two major classes: edge-based models and region-based models. Edge-based models use local edge information to attract the active contour toward the object boundaries. Region-based models aim at identifying each region of interest by using a certain region descriptor to guide the motion of the active contours. However, mostly popular region-based models tend to rely on intensity homogeneity in each of the regions to be segmented. For example, the popular piece-wise constant (PC) models are based on the assumption that image intensities are statistically homogeneous in each region.

Magnetic resonance images are often corrupted by slowly intensity inhomogeneity for the same tissue over the image domain. In the experiment we found that, although the geometric activity curve has obvious advantages, can better overcome the influence of random noise, but, in the structural noise more serious cases, geometric active contour evolution to the boundary will be affected, especially when initial curve is far from the final boundary curve.

In order to solve this problem, in this paper, the multiscale geometric active contour model which is multi-scale edge detection algorithm based on bidimensional empirical mode decomposition is proposed.

In this paper, we propose a novel multiscale active contour model that is able to segment images with intensity inhomogeneity which is multi-scale edge detection algorithm based on bidimensional empirical mode decomposition.

The remainder of this paper is organized as follows. In Second II, we first introduce the BEMD, and then followed by Section 3 with background of active contour methods in MR images segmentation. The proposed method is introduced in Section 4. In Section 5, gives out implementation results and analysis. And last is future work.

2   Bidimensional Empirical Mode Decomposition

2.1   Method of EMD

Huang proposed intrinsic mode function (IMF) and empirical mode decomposition (EMD) in 1998 [7]. EMD is an adaptive and multiscale signal processing tool. The method can analyze non-linearity and non-stationary data well [8]. EMD is a novel data representation and it has better spatial and frequency characteristics than wavelet analysis. 1D EMD with better physical characteristics can be expanded to analyze 2D signal. EMD has already been used in the field of physical geography, biomedicine, mechanical engineering and other fields [9].

In the process of 1D EMD screening, cubic spline function that constructs enve-loping surfaces will be divergent in both ends of the data series and the edges will have large errors. On the other hand, the errors propagate inward in the process of screening and data series are polluted. Data will have boundary effect after Hilbert transformation. For high-frequency IMF components are influenced by the boundary effect of EMD less than low-frequency IMF components [10], in order to improve the result of medical image segmentation, active contour model is proposed to select low-frequency coefficients in this paper. IMF components on each layer include different spatial scale information. Although textures in several spatial scales are different obviously, the method is convenient to extract these textures.

2.2   BEMD Models

For 2D signal, such as image, source image can be decomposed into several 2D IMF components and a residue component by BEMD[11], whose frequencies are from high to low. BIMF meets two constraints: the local mean of the original 2D signals should be symmetric and its own mean is zero; its maximum is positive, minimum is negative. IMF components have the following characteristics: (1) In data set, the number of maximum points set and minimum points is equal to the number of zero crossing points, or their difference is less than 1;

(2) At any point, the mean of envelope constituted by minimum and maximum is close to zero. IMF components are near orthogonal, they represent every frequency of local data and they correspond to high-frequency and low frequency data, the residue component represents development tendency of the original image.

BEMD is a kind of completely self-adaptive decomposition, a large extent image decomposition depends on the characteristics of data itself. It means that if screening stop condition is consistent, the number of BIMF depends on the data characteristics [12].

So, the number of BIMF may be different in different images. The steps of BEMD algorithm are as follows:

1) Initialization, the residue component $R = I$, I is the source image.

2) If the residue R is monotone or it reaches decomposition number of an image, the algorithm stops; Otherwise, make $H = R$ and the screening process starts.

3) The extrema in image P are achieved, maximum points set and minimum points set in the region are searched.

4) The maximum points set and the minimum points set are plane interpolated, and upper enveloping surfaces $U(m, n)$ and lower enveloping surfaces $L(m, n)$ of the image are achieved, the mean value M of the image H is also solved by enveloping surfaces.

$$M(m,n) = (U(m,n) + L(m,n))/2 \tag{1}$$

$$H_k(m,n) = H_{k-1}(m,n) - M(m,n) \tag{2}$$

5) screening process is used for judging the stop condition which is shown in formula (3), if the stop condition is not satisfied, turns to step 3.

$$SD = \sum_{m}^{X} \sum_{n}^{Y} \frac{\left(h_{k-1}(m,n) - h_k(m,n)\right)^2}{h_{k-1}^2(m,n)} \qquad (3)$$

6) If the BIMF $D(m,n)$ = $H(m,n)$, an IMF component is achieved.

7) Function $R(m,n)$ can be expressed by
$R(m,n)$ = $R(m,n)$ − $D(m,n)$,and turns to step 2.

In the above method, the cores of the method are plane interpolation, how to get extrema and screening stop condition.

After J layers BEMD, the final decomposition process can be expressed as:

$$I(m,n) = \sum_{j=1}^{J} D_j(m,n) + R_J(m,n), J \in N \qquad (4)$$

3   Active Contour Methods

The active contour models are classified into two kinds of types, which are parametric active contour models and geometric active contour models. Parametric active contour models represent curves and surfaces explicitly in their parametric forms during deformation. This representation allows direct interaction with the model and can lead to a compact representation for fast real time implementation. Adaptation of the model topology, however, such as splitting or merging parts during the deformation, can be difficult using parametric models. On the other hand, geometric active contour models can handle topological changes naturally [2]. These models represent curves and surfaces implicitly as a level set of a higher dimensional scalar function [3]. Here we have an interest with an image segmentation using geometric active contour models. These models are based on evolution theory and level set method. The evolution theory is to study the deformation process of curves or surfaces using only geometric measures such as the unit normal and curvature.

3.1   Active Contour Model Equation

Define image differentiable function:

$$\Phi = \frac{1}{1 + \left\| \nabla G\sigma * I \right\|^n} \qquad (5)$$

$G\sigma$ is for the Gauss filter represents the standard deviation σ.

Let $C=C(p,t)$ is a family of smooth closed curves, p is curve parameter, t is family parameter. $0 \le p \le 1$, $C(0,t)=C(1,t)$, $C'(0,t)=C'(1,t)$. The traditional Euclidean unit arc length

$$ds = \|C_p\| dp = \left(x_p^2 + y_p^2\right)^{1/2} dp \tag{6}$$

modified as follows

$$ds\phi = \phi ds = \left(x_p^2 + y_p^2\right)^{1/2} \phi dp \tag{7}$$

Then, modified curve length represented:

$$L\phi(t) = \int_0^1 \|C_p\| \phi dp \tag{8}$$

Differential of $L\Phi(t)$ as follow:

$$L\phi'(t) = \int_0^1 \phi_t \|C_p\| dp + \int_0^1 \langle C_{pt}, C_p \rangle \frac{1}{\|C_p\|} dp$$

$$= -\int_0^{L(t)} \langle C_t, [\phi_k - (\nabla\phi \bullet N)] N \rangle ds \tag{9}$$

Therefore, in order to make $L\Phi(t)$ decrease fastest,

$$C_t = \left(\phi - (\nabla\phi \bullet N)\right) N \tag{10}$$

The expansive force added to above formula, get the geometric active contour complete evolution equation

$$C_t = \left(\phi_{(k+v)} - (\nabla\phi \bullet N)\right) N \tag{11}$$

3.2   The Numerical Solution of Geometric Active Contour

Through deduction, geometric active contour level set representation is

$$\Psi_t = \Phi\left(div\left(\frac{\nabla\Psi}{\|\nabla\Psi\|}\right) + v\right)\|\nabla\Psi\| + \nabla\Phi\nabla\Psi \tag{12}$$

Level set evolution equation as following:

$$\Psi_{ij}^{n+1} = \Psi_{ij}^{n} + \nabla t \left\{ \begin{array}{l} \Phi_{ij}\left[\max(v,o)\nabla^{+} + \min(v,0)\nabla^{-}\right] + \\ \Phi_{ij}K_{ij}^{n}\left(D_{ij}^{ox2} + D_{ij}^{oy2}\right)^{1/2} + \\ \left[\begin{array}{l}\left[\max\left(D\Phi_{ij}^{ox},0\right)D_{ij}^{-x} + \min\left(D\Phi_{ij}^{ox},0\right)D_{ij}^{+x}\right] + \\ \left[\max\left(D\Phi_{ij}^{oy},0\right)D_{ij}^{-y} + \min\left(D\Phi_{ij}^{oy},0\right)D_{ij}^{+y}\right]\end{array}\right]\end{array}\right\} \tag{13}$$

$$\nabla^{+} = \left[\begin{array}{l}\max\left(D_{i,j,k}^{-x},0\right)^{2} + \min\left(D_{i,j,k}^{+x},0\right)^{2} + \\ \max\left(D_{i,j,k}^{-y},0\right)^{2} + \min\left(D_{i,j,k}^{+y},0\right)^{2} + \\ \max\left(D_{i,j,k}^{-z},0\right)^{2} + \min\left(D_{i,j,k}^{+z},0\right)^{2}\end{array}\right]^{1/2} \tag{14}$$

$$\nabla^{-} = \left[\begin{array}{l}\max\left(D_{i,j,k}^{+x},0\right)^{2} + \min\left(D_{i,j,k}^{-x},0\right)^{2} + \\ \max\left(D_{i,j,k}^{+y},0\right)^{2} + \min\left(D_{i,j,k}^{-y},0\right)^{2} + \\ \max\left(D_{i,j,k}^{+z},0\right)^{2} + \min\left(D_{i,j,k}^{-z},0\right)^{2}\end{array}\right]^{1/2} \tag{15}$$

4   Multiscale Active Contour Model

As a general boundary extraction algorithm, geometric active contour method theo-retically rigorous, uses a level set representation method, automatic acquisition of topology changes.

Although the geometric active contour method has these advantages, but extraction of medical image boundary, high complexity of image itself makes the evolution of geometric active contour by a certain degree of influence.

In this paper, we proposed a novel multiscale active contour models based on BEMD, the algorithm is as follows:

Image multiscale edge detection based on BEMD transform, multiscale edge ex-traction of image

Set Scale j=J;

On the scale j, computing multiscale potential function ϕ_j, let ϕ_j instead of ϕ in active contour level set *equation* 12,then, According to the equation 13 for geometric active contour evolution;

If active contour curve is not moving in N_i steps, j=j-1.or j=0,turn to step 5.ortherwise turn to step 3;

Continue geometric active contour evolution according equation 13.

Figure 1 is an original MR image for kidney tissue, and the figure 2 is the result of segmentation of figure 1.

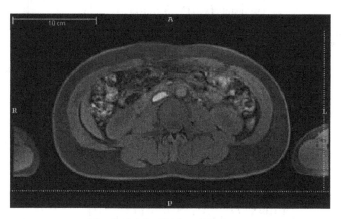

Fig. 1. Original kidney MR image

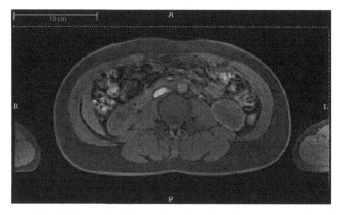

Fig. 2. The result of extraction of medical image boundary

In above expression, multiscale geometric active contour model is proposed. based on multiscale edge robust detection algorithm, potential function image is modified, a multi-scale edge images to calculate a new potential function, a coarse to fine search to extract the object boundary. In the larger scale, multiscale geometric active contour model can overcome the better effect of boundary image delicate objects, smooth evolution to ultimate boundary. At smaller scales, a new potential function can reflect the image boundary objects accurately in place, the activity curve to obtain the evolution speed in the corresponding position. The coarse to fine processing method, in which the accuracy of the boundary curve extraction activities at the same time, to avoid the influence of other objects in the image of the structured noise, not only speed up the curve evolution speed, but also conducive to maintaining activity of normal curve.

5   Conclusions and Future Works

In this paper, we present a new multiscale active contour models that using BEMD for obtain multiscale images The proposed method can obtain more accurate segmentation results from different modalities medical images, however, from the results, we can see the following problem: (1) When there are several objects our method will not get promising results but better than the method proposed in references; (2) For some images such as MIP vessel images, we can segment small branches with filtering preprocessing, but it still exists redundant curves. Due to the two problems, we need further research and in the future, we can extend to three-dimension images.

Ackownledgments. This paper is supported by the following grants: National Natural Science Foundation of China (61103165), Shenzhen Key Laboratory Project (CXB201005260056A), and ShenZhen Distinguished Young Scholars Fund (JC201005260248).

References

1. Kass, M., Witkin, A., Terzopoulos, D.: Snakes: active contour models. Int. J. Comput. Vis. 1(4), 321–331 (1987)
2. Caselles, V., Catte, F., Coll, T., Dibos, F.: A geometric model for active contours in image processing. Number. Math. 66, 1–31 (1993)
3. Malladi, R., Sethian, J.A., Vemuri, B.C.: Shape modeling with front propogation: a level set approach. IEEE Trans. Patt. Anal. Mach. Intell. 17, 158–175 (1995)
4. Li, C., Kao, C.-Y., Gore, J.C., Ding, Z.: Implicit Active Contours Driven by Local Binary Fitting. In: Proceedings of the 2007 IEEE Computer Society Conference on Computer Vision and Pattern Recognition (2007)
5. Li, C., Kao, C.-Y., Gore, J.C., Ding, Z.: Minization of Region-Scalable Fitting Energy for Image Segmentation. IEEE Transactions on Image Processing 10(10) (October 2008)
6. Li, C., Xu, C., Gui, C., Fox, M.D.: Level Set Evolution without Re-initialization: A new Variational Formulation. In: Proceedings of the 2005 IEEE Computer Society Conference on Computer Vision and Pattern Recognition (2005)
7. Chan, T.F., Vese, L.A.: Active Contours without Edges. IEEE Transactions on Image Proceesing 10(2) (Febrauary 2001)
8. Huang, N., et al.: The empirical mode decomposition and the Hilbert spectrum for non-linear and non-stationary time series analysis. In: Proc. R. Soc. Lond. A, vol. 454, pp. 903–995 (1998)
9. Flandrin, P., Rilling, G.: Empirical mode decomposition as a filter bank. IEEE Signal Proc. Lett. 11(2), 112–114 (2004)
10. Cheng, J.S., Yu, D.J., Yang, Y.: Research on the intrinsic mode function(IMF) criterion in EMD method. Mech. Syst. Signal Proc. 20(4), 817–824 (2006)
11. Yushan, Z., et al.: Processing boundary effect of EMD based on AR model. Prog. Nat. Sci. 13(10), 1054–1059 (2003)
12. Nunes, J.C., Guyot, S., Delechelle, E.: Texture analysis based on local analysis of The bi-dimensional empirical mode decomposition. Mach. Vision Appl. 16, 177–188 (2005)

Discovering New Analytical Methods
for Large Volume Medical and Online Data Processing

Hao Lan Zhang[1], Roozbeh Zarei[2], Chaoyi Pang[1,3], and Xiaohui Hu[4]

[1] Center for SCDM, NIT, Zhejiang University, Ningbo, China
[2] College of Engineering & Science, Victoria University, Australia
[3] The Australian E-health Research Centre, CSIRO, Australia
[4] School of Physics & Telecom, South China Normal University, China
haolan.zhang@nit.zju.edu.cn, roozbeh.zarei@live.vu.edu.au,
chaoyi.pang@csiro.au, xiaohui_huhu@sina.com

Abstract. The rapid growth of online data, which include online transaction data, online multimedia data, online social networking data, and son on, has made huge demand for more efficient data reduction and process. Online clustering to detect/predict anomalies from multiple data streams is valuable to those applications where a credible real-time event prediction system will minimize economic losses (e.g. stock market crash) and save lives (e.g. medical surveillance in the operating theatre). This project discovers and develops effective, efficient and accurate methods for online data processing using the Self-Organizing Map (SOM) method. The SOM method is efficient for solving big data problems. The experimental results are illustrated in this paper to demonstrate the efficiency of using SOM for large data analysis based on large volume medical and online transaction data.

Keywords: Self-Organizing Map, Big Data, Incremental SOM, Social Data.

1 Introduction

The arrival of the Big Data age urges researchers to find optimized solutions for dealing with large quantity of data, particularly for online commercial and social data. The ANN techniques and methods have adopted extensively for various application of the data mining, which include SOM. In many cases, medical data associate with time series data. The application of SOM becomes exceptionally important to cluster the time series data as Time series database is very high dimensional.

In multiple data streams, each time series is related to one of multiple attributes of one object/entity that are recorded in the same time period. Real-time systems such as the Internet, sensor networks, remote satellites, surveillance systems and other dynamic environments often generate tremendous amounts of time series data; the volume of data is too large to be stored on disks or scanned multiple times. In many cases, accurate online clustering techniques are required to analyze multiple correlated data streams to alert people about dramatic changes; this is vital to minimize the economic losses and save lives. Consider the following scenario.

Y. Zhang et al. (Eds.): HIS 2014, LNCS 8423, pp. 220–228, 2014.

A medical surveillance system monitors infinite physiological time series data on a patient's blood pressure, heart rate, temperature, and other vital signs in an Intensive Care Unit (ICU)/operating theatre in real time. These multiple correlated time series data include electrocardiogram, arterial blood pressure, non-invasive blood pressure, central venous pressure, intracranial pressure, tidal volume and respiration rate. Generally, such physiological data are high-volume, highly periodic stream data and are rarely stored entirely in databases. Medical professionals usually monitor three kinds of respiratory data: endtidal O2, FIO2 and bronchoalveolar lavage. Obviously, when an anomaly (e.g. deterioration in a patient's condition) occurs, the time series will show significant pattern changes. This project will develop methods that accurately detect such anomalies in time, allowing initiation of timely, high-quality responses (e.g. medical intervention).

Time series data are omnipresent in the factual planet, and there are countless relevance areas ranging from genetic information dispensation to chronological data mining. In broad-spectrum, indispensable sequential succession dealing out techniques are categorized as modeling, clustering, taxonomy, and forecast. Unlike stagnant data, there is a sky-scraping quantity of reliance among time series and the proper treatment of data dependency or correlation becomes critical in time series processing [1].

Assume a collection of j semi-infinite data streams from medical surveillance devices in an operating theatre, producing a value x_{ij}, which is a discrete sequence, for every j^{th} stream and for every i^{th} time-tick. The j stream values at time-tick i can be expressed as: $\{X_{1j}=[x_{11}, x_{12}...,x_{1j}]... X_{ij} = [x_{i1}, x_{i2},..., x_{ij}]\}$. Notice that j may increase with a new time-tick; the number of streams may increase when the streams evolve. X_i, $j+1$ will be the new column-vector of stream values at time i. The time length i will increase as the streams evolve as well, where one new row X_{i+1}, j is added at time $i+1$. Typically, in a collection of j multiple streams, we will do the online clustering based on those multiple data streams.

2   Related Work

The clustering methods developed for handling various static data are classified into five major categories: partitioning methods, hierarchical methods, density based methods, grid-based methods, and model-based methods. Three of the five major categories of clustering methods for static data, specifically partitioning methods, hierarchical methods, and model based methods, have been utilized directly or modified for time series clustering. Time series clustering methods have been divided into three major categories depending upon whether they work directly with raw data, indirectly with features extracted from the raw data, or indirectly with models built from the raw data [2].

Self Organize Map is used in implementing Normalized Longest Common Subsequence [3]. The NLCS method is used widely for the comparison of the character sequences where a novel algorithm is presented which performs better than Euclidean distance because the four cluster validity indices leads the result or output to be generated in higher quality by using SOM based on the experiment on the real life or synthetic data. The algorithm calculates the similarity of time series accurately [4].

The SOM method has been widely used in the field of bio informatics. One of the SOM application used for the online clustering in the gene expression time series is TimeClust. TimeClust is a software package to cluster genes according to their temporal expression profiles. It can be conveniently used to analyze data obtained from DNA micro array time-course experiments. It implements two original algorithms specifically designed for clustering short time series together with hierarchical clustering and Self Organize Maps [5].

Paplinski [6] describes the incremental SOM in categorization of visual objects. Pavlo et al [8] conducted a comparison on several major methods for large-scale data analysis. Erturk and Sengul [7] developed a 3D visualization software for medical data analysis, in particular the human brain electroencephalography (EEG) data.

3   SOM for Large Data Processing

The self-organizing map (SOM) network is an unsupervised learning neural network introduced by Kohonen [8]. It can learn from complex, multidimensional data and transform them into a map of fewer dimensions (a one or two dimensional discrete lattice of neuron units). Each node of the map is defined by a vector W_{ij}. During the training stage, SOM processes the input units in the network and adjusts W_{ij} based on the lateral feedback connections. The SOM map neighboring inputs in the input space to neighboring neurons in the map space by capturing the topological relationships between inputs [8, 9].

The SOM typically has two layers of nodes, the input layer and the Kohonen layer. First layer includes input nodes and second layer includes output nodes. Output nodes are in a two-dimensional grid view. The input layer is fully connected to the Kohonen layer with adjustable weights [8].

The network undergoes a self-organization process through a number of training cycles, starting with randomly chosen weights for the nodes in Kohonen layer. During each training cycle, every input vector is considered in turn and the winner node is determined based on the minimum Euclidean distance between the weight vector and the input vector. Let x be the input and W_{ij} be the weight vector to the nodes. Vector x is compared with all the weight vectors. The smallest Euclidian distance (d_{ij}) is defined as the best matching unit (BMU) or winner node.

$$d_{ij} = \min \| x(t) - w_{ij}(t) \|$$

The weight vectors of the winning node and the nodes in the neighborhood are updated using a weight adaptation function based on the following Kohonen rule:

$$w_{ij}(t+1) = w_{ij}(t) + a(t)\lfloor x(t) - w_{ij}(t) \rfloor, i \in N_c$$

$$w_{ij}(t+1) = w_{ij}(t), i \in N_c$$

Where, for time t, and a network with n neurons: α is the gain sequence ($0 < \alpha < 1$) and N_c is the neighborhood of the winner ($1 < N_c < n$). The basic training algorithm is quite simple:

- Each node's weights are initialized.
- Vector is chosen at random from the set of training data.

- Every node is examined to calculate which one's weights are most like the input vector. The winning node is commonly known as the Best Matching Unit (BMU).
- Then the neighborhood of the BMU is calculated. The amount of neighbors decreases over time.
- Update weights to node and neighbors.
- If N_c, 0 then repeat step 2.

Generating low-dimensional data sets with reassembly function is one of the key issues for efficient data analysis and processing in Big Data environment. Basically, two directions can be considered while reducing the volume of large data sets: (1) reducing data rows (data sets split); (2) reducing data columns (dimensionality reduction). For splitting large data sets, an enhanced UV-decomposition method can be used. The following sections describe the UV-decomposition and incremental SOM methods for improve large data processing efficiency.

3.1   Incremental SOM (iSOM)

In [6], iSOM deals with the situation where the number of nodes per stimulus, $\in$ is approximately constant and in the range [10, 11]. The neuronal node in [6] is identified by its weight vector wk and the position vector vk, both being unity vectors. The initial number of stimuli and nodes start with is $3*\in$. According to the Kohonen "dot-product" learning law the iSOM expression is:

$$\Delta w_j = \eta. \ \Lambda_j. \left(x^T - d_j.w_j \right); \ d_j = w_j. \ x$$

where Λ_j is a neighborhood function, In Paplinski's cases, Gaussian centered on the position of the winning neuron, and d_j is the post-synaptic activity of the jth neuron. $\eta = \exp(-n^2/(2\sigma))$, where σ is selected so that $\eta = 0.5$ for $n = E/2$, E being the number of epochs [6].

3.2   UV-Decomposition for Data Size Reduction

According to UV-Decomposition [12], a sample data table contains 1000 rows and 100 columns can be decomposed into two tables based on as follows:

$$\begin{bmatrix} x_{1,1}x_{1,2}x_{1,3}x_{1,4}.....x_{1,100} \\ x_{2,1}x_{2,2}x_{2,3}x_{2,4}.....x_{2,100} \\ .... \\ x_{1000,1}x_{1000,2}.......x_{1000,100} \end{bmatrix} = \begin{bmatrix} x_{1,1}x_{1,2} \\ x_{2,1}x_{2,2} \\ .... \\ x_{1000,1}x_{1000,2} \end{bmatrix} \times \begin{bmatrix} x_{1,1}x_{1,2}x_{1,3}x_{1,4}.....x_{1,100} \\ x_{2,1}x_{2,2}x_{2,3}x_{2,4}.....x_{2,100}. \end{bmatrix}$$

For a very large data set, UV-decomposition still generates another large data set, particularly for rows. However, the authors observe that it has been a common phenomenon that online data presents a number of normal-distribution-like forms in different groups. The decomposed matrices can be further broken down into smaller data sets based on the number of generated grouping results. In this way, the UV-decomposition can be more efficient for very large data sets.

4   Experimental Results

In this paper we conducted the experimental analysis to evaluate the performance of using SOM in processing large medical data. The following sections illustrate the experimental results.

4.1   Data Set

The breast cancer database used in this study is based on the research carried out at the university of Wisconsin hospitals. The database consists of 635 samples in which 444 samples account for benign and 239 samples account for malignant. Each sample consists of 10 features such as Clump Thickness, Uniformity of Cell Size and Uniformity of Cell Shape. The source of this data set is UCI KDD Archive and other details of this data set are available in [13]. We further analyzed an online transaction data (obtained from an anonymous travel agency's 2012 data).

4.2   Methodology

Our objective is to compare K-means and SOM algorithms in order to select the algorithm with higher accuracy of results. Moreover, the effect of number of neurons on SOM algorithm was taken into account. To compare K-means and SOM algorithms, the breast cancer dataset was clustered to two groups according to K-means and SOM algorithms. The results of both algorithms was compared based on false positive rate, true positive rate, false negative rate, true negative rate, and accuracy. To analyze the effect of number of neurons SOM algorithm, the number of neurons was set to be from 4 neurons to 121 neurons with increased interval ranges. The neurons in the layer of an SOM are arranged originally in physical positions according to hexagonal topology.

4.3   Results and Analysis of UCI KDD Medical Data

Results are summarized in Tables 1 to 2. Tables 1 shows the comparison of results between K-means and SOM algorithms. No significant accuracy was observed in the results of both algorithms according to the table.1. It can be concluded that SOM with a small number of neurons behave in a way that is similar to K-means.

Table 1. Results of K-means and SOM algorithm

Algorithm	FPR	TPR	FNR	TNR	Accuracy
k-means	2.03	92.47	7.53	97.97	96.05
SOM	2.03	92.89	7.11	97.97	96.19

According to the Table.2, it was notice that as the number of neurons increased the higher accuracy results were observed using the SOM algorithm. In addition, larger SOM rearrange data in a way that is fundamentally topological in character.

Table 2. Effect of number of neurons on SOM

Algorithm	FPR	TPR	FNR	TNR	Accuracy
SOM (121 neurons)	2.93	100	0	97.07	98.10
SOM (100 neurons)	2.93	99.58	0.42	97.07	97.95
SOM (81 neurons)	2.7	98.74	1.26	97.3	97.80
SOM (64 neurons)	2.25	96.65	3.35	97.75	97.36
SOM (49 neurons)	2.48	96.65	3.35	97.52	97.22
SOM (36 neurons)	3.38	98.33	1.67	96.62	97.22
SOM (25 neurons)	2.7	97.07	2.93	97.3	97.22
SOM (16 neurons)	3.38	98.33	1.67	96.62	97.21
SOM (9 neurons)	3.6	99.58	0.42	96.4	97.51
SOM (4 neurons)	2.7	95.82	4.18	97.3	96.78

4.4 Results and Analysis of the Online Transaction Data

The online transaction data is shown in Fig 1.

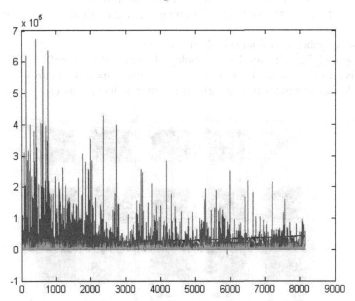

Fig. 1. Raw Online Transaction Data

After the SOM clustering and learning process, the variance accumulative contribution rate exceeds 96% as shown in Fig 2.

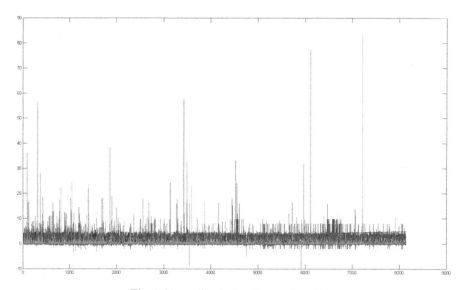

Fig. 2. Normalize Online Transaction Data

The SOM Configuration is set as below:

- Dimensions=[15 15] (Row vector of dimension sizes)
- CoverSteps=100 (Number of training steps for initial covering of the input space)
- InitNeighbor=3 (Initial neighborhood size)
- TopologyFcn= hextop(Layer topology function =hexagonal)
- DistanceFcn=linkdist (Neuron distance function= *link distance* (the way to calculate distances from a particular neuron to its neighbor))

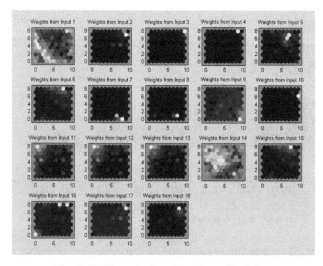

Fig. 3. SOM results based on Normalized data

5   Conclusion

This research reviews and clarifies the procedures and techniques used in dealing with large volume data sets. SOM is an artificial neural network which contains special property of creating internal representation with spatial organization of input signals and their abstractions. The UV-Decomposition method is efficient for splitting large data sets.

In this paper we present a survey on SOM and its applications. The SOM-based methods have certain limitations on generating analytical results based on high dimensional data sets when millions or trillions of neurons are required. The incremental SOM is efficient for dealing with large data sets including medical data and image processing. For the highly dimensional multipurpose time series database suppose if we want to use same online clustering method for the pattern recognition as well as semantics then we need to improve the SOM technique so that SOM can capture the clustering method quickly. The combination of iSOM and UV-decomposition method could improve the analytical results. Finally, the experimental results review that the SOM based method can improve the analytical performance.

Acknowledgements. This work is partially supported by Zhejiang Philosophy and Social Science Project Grant (No. 11JCSH03YB, China), Ningbo Nature Science Grant (No. 2012A610060, 2012A610025), Ningbo Soft Science Grant (No. 2012A10050), Ningbo Smart City Grant (2013), and National Nature Science of China Grant (No. 61272480).

References

[1] Yang, Y., Chen, K.: Time series clustering via rpcl network ensemble with different representations. IEEE Transactions on Systems, Man, and Cybernetics, Part C 41(2), 190–199 (2011)

[2] Rani, S., Sikka, G.: Recent techniques of clustering of time series data: A survey. International Journal of Computer Applications 52(15), 1–9 (2012)

[3] Nie, D., Fu, Y., et al.: Time series analysis based on enhanced NLCS. In: Proc. of ICIS 2010, pp. 292–295. IEEE (2010)

[4] Alahakoon, D., Halgamuge, S.K., Srinivasan, B.: Dynamic Self-organizing Maps with Controlled Growth for Knowledge Discovery. IEEE Transaction on Neural Networks 11(3), 601–614 (2000)

[5] Magni, P., Ferrazzi, F., Sacchi, L., Bellazzi, R.: Timeclust: a clustering tool for gene expression time series. Bioinformatics 24(3), 430–432 (2008)

[6] Papliński, A.P.: Incremental Self-Organizing Map (iSOM) in Categorization of Visual Objects. In: Huang, T., Zeng, Z., Li, C., Leung, C.S. (eds.) ICONIP 2012, Part II. LNCS, vol. 7664, pp. 125–132. Springer, Heidelberg (2012)

[7] Erturk, K.L., Sengul, G.: Three-Dimensional Visualization with Large Data Sets: A Simulation of Spreading Cortical Depression in Human Brain. Journal of Biomedicine and Biotechnology 2012, 1–7 (2012)

[8] Kohonen, T.: Self-Organized Formation of Topologically Correct Feature Maps. Biological Cybernetics 43(1), 59–69 (1982)

[9] Pavlo, A., Paulson, E., et al.: A Comparison of Approaches to Large-Scale Data Analysis. In: SIGMOD 2009. ACM Publication (2009)

[10] Shah-Hosseini, H., Safabakhsh, R.: TASOM: A New Time Adaptive Self-Organizing Map. IEEE Trans. Syst. Man Cyber. B 33(2), 271–282 (2003)

[11] Shah-Hosseini, H., Safabakhsh, R.: Binary Tree Time Adaptive Self-Organizing Map. Neurocomputing 74, 1823–1839 (2011)

[12] Stewart, G.W.: On the Early History of the Singular Value Decomposition. SIAM Review 35(4), 551–566 (1993)

[13] Wolberg, W.H., Street, W.N., Mangasarian, O.L.: Breast Cancer Wisconsin (Diagnostic) Data Set (2013) (Online Source accessed on November 1, 2013)

Water Molecules Diffusion
in Diffusion Weighted Imaging

Fan Zhang[1,2], Zhiwei Cao[2], Xinhong Zhang[3], and Kui Cao[1]

[1] Institute of Image Processing and Pattern Recognition,
Henan University, Kaifeng 475001, China
[2] School of Computer and Information Engineering,
Henan University, Kaifeng 475001, China
[3] Software School, Henan University, Kaifeng 475001, China
zhangfan@henu.edu.cn

Abstract. In the studying of fibers microstructure of brain white matter, many reconstruction methods have been proposed to interpret the diffusion-weighted signal. Those methods can be categorized into model-based and model-free methods. In this paper, the diffusion configuration of water molecules are discussed, and two questions are put forward to analyze the performance of the current algorithms about diffusion configuration.

Keywords: diffusion weighted MRI, diffusion configuration, fibers microstructure.

1 Introduction

In diffusion weighted MRI, it is now generally accepted that microscopic boundaries of diffusion in the brain coincide with the local orientations of white matter (WM) fiber tracts. The diffusion MRI as a tool for modeling intravoxel diffusion has inspired a number of promising applications in which white matter connectivity can be evaluated in both health and disease [1]. The diffusion MRI is now widely used to characterize regional anisotropy and orientation of WM throughout the brain, and the fiber pathways can be 3D delineated by tractography algorithms. In the diffusion weighted MRI, images are acquired using the Stejskal-Tanner pulsed gradient spin-echo method [2]. It describes measured signal intensity $S(\mathbf{g}_i)$ in the presence of a diffusion sensitizing gradient in direction $\mathbf{g}_i$ as a function of unweighted intensity $S(0)$, the apparent diffusion coefficient (ADC) $D(\mathbf{g}_i)$, and an acquisition constant b:

$$S(\mathbf{g}_i) = S(0) \exp\left(-b \cdot D(\mathbf{g}_i)\right), \tag{1}$$

where $b = \gamma^2 G^2 \delta^2 (\Delta t - \delta/3)$ is b-value. γ is the gyromagnetic ratio, δ is the duration of the diffusion gradient pulses, and G is the strength of the diffusion gradient. The apparent diffusion coefficient $D(\mathbf{g}_i) = \mathbf{g}_i^T \mathbf{D} \mathbf{g}_i$, $\mathbf{D}$ is diffusion tensor.

Y. Zhang et al. (Eds.): HIS 2014, LNCS 8423, pp. 229–236, 2014.

In diffusion tensor imaging (DTI) images, diffusion tensor is used to describe the diffusion profile of water molecules [3]. Diffusion tensors can be modeled as ellipsoids with the eigenvectors describing the major and minor axes of the ellipsoid and the associated eigenvalues scaling these axes. Isotropic diffusion profiles result in spherical tensors while anisotropic diffusion profiles produce linear tensors (ellipsoid). The parameters which describe these tensors are obtained from DWI images. Fig. 1 shows the diffusion profiles of water molecules according to diffusion tensor imaging. (a) is spherical case, (b) and (c) are linear case and planar case respectively.

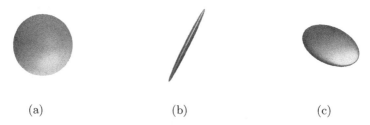

(a)   (b)   (c)

Fig. 1. Diffusion ellipsoids of water molecules according to diffusion tensor imaging. (a) Spherical case. (b) Linear case. (c) Planar case.

The diffusion ellipsoids of water molecules are accepted widely, especially in diffusion tensor imaging. Fig. 2 shows the diffusion profiles in a voxel. Assuming the box in Fig. 2 denotes a voxel, the diffusion profile of water molecules is a sphere if no any nerve fibers in this voxel, which is shown in Fig. 2(a). If there is one fiber or a bundle of fibers in a voxel, the diffusion profile of water molecules is a narrow ellipsoid (linear case), which is shown in Fig. 2(b). One tensor DTI model can only map a single orientation inside a voxel, so it is limited to characterize the complexity of white matter structure within a voxel. That is to say, one tensor DTI algorithms are in principle not able to resolve more than one orientation of fibers per voxel.

In voxel, the ellipsoid tensor may not corresponds only to one fiber, it may describes more than one fiber, which is shown as Fig. 3. The reason is that fibers usually appear as bundles, and we can not measure each fibers separately by now.

To overcome the limitation of DTI, several reconstruction methods have been proposed to interpret the diffusion-weighted signal in the studying of fibers microstructure. Those methods can be categorized into model-based and model-free approaches [4]. One of the simplest model-based method is diffusion tensor imaging, which describes a Gaussian estimate of the diffusion orientation and strength at each voxel. To handle more complex diffusion patterns, several model-based methods have been introduced, such as higher-order tensors [5], two tensors or multi-tensors tractography [6].

In this paper, we will put forward two questions to analyzes the performance of the current algorithms about diffusion configuration. The first question is about the diffusion profile of water molecules. The second question is about the

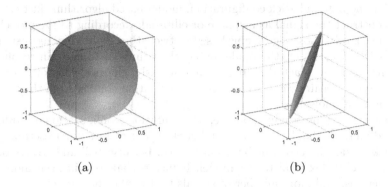

(a)   (b)

Fig. 2. Diffusion profiles in a voxel according to diffusion tensor imaging

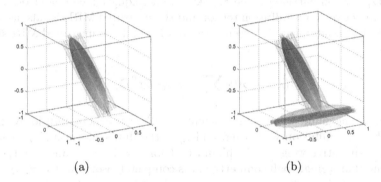

(a)   (b)

Fig. 3. Ellipsoid tensor may corresponds to a fiber or a bundle of fibers. (a) One orientation of fiber bundle. (b) Two orientations of fiber bundles.

location of fibers in voxel. The remainder of this paper is organized as follows: Section 2 analyzes the the diffusion profiles in voxel. In Section 3, the location of fibers is discussed. Finally, Section 4 concludes the paper.

2   What the Diffusion Profile Looks Like in Voxel?

In diffusion tensor imaging, the Gaussian diffusion profiles in voxel are widely accepted, which is shown in Fig. 2. Many reconstruction methods are designed and realized based on this model. The diffusion profile of water molecules is a sphere if there are no any nerve fibers in this voxel. If there is one fiber or a bundle of fibers in a voxel, the diffusion profile of water molecules is a narrow ellipsoid.

The diffusion configuration of water molecules in voxel is complex. We can not count on describing them precisely just by the sample tensor model. The current model-based reconstruction methods just give a sample tensor output (sphere or ellipsoid) no matter how complex the DWI signals are. Even the signal looks like the ball-and-stick configuration, model-based algorithms just estimate and reconstruct the signal as a sphere or ellipsoids according to the model they based. The model those algorithms based restricts the results they reconstructed. Given a DWI signal set, the model-based algorithms of course can reconstruct the signal and can tract the fibers, but obviously, the positions of fibers may be inaccurate, because they ignore many information coming from the isotropic diffusion water molecules.

According to the analysis above, the diffusion configuration of diffusion weighted imaging should be as ball-and-stick. What can we do? Describing ball-and-stick model directly will be a hard work, because ball-and-stick model is much more complex than tensor model. It means that we will need more complex functions, and more number of signals to describe this model.

Multi-tensor models assume k diffusion compartments with little or no exchange during measurement time, each parametrized by a symmetric diffusion tensor $\mathbf{D}_j$ per compartment. The Stejskal-Tanner equation can describes the relationship between one diffusion tensor and the measured MRI signals, as shown in Eq. 1. The relationship between k tensors $\mathbf{D}_j$ and the measured MRI signals $S(\mathbf{g}_i)$ is,

$$S(\mathbf{g}_i) = S(0) \sum_{j=1}^{k} f_j \exp(-b\mathbf{g}_i^T \mathbf{D}_j \mathbf{g}_i), \tag{2}$$

where k is the number of compartments, $S(0)$ is the non diffusion-weighted signal, b is the diffusion weighting, and $\mathbf{g}_i$ is the diffusion-sensitizing gradient. f_j are non-negative weights which sum to 1 for $j = 1, \cdots, k$ and $i = 1, \cdots, n$. Assuming that a single ball compartment is completely isotropic ($\lambda_1 = \lambda_2 = \lambda_3$), the remaining stick compartments are perfectly linear ($\lambda_1 = \lambda_2 = 0$). For n fibers or n bundles of fibers, this leads to $k = n + 1$ compartments, where n denotes the number of sticks, and the one denotes the ball.

Spherical deconvolution algorithm can be used in tensor decomposition [7]. The measured signal $S(\theta, \varphi)$ is expressed as the convolution of a orientation density function $F(\theta, \varphi)$ with an axially symmetric response function $R(\theta)$,

$$S(\theta, \varphi) = F(\theta, \varphi) * R(\theta), \tag{3}$$

where θ and φ are polar and azimuth angles respectively. After $S(\theta, \varphi)$ has been measured, the response function $R(\theta)$ is estimated from voxels. The distribution $F(\theta, \varphi)$ is then obtained by spherical deconvolution.

3   What Is the Location of Fibers in a Voxel?

As the analysis above, model-based algorithms can not work well in ball-and-stick model. How about the model-free algorithms? They usually decompose diffusion signal into spherical or radial functions, which seem more suitable for ball-and-stick model. In this section we will discuss the performance of model-free algorithms in ball-and-stick model.

Model-free methods, also called q-space imaging methods, are based on the Fourier transform relation between the diffusion MR signals and the underlying diffusion displacement. The aim of model-free methods is to resolve the problem of fibers crossing, so they focus on the angular resolution of signals. These methods tackle this problem by acquiring the orientation distribution function (ODF) of the diffusion displacement.

Measured image intensities $S(\mathbf{q})$ are linked to $p(\mathbf{r})$, the displacement probability function of water molecules, via the following Fourier transform,

$$S(\mathbf{q}) = S(0) \int p(\mathbf{r}) \exp(i\mathbf{q} \cdot \mathbf{r}) d\mathbf{r}, \tag{4}$$

where the diffusion wavevector is defined as $\mathbf{q} = (2\pi)^{-1}\gamma\delta\mathbf{g}$, and γ is the gyromagnetic ratio, δ is the diffusion gradient duration and $\mathbf{g}$ is the diffusion gradient vector. $S(0)$ denotes the baseline image without any gradient. Assuming a simple one-tensor Gaussian diffusion model, the diffusion process of water molecules can be indicated by a displacement probability function $p(\mathbf{r})$ of molecules displaced by $\mathbf{r} \in \mathbb{R}^3$ within a specified time Δt [8,9].

The orientation distribution function can be calculated by radial integration to the displacement probability function in q-space imaging [10,11].

$$\psi(\mathbf{u}) = \frac{1}{Z} \int_0^\infty p(\alpha\mathbf{u}) d\alpha, \tag{5}$$

where $\mathbf{u}$ is the direction vector on the unit sphere $\mathbb{S}^2$, Z is a dimensionless normalization constant and ψ is the ODF.

The ODF at a direction $\mathbf{u}$ can be calculated by integrating the signal over equator in q-space perpendicular to $\mathbf{u}$ by Funk-Radon transform (FRT). The Funk-Radon transform corresponds to the Fourier Transform on the sphere.

$$\psi(\mathbf{u}) = \oint_{\mathbf{q} \perp \mathbf{u}} S(\mathbf{q}) d\mathbf{q}. \tag{6}$$

In another implementation method, both the signal and the ODF were decomposed into the spherical harmonic (SH) basis set, and the ODF can be measured and reconstructed on a sphere. One can decompose a function U on a sphere into spherical harmonics as follows:

$$U(\theta, \varphi) = \sum_{l=0}^{L} \sum_{m=-l}^{l} u_{lm} Y_{l,m}(\theta, \varphi), \tag{7}$$

where $Y_{l,m}(\theta, \varphi)$ are the spherical harmonics at elevation θ, azimuth φ and u_{lm} are the spherical harmonics coefficients. The spherical harmonics $Y_{l,m}(\theta, \varphi)$ are defined by,

$$Y_{l,m}(\theta, \varphi) = \sqrt{\frac{(2l+1)(l-m)!}{4\pi(l+m)!}} P_l^m(\cos(\theta)) e^{im\varphi}, \tag{8}$$

where P_l^m are the associated Legendre polynomials.

So in model-free algorithms, the ODF of diffusion signal are radially reconstructed in q-space (DSI and QSI algorithms), or the ODF is reconstructed directly in the spherical shells (QBI and GQI algorithms), as shown in Fig. 4. In model-free algorithms, we can find the fibers directions just by finding the directions of ODF peaks in q-ball. Fig. 5 is an example of signal reconstruction by model-free algorithms.

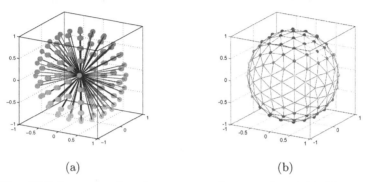

(a)   (b)

Fig. 4. The ODF is measured and reconstructed on a sphere. (a) The vertexes of four-order tessellated icosahedron. (b) Four-order spherical tessellated icosahedron.

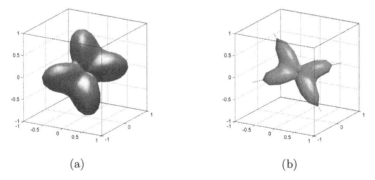

(a)   (b)

Fig. 5. Signal reconstruction according to model-free algorithms. (a) The probability density function (PDF) of diffusion. (b) The orientation distribution function (ODF) of diffusion.

Because model-free algorithms using radial reconstruction or spherical reconstruction to capture both radial and angular information of diffusion signals, they seem more suitable for describing ball-and-stick model. But those algorithms must assume that there is a center of radial propagator or a center of sphere, the center usually is the center of voxel, and accordingly, they have to assume that all fibers or fiber bundles pass through this center, as shown in Fig. 5. Model-free algorithms restrict the location of fibers. That is to say, model-free algorithms just provide direction information of fibers, ignore or can not provide useful location information of fibers.

In ball-and-stick model, tensor is decomposed by spherical deconvolution. We notice that the $R(\theta)$ and the reconstructed ODF $F(\theta, \varphi)$ are axially symmetric function in Eq. 3, which means that sticks are restricted that passing the center of ball or the center of voxel, and result in can not resolve the fibers location problem well.

4 Conclusions

In this paper, we discuss diffusion configuration of water molecules in diffusion weighted imaging, and two questions are put forward to analyzes the performance of the current algorithms about diffusion configuration. The first question is about the diffusion profile of water molecules. The second question is about the location of fibers in voxel. We find that, firstly, most of model-based algorithms ignore many information coming from the isotropic diffusion water molecules when they estimate and reconstruct the signal. Which will lead to a inaccurate estimation. Secondly, model-free algorithms just provide direction information of fibers, ignore or can not provide location information of fibers. So unfortunately, neither model-based methods nor model-free methods can resolve those two questions very well. This paper just put forward questions but not give solution. How to resolve those questions is still a open problem, and it may be an interesting direction in the future research.

References

1. Kubicki, M., McCarley, R., Westin, C.F., Park, H.J., Maier, S., Kikinis, R., Jolesz, F.A., Shenton, M.E.: A review of diffusion tensor imaging studies in schizophrenia. Magnetic Resonance Imaging 41(1-2), 15–30 (2007)
2. Stejskal, E., Tanner, J.: Spin diffusion measurements: spin echoes in the presence of a time-dependent field gradient. Journal of Chemical Physics 42, 288–292 (1965)
3. Bihan, D.L., Mangin, J.F., Poupon, C., Clark, C.A., Pappata, S., Molko, N., Chabriat, H.: Diffusion tensor imaging: concepts and applications. Magnetic Resonance Imaging 13, 534–546 (2001)
4. Yeh, F.-C., Wedeenb, V.J., Tseng, W.Y.I.: Estimation of fiber orientation and spin density distribution by diffusion deconvolution. NeuroImage 55, 1054–1062 (2011)
5. Barmpoutis, A., Hwang, M., Howland, D., Forder, J., Vemuri, B.: Regularized positive-definite fourth order tensor field estimation from DW-MRI. Neuroimage 1, 153–162 (2009)
6. Rathia, Y., Kubickia, M., Bouixa, S., Westinc, C.F., Goldsteina, J., Seidmane, L., Gatelye, R.M., McCarleyd, R.W., Shenton, M.E.: Statistical analysis of fiber bundles using multi-tensor tractography: application to first-episode schizophrenia. Magnetic Resonance Imaging 29, 507–515 (2011)
7. Schultz, T., Seidel, H.P.: Estimating Crossing Fibers: A Tensor Decomposition Approach. IEEE Transactions on Visualization and Computer Graphics 14(6), 1635–1642 (2008)

8. Fonteijn, H.M.J., Verstraten, F.A.J., Norris, D.G.: Probabilistic Inference on Q-ball Imaging Data. IEEE transactions on medical imaging 26(11), 1515–1524 (2007)
9. Leow, A.D., Zhu, S., Zhan, L., McMahon, K., de Zubicaray, G.I., Meredith, M., Wright, M.J., Toga, A.W., Thompson, P.M.: The tensor distribution function. Magnetic Resonance in Medicine 61(1), 205–214 (2009)
10. Rathia, Y., Michailovichb, O., Shentona, M.E., Bouix, S.: Directional functions for orientation distribution estimation. Medical Image Analysis 13, 432–444 (2009)
11. Tuch, D.S., Reese, T.G., Wiegell, M.R., Wedeen, V.J.: Diffusion MRI of complex neural architecture. Neuron 40(5), 885–895 (2003)

Feasibility Study of Signal Similarity Measurements for Improving Morphological Evaluation of Human Brain with Images from Multi-Echo T2-Star Weighted MR Sequences

Shaode Yu[1], Xuyin Cheng[2], and Yaoqin Xie[1]

[1] Shenzhen Institutes of Advanced Technology, CAS, China. 518055, Shenzhen, China
[2] Anqing First People's Hospital, China. 246004, Anqing, China
{sd.yu,yq.xie}@siat.ac.cn, chengxuyin0701@gmail.com

Abstract. Signal correlation measurement has been widely used for segmenting specific tissues, localizing abnormal regions and analyzing functional areas in dynamic imaging modalities. In this paper, we discussed the feasibility of similarity mappings derived from six signal coefficient measurements in improving morphological evaluation of human brain. These images are from a digital phantom and four normal volunteers scanned by multi-echo T2-star weighted MR sequences. Simulation studies have shown that similarity mappings from cross-correlation, normalized cross-correlation, mean square error and cubed sum coefficient are not helpful in distinguishing the reference region from its surrounding tissues. Clinical experiments were focused on similarity coefficient mapping (SCM) and improved SCM (iSCM). Final results have demonstrated comparative capacity of SCM and iSCM in improving image quality from quantitative metrics and visual analysis.

Keywords: Signal correlation measurement, similarity mapping, morphological evaluation, multi-echo T2-star weighted MR sequences.

1 Introduction

Health information science is highly cross-discipline which involves information science, computer science and health care, and its fundamental purpose is to use these recorded information for early detection and diagnosis of disease or cancer. These information mainly comes from medical images. As a non-invasive imaging technique, multi-echo T2-star weighted magnetic resonance imaging (MRI) has played an important role in information analysis and clinical diagnosis with various superior features, such as high contrast of soft tissues [1]. Meanwhile, multi-echo T2-star weighted MRI is able to reveal functional and morphological characteristics by taking advantage of differences in tissue properties [2–4]. It is also capable of acquiring a large number of medical images for specific applications in a very short period of time [1–5].

Mapping extraction is quite a useful tool in medical image analysis for specific messages. It can localize regions with similar behavior from dynamic image

Y. Zhang et al. (Eds.): HIS 2014, LNCS 8423, pp. 237–247, 2014.

series [4–10]. These dynamic images may come from CT and MRI for probing structural, functional or physiological information. Similarity mappings are usually derived from pixel-wise analysis of signal correlation, and signals in dynamic medical imaging relate to time-resolved data sets about a stationary anatomical structure. The whole procedure consists of three steps [8]. First it defines a reference signal from a region of interest (ROI) for different purposes, such as localizing functional areas or segmenting specific tissues. The reference signal is a time-resolved intensity vector which is usually acquired by averaging gray values in the ROI from each original image for robustness. Then signal correlation is measured between the time-resolved intensity distributions of one position with the reference signal. Finally a similarity mapping is constructed by pixel-wise analysis, and pixel values in the mapping show the similarity to the reference signal. In this way, the whole image sequence is mapped into a single image which reduces time cost in image analysis and diagnostic interpretations, which releases patients and doctors.

The constructed similarity mapping is itself an image, where the pixel values on the mapping show specific correlations of temporal behaviors between signals and the reference signal [4–9]. There are many ways to measure signal correlation. Cross-correlation (CC) [6, 7] and normalized cross-correlation (NCC) [8] are helpful in identifying functional regions and localizing tissue structures in contrast-agent-based dynamic MRI. While [9] disproved the effectiveness of CC and NCC in the oncological dynamic PET study, and revealed that mappings from cubed sum coefficient (CSC) provide the best parametric images. In addition, mean square error (MSE) [10] is also applied to measure signal correlation. These MSE-based mappings were capable of mapping vascular behavior to detect potential multiple sclerosis and calculating relative blood volume to analyze vessel function.

As we know, dynamic imaging involves contrast agents, because contrast agents enable medical images to illustrate invisible hemodynamic messages about tissue differences and local pharmacokinetics [8–10]. But there are still many open questions about contrast agent usage, such as hypersensitivity [11] and renal function reduction [12]. Meanwhile, image quality of these derived mappings is very sensitive to the choice of reference signal [4, 9]. In addition, the image quality of derived maps is very sensitive to the choice of reference signal. With different reference signals, contrast values of several methods [9] widely range from 0.0 to 54.0 in PET studies, and contrast values of tissue similarity maps [4] range from 0.03 to 2.00. To tackle these problems, similarity coefficient mapping (SCM) was proposed to release contrast agent [4]. It generalizes signal response to time course with signal response to time-of-echo (TE) in multi-echo T2-star weighted MR sequence. SCM is able to improve image quality and morphological evaluation, but different tissues are with different sensitivities to that reference signal, so improved SCM (iSCM) was proposed and reference signal is adaptive for better image quality [5]. In this paper, we discussed the feasibility of six signal correlation coefficients (CC, NCC, CSC, MSE, SCM and iSCM) in improving morphological evaluation of human brain with images from multi-echo

T2-star weighted MR sequences. For fairness and consistency, all coefficients are transformed to similarity measurement, which means that pixel values close to 1 shows much similar to the reference signal. The results were validated by simulated digital phantom and 16 series of clinical data sets from four volunteers, and compared by signal-to-noise ratio (SNR) and morphological analysis.

2   Methods

Many methods have been proposed to measure signal correlations with images from different modalities [4–10]. To a stationary subject, we assume that a image series are acquired by n-echo T2-star weighted MRI. Let $I = \{I_1, I_2, ..., I_n\}$ be spatially registered with ascending TE values. For any position (i, j), there exists a row vector of pixel intensities $V_{ij} = \{V_{ij1}, V_{ij2}, ..., V_{ijn}\}$. Then we delineate a region of interest (ROI) and average these pixel intensities as a reference signal $R = \{R_1, R_2, ..., R_n\}$. For specific purpose, different regions or tissue are delineated out as the ROI, i.e., the reference signal.

In previous researches, renal cancer was sketched out as the ROI to improve morphological evaluation with images from multi-echo T2-star weighted MRI [4]. [7] took lesion area as the reference signal to detect potential lesions in CT perfusion imaging. [8] delineated renal cortex and medulla of a rabbit, ischemia of a dog heart, human lung tumor and focal ischemia of a cat's brain as ROI respectively in dynamic MRI experiments. [9] outlined lesion area to localize potential lesion regions in PET studyies.

Pixel values on these derived mappings are with different meanings and different ranges. For fairness and consistency, we re-scaled these values in MSE-based, SCM-based and iSCM-based mappings to [0, 1] with equation 4 to 6, respectively. As to CC-based, NCC-based and CSC-based mappings, we take absolute values of pixel intensities with equation 1 to 3.

$$CC_{ij} = \left\| \frac{V_{ij} R^T}{\sqrt{(V_{ij} V_{ij}^T)(RR^T)}} \right\|. \tag{1}$$

$$NCC_{ij} = \left\| \frac{(V_{ij} - \mu_{ij})(R^T - \mu_R)}{\sqrt{((V_{ij} - \mu_{ij})(V_{ij}^T - \mu_{ij}))((R - \mu_R)(R^T - \mu_R))}} \right\|. \tag{2}$$

$$CSC_{ij} = \left\| \frac{((V_{ij} - \mu_{ij})(R^T - \mu_R))^3}{\mu_R^2 \sqrt{((V_{ij} - \mu_{ij})(V_{ij}^T - \mu_{ij}))((R - \mu_R)(R^T - \mu_R))}} \right\|. \tag{3}$$

$$\begin{cases} MSE_{ij} = \frac{1}{n}(V_{ij} - R)(V_{ij} - R)^T; \\ MSE_{ij} = \left\| \frac{(MSE_{ij} - max(MSE))}{max(MSE)} \right\|. \end{cases} \tag{4}$$

$$\begin{cases} SCM_{ij} = \frac{\overline{V_{ij} R^T}}{\overline{RR^T}}; \\ SCM_{ij} = \|(\overline{SCM}_{ij} - 1)\|; \\ SCM_{ij} = \left\| \frac{(SCM_{ij} - max(SCM))}{max(SCM)} \right\|. \end{cases} \tag{5}$$

$$\begin{cases} iSCM_{ij} = \frac{\overline{V_{ij}R^T} - \overline{V_{ij}} \times \overline{R}}{\overline{RR^T} - \overline{R} \times \overline{R}}; \\ iSCM_{ij} = \|(iSCM_{ij} - 1)\|; \\ iSCM_{ij} = \|\frac{(iSCM_{ij} - max(iSCM))}{max(iSCM)}\|. \end{cases} \tag{6}$$

In these equations, V_{ij} is a n-dimensional row vector. R is the reference signal with average pixel values from delineated ROI. A^T means to transform the row vector A to its column format. u is the mean value of corresponding vector, and $\overline{A}$ stands for the procedure of calculating mean value in vector A. $\|A\|$ is an absolute value of scalar A. $max(A)$ finds the maximum value in vector or array A. By a point-wise calculation, all points make up the mappings with pixel values ranging from $[0, 1]$. The effect of the number of echoes is previously discussed and in this paper n is 12. In clinical applications, if possible, larger n leads to higher perceived image quality with higher SNR [4].

3 Experiments and Results

3.1 Evaluation Metrics

SNR is to measure image quality $SNR = \frac{\overline{ROI}}{std(Air)}$. Operator $std(Air)$ denotes the standard deviation of pixel values in the air area, and air area is manually delineated. For each ROI in original image series, there exist a maximum (SNR-max). Taking SNRmax as an baseline, SNR improvement in derived mappings are evaluated with an factor $R_{map} = \frac{SNR_{map}}{SNR_{max}}$. Rmap is for validating mappings' capacity in SNR enhancement. SNR of mappings from different image sequences with same reference signal are statistical analyzed. Visual morphological analysis is also demonstrated.

3.2 Simulation Study

Simulated Brain Phantom. Firstly, simulation study is to evaluate the feasibility of these six methods. A digital phantom of normal human brain is borrowed from BrainWeb [13]. We simplified it to four tissues, cerebra-spinal fluid (CSF), white matter (WM), grey matter (GM) and MEAT. Tissues of skull, muscle, fat and skin are merged into MEAT, and glial matter is merged into GM. Outside the phantom is air circumstance. The size of brain phantom is 255×255. Figure 1 shows spatial distributions of the digital phantom.

Imaging parameter values of relative proton density and T2-star are 1.00 and 58ms for CSF, 0.86 and 69ms for GM, 0.77 and 51ms for WM, 0.77 and 61ms for MEAT. In simulation study, the whole region of CSF is averaged as the reference signal, and then the whole WM. We took no considerations of T1 values, neither intensity in-homogeneity nor artifacts. Image series are simulated with $I_i = \rho e^{TE_i/T2^*}$ [14]. TE values range from 2.61ms to 38.91ms with equal interval of 3.3ms. These 12 frames construct a image series. Finally these frames were corrupted with 5% Rician noise [15].

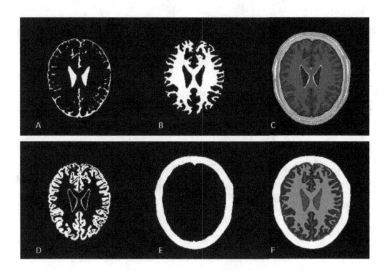

Fig. 1. Simplified human brain phantom. Simplified phantom (F) contains only CSF (red), WM (green), GM (blue) and MEAT (white). Spatial distributions of CSF, WM, GM and MEAT are shown in (A), (B), (D) and (E). Original digital phantom is (C).

The Racian noise was built from white Gaussian noise in the complex domain:
- $I_r = I + \eta_1, \eta_1 \backsim \mathcal{N}(0, \sigma_n)$
- $I_i = \eta_2, \eta_2 \backsim \mathcal{N}(0, \sigma_n)$

where I is the noise-free image, and I_r is the real part and I_i is the imaginary component, and σ_n is the standard deviation of the added white Gaussian noise. The noisy image is computed as

$$Img = \sqrt{I_r^2 + I_i^2}. \tag{7}$$

Rmap Analysis in Simulation Study. Figure 2 shows Rmap values of different regions in derived mappings by taking CSF and WM as reference signal. By experiments, to different levels of Racian noise ranging from 1% to 10%, the results are similar to Figure 2. By comparison, we obtain the conclusion that derived mappings based on CC, NCC and MSE measurements are not effective in improving SNR, and this conclusion is the same to [9]. It means that application fields based on CC, NCC and MSE are only suitable for specific usage. Rmap values from CSC-based mappings are much higher than Rmap from other five methods but fluctuate wildly respecting to different reference signals. Rmap values from SCM-based and iSCM-based mappings show comparative and stable capacity in improving SNR.

Visual Analysis in Simulation Study. Mappings derived from CC, NCC and MSE are high sensitive to the selection of reference signal [4, 9], and this phenomenon is also discovered in our simulation study. For convenience, we

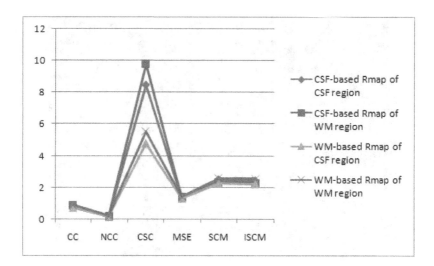

Fig. 2. Quantitative results of Rmap in simulation study. Ineffectiveness of CC, NCC and MSE is shown by comparing Rmap values. Rmap based on CSC are much higher but fluctuate wildly, and Rmap values from SCM and iSCM show comparative capacity.

only illustrate mappings derived from CSC, SCM and iSCM in Figure 3. (A, B, C) are original images from image sequence. (D, E, F) are derived from CSC, SCM and iSCM with CSF as the reference signal, and (G, H, I) are from CSC, SCM and iSCM with WM as the reference. From (A, B, C), image quality decreases. In clinical usage, proper MR images are acquired by setting imaging parameters with empirical values. When taking CSF as the reference signal (the middle row), pixel intensities in CSF region in derived mappings from SCM (E) and iSCM (F) are higher than other pixel values, because these pixels are much similar to the reference signal. Higher SNR from CSC-based images in Figure 2 does not support visual quality. When taking WM as the reference signal (the bottom row), pixel intensities in WM region in derived mappings from SCM (H) and iSCM (I) are higher than other pixel values. Mappings from CSC don't demonstrate this kind of message which implies that CSC may be helpful in potential applications, such as in oncology PET studies [9], but it is not applicable in all situations.

3.3   Clinical Cases

All clinical MR imaging was on a 3 Tesla scanner (Siemens) with GRE sequence (FA: 15°; FOV: 220mm×220mm; Matrix size: 384×384; Slice thickness: 3.0mm; TR: 200ms; Slice gap: 0.9mm). TE values is same to those in simulation studies ranging from 2.61ms to 38.91ms with equal interval of 3.3ms. Each of these four volunteers (aged 24.75±3.10) is scanned 4 paralleling cross-sections, and we obtained 16 groups of MR images. In clinical cases, we also delineated CSF and WM as ROIs, and air area are outlined for calculating SNR values. Both ROIs

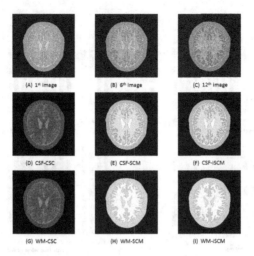

Fig. 3. Visual analysis of derived mappings in simulation study. Visual analysis of original images and mappings from CSC, SCM and iSCM based on different reference are illustrated. The 1st, 6th and 12th frame are shown in (A, B, C). Mappings from CSC (D), SCM (E) and iSCM (F) are taking CSF as reference signal, and mappings from CSC (G), SCM (H) and iSCM (I) are generated by taking WM as the reference.

of CSF and WM are with the same size of 6pixels×6pixels, and delineated air area is 60 pixels×60 pixels. In clinical cases, we only consider mappings derived from SCM and iSCM methods.

Objective Metrics for Clinical Cases. Image quality from MRI is subject to many factors, such as motion artifacts, partial volume effects, magnetic inhomogeneity and noise. Our simulation study considers only Racian noise. To demonstrate the feasibility of SCM and iSCM in clinical cases, we carried these two methods out on 16 series of clinical images from 4 volunteers. Since these two methods are insensitive to the choice of reference signals which is proved in simulation study, we analyzed the SNR from different tissue areas (CSF and WM regions) regardless of reference signals.

Figure 4 shows quantitative analysis of SNR and Rmap from these 16 image series from four volunteers. SNRmax, SNR from SCM and iSCM in CSF region and WM region are shown in Figure 4.(A,C), respectively. Correspondingly Rmap values are in Figure 4.(B,D). In (A), SNRmax from these 16 series are less than 60 in CSF regions. And in (C), all SNRmax are less than 55 in WM regions. It is easily observed that SNR from SCM and iSCM are much higher than corresponding SNRmax in original MR sequences. The quantitative improvement is shown in (B) and (D). On the one hand, regardless of reference signals, SNR values are positively enhanced by SCM and iSCM methods with Rmap ranging from 2.0 to 3.2 times. On the other hand, iSCM has demonstrated competitive capacity as SCM method in improving SNR.

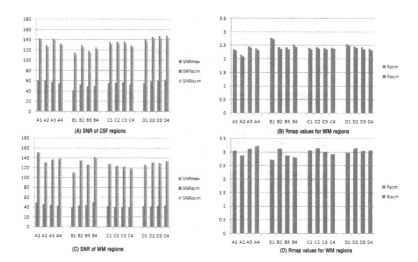

Fig. 4. Analysis of SNR and Rmap in 16 clinical cases from four volunteers. SNRmax, SNR of SCM and iSCM in CSF region is shown in (A) and those SNR values in WM region are illustrated in (C). Corresponding Rmap values are shown in (B) and (D).

Visual Analysis for Clinical Cases. In Figure 5, (A, B, C, D, G) are five original images from one series. With ascending TE values, MR images show anatomical structure with different emphasis which can be observed from (A) and (D). Comparing to image (A), image (C, D, G) indicate much details about anatomical textures and structures. In (D), green ROI is WM, red ROI is CSF, and pink region is delineated air ares. Derived mappings from SCM and iSCM are very close in perceived image quality in (E, F) and (H, I) based on different reference signals.

4   Discussion

Medical imaging technologies have been imposing valuable meanings on signal correlation measurement for clinical usage, such as mapping extraction discussed in this paper. These mapping extraction methods need to manually define a ROI to form a reference signal, and generate similarity mappings based on a pixel-wise calculation. CC-, NCC- and MSE-based methods are used in dynamic imaging for specific tissue localization and segmentation, such as lesion, ischemia and etc. CSC-based method has been proved effective in oncology PET studies. SCM and iSCM replaces the signal response to time course in dynamic imaging with signal response to one imaging parameter changes and involve no contrast agents. In simulation study, we find that CC-, NCC-, MSE- and CSC-based methods are not suitable for analyzing signals from MRI either for its low improvement in SNR or wild fluctuation in Rmap. Quantitative results from SCM and iSCM show that SNR is enhanced from 2.0 to 2.5 times than the maximum SNR in original images in simulation study, and 2.0 to 3.5 times in clinical study.

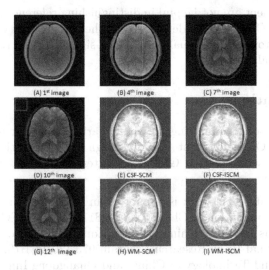

Fig. 5. Visual analysis of mappings from one clinical series. Original images, mappings from SCM and iSCM based on different references are illustrated. The 1st, 4th, 7th, 10th, 12th frame are shown in (A, B, C, D, G), respectively. Mappings from SCM (E) and iSCM (F) are taking CSF (red square in D) as the reference signal, and mapping from SCM (H) and iSCM (I) are generated by taking WM (green square in D) as the reference. Delineated pink square is for calculating SNR values.

Since these methods are targeted to the same section of an object, the anatomical structures in the image sequences should remain stationary. If relative motion occurs, accurate spatial registration becomes necessary. Meanwhile, correct delineation of reference signal is crucial before calculating mappings, because inaccurate delineation may result in uncertainty and errors. These results from inaccurate delineation are far away from the initial research purpose. In addition, by experiments, it has been verified that there is no need to process these image sequences by de-noising, correcting in-homogeneity or fitting the reference signal to mono-exponential function. Using these mapping techniques, image quality is improved with suppressed noise, but this kind of de-noising property doesn't mean the reduction of partial volume effects nor intensity in-homogeneity nor artifacts. These two methods, SCM and iSCM can be straightly applied to other MRI sequence, such as T1 and T2 weighted weighted MRI, or extended to other image sequences from functional MRI, CT and PET.

5   Conclusion

In this paper, we discussed the feasibility of six signal similarity coefficients in improving morphological evaluation of human brain with images from multi-echo T2-star weighted MR sequences. Simulation studies have shown that mappings from cross-correlation, normalized cross-correlation, mean square error and cubed sum coefficient are not helpful in distinguishing reference region from surrounding tissues. Clinical cases demonstrated the comparative capacity of SCM and iSCM in improving image quality by region signal-to-noise ratio and visually morphological analysis.

6 Abbreviations

MRI, magnetic resonance imaging; SCM, similarity coefficient mapping; iSCM, improved SCM; ROI, region of interest; SNR, signal-to-noise ratio; CSF, cerebral-spinal fluid; WM, white matter; GM, grey matter.

Acknowledgment. This work is supported in part by grants from National Natural Science Foundation of China (NSFC: 81171402), NSFC Joint Research Fund for Overseas Research Chinese, Hong Kong and Macao Young Scholars (30928030), National Basic Research Program 973 (2010CB732606) from Ministry of Science and Technology of China, and Guangdong Innovative Research Team Program (No. 2011S013) of China.

References

1. Chavhan, G.B., Babyn, P.S., Thomas, B., et al.: Principles, techniques, and applications of T2*-based MR imaging and its special applications. RadioGraphics 29(5), 1433–1449 (2009)
2. Tardif, C.L., Bedell, B.J., Eskildsen, S.F., et al.: Quantitative magnetic resonance imaging of cortical multiple sclerosis pathology. Multiple sclerosis international (2012)
3. Mamisch, T.C., Hughes, T., Mosher, T.J., et al.: T2 star relaxation times for assessment of articular cartilage at 3 T: a feasibility study. Skeletal Radiology 41(3), 287–292 (2012)
4. Wang, H.Y., Hu, J., Xie, Y.Q., et al.: Feasibility of similarity coefficient map for improving morphological evaluation of T2* weighted MRI for renal cancer. Chinese Physics B 22(3), 8702 (2013)
5. Yu, S.D., Wu, S.B., Xie, Y.Q.: Automatic mapping extraction from multi-echo T2-star weighted magnetic resonance images for improving morphological evaluations in human brain. Comput. Math. Methods Med. 2013 (2013)
6. Lo, E., Rogowska, J., Bogorodzki, P., et al.: Temporal correlation analysis of penumbral dynamics in focal cerebral ischemia. Journal of Cerebral Blood Flow and Metabolism 16(1), 60–68 (1996)
7. Zhu, F., Rodriguez, G.D., Carpenter, T., et al.: Lesion Area Detection Using Source Image Correlation Coefficient for CT Perfusion Imaging. Journal of Biomedical and Health Informatics 17(5), 950–958 (2013)
8. Rogowska, J., Preston Jr., K., Hunter, G.J., et al.: Applications of similarity mapping in dynamic MRI. IEEE Transactions on Medical Imaging 14(3), 480–486 (1995)
9. Thireou, T., Kontaxakis, G., Strauss, L.G., et al.: Feasibility study of the use of similarity maps in the evaluation of oncological dynamic positron emission tomography images. Medical & Biological Engineering & Computing 43(1), 23–32 (2005)

10. Haacke, E.M., Li, M., Juvvigunta, F.: Tissue similarity maps (TSMs): A new means of mapping vascular behavior and calculating relative blood volume in perfusion weighted imaging. Journal of Magnetic Resonance Imaging 31(4), 481–489 (2013)
11. Brockow, K.: Contrast media hypersensitivity - scope of the problem. Toxicology 209(2), 189–192 (2005)
12. Tepel, M., Van der Giet, M., Schwarzfeld, C., et al.: Prevention of radiographic-contrast-agent-induced reductions in renal function by acetylcysteine. The New England Journal of Medicine 343(3), 180–184 (2000)
13. Collins, D.L., Zijdenbos, A.P., Kollokian, V., et al.: Design and construction of a realistic digital brain phantom. IEEE Transactions on Medical Imaging 17(3), 463–468 (1998)
14. Haacke, E.M., Brown, R.W., Thompson, M.R., et al.: Magnetic resonance imaging: physical principles and sequence design. Wiley-Liss, New York (1999)
15. Coupe, P., Manjon, J.V., Gedamu, E., et al.: Robust Rician noise estimation for MR images. Medical Image Analysis 14(4), 483–493 (2010)

Multi-agent Based Clinical Knowledge Representation with Its Dynamic Parse and Execution

Yumin Hu[*], Liang Xiao, Xing Liu, Jianzhou Liu,
Zhenzhen Yan, Qiuju Wei, and Haifeng Chen

Department of Computer Science, Hubei University of Technology,
Wuhan 430068, Hubei,
People's Republic of China
48453626@qq.com
Department of Computer Science, Hubei University of Technology,
Wuhan 430068, Hubei, People's Republic of China
min_rly1124@163.com

Abstract. In contemporary society, the acquirement, storage, transmission and management of information in medical are the main content of medical information technology. The clinical decision support system (CDSS) and related technology have been improved rapidly in recent years. In this paper, we use Triple assessment (a method of treatment about breast cancer) as an example. Through the definition of knowledge tag set, this article converts the basing on the evidence-based, widely accepted clinical knowledge to an XML document, and implement a Rules Execution Engine to make clinical decisions according to this XML document. Interface Generation Engine dynamically generates some detected information that doctors need to ask in this decision-making process. So we can capture the needed data in the process of diagnosis simply and quickly. The electronic health records (EHRs) are standard because of the storage of the data.

Keywords: clinical decision support system (CDSS), Triple assessment, XML, Rules Execution Engine, Interface Generation Engine.

1 Introduction

Clinical guidelines (CGLs) are a set of clinical knowledge based on the evidence-based clinical guidelines which are accepted by the large number of doctors and patients. Using the CGLs can help to the accuracy and security of clinical decisions. Thus, they are of great guiding importance to the clinical decisions that the doctors make during the process. Although their importance is generally recognised by the doctors, they are not very convenient when making the clinical decisions. On the one hand, publishing of the CGLs are usually based on the text, which makes it hard to be processed[1]. On the

---

[*] Corresponding author.

Y. Zhang et al. (Eds.): HIS 2014, LNCS 8423, pp. 248–260, 2014.
© Springer International Publishing Switzerland 2014

other hand, there is no unified standard for the CGLs to be converted to machine-executable. If CGLs are structured and standardized in form, they will be more widely and efficiently used to improve the medical effect in the CDSS.

Recent years, much progress have been made in the structured expression of CGLs, much predominant of which is PROforma[2], a executable process modeling language proposed by professor John Fox Proforma. At present the language has been used in many CDSSs.

PROforma is a formal knowledge that is capable of capturing the structure and content of a CGL in a form which can be interpreted by a computer. The language forms the basis of a method and a technology to develop and publish executable CGLs. Applications using PROforma software are intended to support the management of medical procedures and clinical decisions that make at the point of care[3]. In PROforma, a guideline application is modelled as a set of tasks and data items. The notion of a task is central - the PROforma task model divides from the keystone (generic task) into four types: plans, decisions, actions and enquiries. A PROforma Decision has a small set of standard attributes, consisting of Candidates (decision options under consideration); Arguments (logical conditions used to generate reasons that argue for or against a candidate); and decision rules that can be used to make recommendations to clinical users, or commitments if the decision making process operates autonomously.

Though the PROforma can accurately convert CGLs based on the text into executable machine and is a standard form of files, it can't perform in a distributed environment. As a result, there are several shortcomings. First, it is not easy to extend and maintain when CGLs change. Second, user cannot connect to the resources needed fast and conveniently. Third, it do not meet the reality. Doctors from different departments make the decisions in their own offices and could not synchronize data operation. Thus, the system synergy degree is very low.

In this article, we put forward a method that apply the XML to CGLs, and make sure that CDSSs don't need restart from the software requirements analysis to the preliminary and detailed design step by step due to the changes of CGLs. Converting the CGLs to standardized and machine-executable XML documents, then we can parse the rules, design and implement a Rules Execution Engine for the doctor's clinical decision making. With the structured rules and the Rules Execution engine, CDSSs must have the support of necessary data. So each agent must be equipped with the corresponding interface to collect data, and it can instruct the doctor ask patients questions, so as to provide test results. This part of content will be detailed in section 4.

2   Approach Overview

With the rapid development of medical information, the process of clinical decision support is in urgent need for the structured CGLs. Therefore, our primary goal is to transform CGLs based on the text into unified standard, machine-executable files. In this article, we use XML for clinical knowledge representation, the reason of using XML is:1) extensible Markup Language XML is a Standard Generalized Markup Language (Standard Generalized Markup Language, SGML). Using a series of simple tag to describe data, and these markers can be established by convenient ways. XML allows people and computers to access, reuse and modify information from the document[4]; 2) the elements in the XML document has a good hierarchy, so it is easy to understand; 3) XML allows users to create suitable tags for their own, which can be applied to many different platforms. Creating an XML document does not need too much skill, so the XML document is easy to extend and maintain. Since XML is simplicity, cross-platform and strong adaptability, it is easy to read and write data in any application. XML quickly became the only common language of data exchange. If you want get more detailed description about this part, please refer to the fourth part of Fig. 3 and Fig. 4.

Another goal is to design and implement a Rules Parser Engine, to parse structured knowledge, applied to the clinical decision making. In the development of Rules Parser Engine, we use JDOM to read, write, and manipulate the XML document. JDOM is an object model, which is a tree structure and have an open source API, based on Java[5] using pure Java technology to analyze, build, process, and serialize the XML document. XML document is expressed as a tree by JDOM, including elements, attributes, processing instructions, etc. The data of this tree may come from the Java program's direct volume, calculation results, or library database which does not belong to the XML library. JDOM only uses a concrete class instead of using an interface, this simplifies the API in some respects, and the API uses the class of Collections a lot. They are more convenient to be used by Java developers who are already familiar with these classes. So when use the XML to show the CGLs, even CGLs change, only change the XML document's content instead of its structure. It is different from the traditional software engineering. In traditional software engineering, the project must be restarted if the requirement is changed. As long as the structure of an XML document has not changed, the development of the parser engine by JDOM does not have to make a code change, which gives us a good scalability.

A third important goal is to develop a Production Rules (PRs) Execution Engine. It is used to perform the CGLs that machine can perform and is converted from the first goal. To accomplish this goal, we introduced the thought of multi-tree storage in data structure, which can construct the nodes in the XML of CGLs into a node tree of multi-tree structure. And it can also initialize a queue to store the leaf nodes of the tree and determine whether each branch of the tree is the pathway in order. Then the results will be recorded in the decision support queue or decision against queue. Finally we calculate weights and give the optimal decision. The design and implementation of the PRs Execution Engine will be described in 4.2 on focus.

The final goal is to design and implement a Interface Generation Engine that bases on rules. In order to achieve this goal, we parse rules using JDOM as well,in which we parse out all the conditions necessary for the execution of the rules. Because the conditions there will have a recurring phenomenon, we need to use hash table algorithm to remove repeat conditions. Thus give the information which should be displayed in the human-computer interaction interface dynamically. This part will be in the back of the 4.3 to make a detailed explanation.

In order to complete the above goal, we will design the system framework as shown in Fig. 1:

The first layer is: 1) Rules: define CGLs as a normalized XML document which consists of a sequence of tag set, including the Behavioural Rules (BRs) and the Production Rules (PRs)[10].

The second layer is four service components: 2) Behavioural Rules Service. 3) Production Rules Service: the service includes three main operations, i) return PRs, and combined with the 4) EHR Web Service together to derive new knowledge (selectPRs); ii) the accumulation of large amounts of data in the process, will produce a new PRs (insertPRs); iii) newly generated knowledge corresponding modifications to the PRs (updatePRs). 4) Electronic Health Records (EHR) Web Service: to preserve EHRs in the form of XML and build index according to the patient's id in the database, find the corresponding EHR of the patient by his/her id number. 5) Dynamic Interface Service: the definition of attributes in the XML of the EHR, fields of rules and so on needs a set of standards to constraint, the description of the patient's information data can provide data source for the dynamically generated interface, and constraint the data.

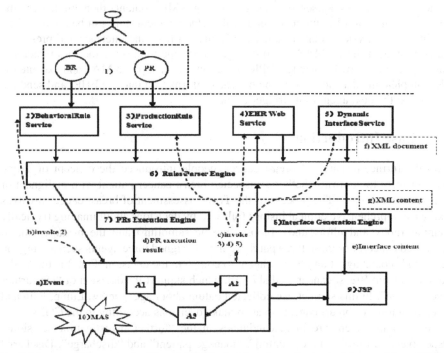

Fig. 1. The overall framework of the project (Dotted line shows the control flow and the solid line shows the data flow)

The third layer includes a native component: 6) Rules Parser Engine: used to do some adding, deleting, modification and query operation on the XML document which was downloaded from all kinds of service of the second layer.

The fourth layer includes two local components, respectively is: 7) the PRs Execution Engine : rules and services are invoked by the Agent, access to rules which will be executed, call the EHR Web Service, get the existed patient's data, execute the PRs, use the existed knowledge to derive additional knowledge, this can help do further decisions for BRs. 8) Interface Generation Engine : call the Production Rules Service, EHR Web Service, Dynamic Interface Service, generate the problem which will be showed in the interface, which include the problem description, options, the default value and so on.

The fifth layer includes: 9) The JSP interface: display the content which is generated by Interface Generation Engine, for human-computer interaction. 10) MAS (Multi-Agent System): at each agent's execution, first of all, BRs matching, find the BR which can handle the current event, the execution BR processes the message, then come to a conclusion and send to receiver that should meet the conditions, then trigger the next agent to perform the corresponding BR for patient's next treatment.

When a)Event (Fig. 1:a)) trigger agent, agent calls Behavioural Rules Service (Fig. 1:b)invoke 2)), download BR XML document which can be matched (Fig. 1:f) XML document)), and execute the BR according the the Rules Parser Engine, then call the Production Rules Service, EHR Web Service, Dynamic Interface Service (Fig. 1:c) invoke 3)4)5)), download the appropriate XML document as the same (Fig. 1:f), implement the Rules Parser Engine, generate g)XML content, then implement the Interface Generation Engine to generate e)Interface content, this can be displayed by JSP interface, physicians enter patient's information from the interface and present to the current agent in the MAS , then the agent continue to execute the PRs Execution Engine, generate new knowledge d)PR execution result, apply to MAS and execute the BR, complete the decisions, store the patient's information into the EHR, and send the decision to the next agent as its trigger event.

3   Case Introduction

With the further research of breast cancer, people introduced the concept of Triple assessment[6] to confirm whether a suspected breast cancer patient with malignant or benign breast disease. The process of the Triple assessment of breast cancer involves taking a comprehensive clinical history followed by decisions about imaging (typically mammography and ultrasound); biopsy (needle sampling) and the management of confirmed cancer. For these three parts, we have designed three agents such as surgeon agent, radiologist agent and biopsy agent to complete the decision. Fig. 2 is the CGLs fragments from Breast cancer CGLs[7,8,9], which support the decision of "Do further investigation". In this snippet, we collected datum about age, gender, Lump, Pain and other symptoms of breast cancer, so as to make decisions according to the CGLs.

For example, there are three candidates in the "further investigation decision": respectively "do further investigation", "manage patient" and "discharge". Discharge option is recommended, when both of the two others are not. If there is a "New lump in preexisting nodularity" and no condition supports the decision "manage patient", the weight of "do further investigation" will be increased by 1. In addition, the weight for "manage patient" will be set to 0, which is lower than the weight for "do further investigation". Hence, the decision, do further investigation, is recommended.

Symptoms and warning signs that are suspicious and warrant urgent investigation
Lump
o any new discrete lump
o new lump in pre-existing nodularity
o asymmetrical nodularity that persists at review after menstruation
Pain
o if associated with a lump
o unilateral persistent pain in post-menopausal women
Pain: Unilateral persistent mastalgia without palpable abnormality: clinical examination only.
Localised areas of painful nodularity: mammography (if > 35 years old) and/or ultrasound
All focal lesions: FNA
Other potential signs of cancer
o ulceration
o skin nodule
o skin distortion
o breast abscess or inflammation not settling after one course of **antibiotics**
o nipple discharge especially if age >50, or bloodstained
o nipple eczema unresponsive to topical steroids
o recent (<3month) nipple inversion
Physical Examination
o An appropriate examination should be performed prior to referral
o The aspiration of a lump in a patient with a history of multiple cysts should only be performed by a General Practitioner who has the necessary skills. Aspiration of solid lumps should not be attempted as it may affect imaging and delay diagnosis or even lead to mis-diagnosis.

Fig. 2. The CGLs fragments from Breast cancer CGLs

4   Design and Implementation

In this project, I majorly focus on four parts. They are Rules Definition, PRs Execution Engine, Interface Generation Engine and information acquisition JSP interface based on rules. These four parts applied in the breast cancer Triple assessment example will be introduced following.

4.1   Definition of Rules

In this section, the CGLs will be defined as executable XML documents with unified standard, which includes two parts, Behavioural Rules (BRs) and Production Rules (PRs). BRs, which are abstracted, are used for guiding the agent to make appropriate decisions. On the contrary, PRs pay more attention to the definition of logical relations which are more detailed. By performing PRs, some new knowledge can be derived from the existing knowledge to guide the agent's behavior.

Definition of Behavioural Rules (BRs)

BRs are norms that defined based on the specific demands and CGLs. Moreover, BRs will standardize the CGLs. It guides the agent's behavior decisions. BRs has decent universality and expandability, so there is no need for redeveloping the entire system when the CGLs changed. BRs is a collection of series tag set, such as role, protocol, component, processing, event and decisionTree. As shown in Fig. 3, role guiding this behavior should be acted by surgeon agent first; protocol describes which agent character takes the responsibility to solve one particular problem; component defines the two service components, Patient and Decision and one local component, Examination. Agent can make trade-off from function, performance, cost and other properties to select the optimal components; processing stipulates that the agent invokes corresponding component to do one operation, such as invoking EHR Web Service, submitting the ID number and obtaining the EHR of this patient, invoking Production Rules Service and deriving additional knowledge based on existing knowledge to make further decision; event triggers agent execution rules; decisionTree defines the behavior need to be acted corresponds to different conditions. For instance, in order to satisfy the condition, decision.getRecommendation(processingResult).equals("do further investigation"), surgeon agent need to do further processing for the patient instead of transferring treatment to other agents.

```
▾<behaviouralRule>
    <role>SurgeonAgent</role>
    <protocol name="TripleAssessment"/>
  ▾<component>
      <type>Patient</type>
      <instance>patient</instance>
    </component>
  ▾<component>
      <type>Examination</type>
      <instance>examination</instance>
    </component>
  ▾<component>
      <type>Decision</type>
      <instance>decision</instance>
    </component>
  ▾<event>
      <sender>PatientAgent</sender>
    ▾<message>
        <type>java.io.FileInputStream</type>
        <content>patient.symptomReportInXml(patient, "/patient.xml")</content>
      </message>
    </event>
  ▾<processings>
      <processing>examination.setPatient(thisPatient)</processing>
    ▾<processing>
        decision.judgePR("further_investigation_PR", examination.getPatient())
      </processing>
      <processing>decision.setPatient(thisPatient)</processing>
    </processings>
  ▾<decisionTree>
    ▾<branch>
      ▾<condition>
          decision.getRecommendation(processingResult).equals("do further investigation")
        </condition>
      ▾<action>
          <content>decision.getFurtherDetails()</content>
        </action>
      </branch>
    ▸<branch>...</branch>
    ▸<branch>...</branch>
    </decisionTree>
  </behaviouralRule>
```

Fig. 3. The BR of Triple assessment

Definition of Production Rules (PRs)

PRs is one kind of detailed definitions of the logical relations in CGLs. It can derive additional knowledge based on existing knowledge, which is the condition of BRs and promotes the BRs make correct decision. In order to process these rules easier, there is a <conditions> tag defined to involve all the required conditions in the decision branches.

This tag defines a type attribute and a <condition> element. Type attribute can take OR, AND and NULL three kinds of value. The default value for type attribute is NULL. It defines the logical relations between all <condition> sub-elements. Similarly, there is a conType attribute and a <con> element defined in the <condition> tag. ConType can take the same three values as type attribute, but the default value for conType is AND. The sub-element of <con> tag has String data type. It defines the name of condition attribute. For instance, the value of this attribute is age and there is a key attribute which guarantees the age must greater than or equal to 35. No matter how complicated the CGLs is, it can be transformed into this kind of tag set. As shown in Fig. 4, it illustrates the PRs for the Triple assessment case. There are three attribute conditions, latestExamination_painOrTenderness, latestExamination_painOrTenderness_cyclicity and latestExamination_painOrTenderness_locality, in the fourth <condition> tag in the figure. The relation between these three attribute conditions is AND. Hence, if the condition changed in this situation, latestExamination_painOrTenderness AND (latest Examination_painOrTenderness_cyclicity OR latestExamination_painOrTenderness_ locality) , there is no need to doubt the universality of the tag set. All we need to do is to split the CGLs into two sub-condition, (latestExamination_painOrTenderness AND latestExamination_painOrTenderness_cyclicity) and (latestExamination_painOr Tenderness AND latestExamination_painOrTenderness_locality). Although it might leads to the increasing space requirement, it is more convenient in the process of resolution or executing rules.

```
<productionRule id="1" name="further_investigation_PR ">
  <role>SurgeonAgent</role>
  <protocol name="TripleAssessment">...</protocol>
  <component>...</component>
  <component>...</component>
  <processings>...</processings>
  <decisionTree>
    <branch>
      <conditions type="OR">
        <condition conType="AND">
          <con key=">=35">age</con>
          <con key="elevated">familyHistoryRisk</con>
        </condition>
        <condition conType="AND">
          <con key="yes">latestExamination_lump</con>
        </condition>
        <condition conType="AND">
          <con key="yes">latestExamination_nippleDischarge</con>
          <con key="yes">latestExamination_nippleDischarge_bloodStained</con>
        </condition>
        <condition conType="AND">
          <con key="yes">latestExamination_nippleDischarge</con>
          <con key="large">latestExamination_nippleDischarge_volume</con>
          <con key="!=yes">currentlyLactating</con>
        </condition>
        <condition conType="AND">
          <con key="yes">latestExamination_nippleInversion</con>
          <con key="recent">latestExamination_nippleInversion_onset</con>
        </condition>
        <condition conType="AND">
          <con key="yes">latestExamination_nodularity</con>
          <con key="localised">latestExamination_nodularity_locality</con>
        </condition>
        <condition conType="AND">...</condition>
        <condition conType="AND">...</condition>
        <condition conType="AND">...</condition>
      </conditions>
      <action>
        decision.setRecommendation("do further investigation")
      </action>
    </branch>
    <branch>...</branch>
    <branch>...</branch>
  </decisionTree>
</productionRule>
```

Fig. 4. The PR of Triple assessment

4.2   PRs Execution Engine

When the Rules Parser Engine processes the content "decision.judgePR("further_ investigation_PR", examination.getPatient())", it triggers the execution of Production Rules Service and provides the patient's data, which could get from EHR by executing "examination.getPatient()" as the service's parameters. The service uses PRs Execution Engine to process a PR named "further_investigation_PR" and return the process result according to the match of patient's information.

The PRs Execution Engine processes each tag <branch> in the selected PR as a multi-tree. The following procedures, using the first tag <branch> in the element "decision Tree" as an example, describe how a multi-tree is constructed: 1) Create the root element of the tree and set content in the tag <action> as the elements' value; 2) Create the child nodes of the root element. The number of the child nodes is the same as the number of tag <condition> in the branch. During the construction, every tag <condition> is processed as a new independent branch of the multi-tree. Assign the content in the first tag <con> in each element "condition" as the child nodes' values sequentially; 3) If there is more than one tag <con> in one element "condition", then create a new node as the node's child node. The node is created in step 2 and the value of which is the content in the first tag <con> in this element "condition"; 4) If there is more than two tag <con> in one element "condition", then create a new node, the value of which is the content in the third tag <con>, as the node's child node. The node is created in step 3; 5) If there is more than three tag <con> in one element "condition", then create new nodes and do the things just like step 3 and step 4. Thus how a multi-tree is constructed.

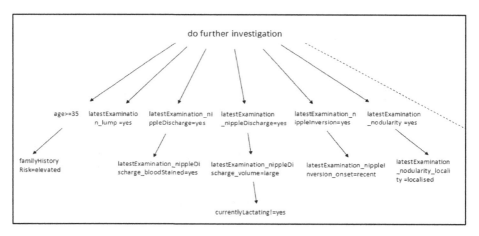

Fig. 5. The node tree generating based on the first decision branch of the PR

Create and initialize a produce queue (produceList), a decision support queue (supportList) and a decision against queue (againstList). Push all the leaf nodes in the node tree such as "familyHistoryRisk = elevated", "latestExamination_lump = yes", "latestExamination_nippleDischarge_bloodStained = yes" and so on into the produceList and set 1 as the leaf nodes' weight. Pop nodes from the produceList by the first in first out (FIFO) order, and then analyze them one by one. If the attribute value of one node equals the value that stored in the EHR, which could be found by the node's attribute name, then analyze the node's parent node. For example, take out the first node "familyHistoryRisk = elevated" as the current node, equals to the familyHistoryRisk attribute value "elevated" obtained from the EHR, so continue to judge its parent node "age > = 35", read the age attribute has a value of 37, therefore this branch is a pathway. Then recording the current node "familyHistoryRisk = elevated" into supportList and give it a weight of 1; Continue to take out the next node "latestExamination_lump = yes", equals to the latestExamination_lump attribute' value "no" obtained from the EHR, so the node does not meet and put the current node latestExamination_lump = yes in the againstList with the weight of 1; After finishing the tree traversal, with the weight of the supportList minus the weight of the againstList, which draw a candidate "do further investigation" of the weights, In this way, calculating the weight of the remaining two candidates "manage patient" and "discharge". For example, the execution result is: the weight of "do further investigation" is 3, the "manage patient" weight of 1, the weight of "discharge" is 0, which is provided to BRs to make the best decisions, the basic algorithm is shown in Fig. 6.

```
list //produce list
solution() {
    for(each list) {
        if(next(list.next())) {
            //add to decision support list
            supportList.add(this);
        }else{
            //add to decision against list
            againstList.add(this);
        }
    }
}

boolean next(ele) {
    if(ele == root)
        return true;
    if(ele.choose==false)
        return false;
    else
        return next(ele.next());
}
```

Fig. 6. The basic algorithm implementation Rules Execution Engine

4.3   The Information Collection Based on the Rules

In the decision making process, when insufficient data provided by the EHR, the clog is derived, and, in turn, influence the decision. Therefore, according to the actual situation of decision rules are derived. We extract the necessary attributes, make decisions in the List, use hash table to heavy algorithm[11], and remove duplicate attribute, and then call the Dynamic Interface Service, access to the specification of these caption, type and so on. Specific practices we are on the page display attributes of caption, complete decision-making which is the doctors need to ask the question to the patients and to enter test results, such as: when the attribute value is currentlyLactating, page shows the problem is "Is the patient currently lactating?"; Then determine the attribute types, the value of the attribute consistent with the read values in the XML document, defaults and options are given a problem; This, in turn, generate problems, was formed based on the rules of driving dynamic human-computer interaction interface, as shown in Fig. 7.

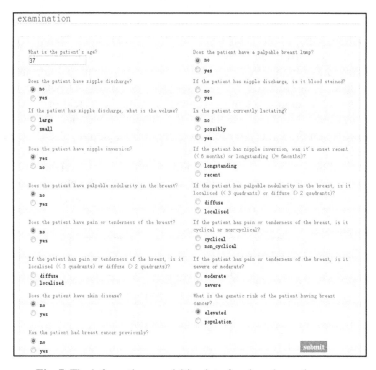

Fig. 7. The information acquisition interface based on rules

Dynamically generated based on the rules of the information acquisition interface, using the GatewayAgent[12] middleware save all the informations collected by information-collecting page in a Patient object which contains the ID number of patients, and the name of save all the attribute name of LIST set, as well as entities corresponding to the attribute name attribute value List collection value, and then sends the object to the Agent, and Agent modify the existing EHRs or create a new EHR, and call the corresponding method of EHR Web Service to update the Patient's EHRs.

5   Conclusion

Through this study, we completed the transform based on evidenced-based CGLs into structured knowledge, and defined a serious of tag set for storage in standard format. Design and implementation of a fast, easy Rules Execution Engine, doctors can make clinical decision quickly and efficiently, improve medical efficiency and medical effect.

There are some achievements on structured CGLs: EON[13], GLIF (Guideline Interchange Format)[14], Asbru[15] and PROforma, the most influential is proposed by John Fox. PROforma is a computer-executable clinical process representation language. The language recognizes the complexity of computation in medicine, draws on work in Knowledge Engineering, Software Engineering, AI, and cognitive science for its theoretical foundation, and adopts a multi-paradigm form of computing, so it's the most influential in the existing research results[10]. Though PROforma can transform the CGLs based on pure text into standard format, executable documents, it also has some disadvantages, such as its legibility is not strong and it has limitations which does not support the execution in a distributed environment.

This paper presents using XML to structure the CGLs and divides into unified structure XML document by different decision, different execution agent. It avoids like PROforma containing all clinical decision support information. Thus this method is more readable and easier to understand and more easier to modify when CGLs changes, avoiding multiple proxy to invoke the same file at the same time call queue and even conflict, it can better support the distributed implementation of the system.

While using the standardized XML represent CGLs for its apply in the CDSS has more support, the application of multi agent system with distributed environment still has some shortcomings. For example, in the progress of the definition of the rules of behavior, combined with description of the messages between the agent in JADE[16] API, to label for further environment; study and learn more tree heap sort algorithm , adjust the node tree to advance the property appear more frequently, avoid to traverse the nodes make repeated judgment, so as to improve the decision-making efficiency.

Acknowledgments. This work is supported by the National Science Foundation of China under Grant Number 61202101 and 61151001.

References

1. Dufour, J., Bouvenot, J., Ambrosi, P., Fieschi, D., Fieschi, M.: Textual Guidelines Versus Computable Guidelines: A Comparative Study in the Framework of the PRESGUID Project In Order to Appreciate the Impact of Guideline Format on Physician Compliance. In: AMIA Annual Symposium Proceedings, USA, pp. 219–223 (2006)
2. Fox, J., Rahmanzadeh, A.: Disseminating medical knowledge: The PROforma approach. Artificial Intelligence in Medicine, 157–181 (1998)
3. Sutton, D.R., Fox, J.: The Syntax and Semantics of the PROforma guideline modelling language. J. Am. Med. Inform. Assoc. 10(5), 433–443 (2003)
4. Laurent, S.S.: XML: A primer. M&T Books, Foster City (1999)
5. Hunter, J.: JDOM makes XML easy. In: Sun's 2002 Worldwide Java Developer Conference (2002)

6. Patkar et al: Triple assessment for suspected breast cancer. British Journal of Cancer (2006), `http://www.openclinical.net/demos/triple-assessment-guideline-for-secondary-care.htmloriginal`

7. Breast Cancer Clinical Guidelines Breast NSSG on behalf of NECN (2011)

8. North Trent Breast Cancer Group. Referral and Management Guidelines for Breast Cancers within North Trent (2012)

9. Non-operative Diagnosis Subgroup of the National Coordinating Group for Breast Screening Pathology. NHSBSP Publication No 50 (2001)

10. Xiao, L., Fox, J., Zhu, H.: An Agent-Oriented Approach to Support Multidisciplinary Care Decisions. In: Eastern European Regional Conference on Engineering of Computer Based Systems (ECBS-EERC), pp. 8–17 (2013)

11. Guha, R.V.: Pass-through architecture via hash techniques to remove duplicate query results: U.S. Patent 6,081,805 (June 27, 2000)

12. Suguri, H., et al.: Assuring interoperability between heterogeneous multi-agent systems with a gateway agent. In: Proceedings of the 7th IEEE International Symposium on High Assurance Systems Engineering. IEEE (2002)

13. Samson, W.T., Mark, A., Musen: Modeling data and knowledge in the EON guideline architecture. Studies in Health Technology and Informatics 1, 280–284 (2001)

14. Boxwala, A.A., et al.: GLIF3: A representation format for sharable computer-interpretable clinical practice guidelines. Journal of biomedical informatics 37(3), 147–161 (2004)

15. Miksch, S., Shahar, Y., Jhnson, P.: Asbru:A task-specific,intention-based, and time-oriented language for reprensenting skeletal plans. In: Proceedings of the 7th Workshop on Knowledge Engineering: Methods & Languages (KEML-1997), Open University, Milton Keynes (1997)

16. Friedman-Hill, E.: Jess, the rule engine for the java platform (2003)

17. Bellifemine, Fabio, et al.: JADE—a java agent development framework. In: Multi-Agent Programming, pp. 125–147. Springer, US (2005)

Research on Applications of Multi-Agent System Based on Execution Engine in Clinical Decision-Making

Zhenzhen Yan[*], Liang Xiao, Jianzhou Liu, Xing Liu, Yumin Hu,
Qiuju Wei, and Xusong Liu

Department of Computer Science,
Hubei University of Technology, Wuhan 430068, Hubei,
People's Republic of China
48453626@qq.com, healthcloud@126.com, 791282452@qq.com

Abstract. Medical errors have become a common concern of social problems. One important reason is the lack of clinical experience. Clinical guidelines are the solution to this problem; however, they are always kept being updated. Let the system adapt to the changing clinical guidelines is a challenging idea. In this paper we propose MAS (Multi-Agent System) based on the Execution Engine can achieve this goal. In the MAS, clinical guidelines are mapped into rules, which are stored in the rule repository and could be processed by the Execution Engine, to guide agents' behaviors. Rules in the system are configurable and Execution Engine can always obtain the latest data at runtime without interrupting system running, so it implements the system's adaptability. Agents, which could be deployed in distributed environments [2], simulate doctors' roles to do aided diagnosis by collaborations which implements data sharing and improves the accuracy of decision-making greatly.

Keywords: Multi-Agent System · Adaptability · Clinical guidelines · Execution Engine · Clinical Decision Making.

1 Introduction

It is well known that human doctors can make mistakes in diagnosis especially in the treatment of complex diseases. In 1999, IOM (U.S. National Institute of Medicine) published a landmark report "To err is Human" (people will make mistakes) [3], the report showed that: first, the quantity of medical errors is huge; second, most medical errors are caused by human factors which can be avoided by means of a computer system[14]. Therefore, improving the quality of care, control ling medical errors, improving patient safety are feasible and imminent.

However, doctors diagnosing the disease is still in the stage of using traditional experience in current medical procedures, they mainly depends on the experience, the diagnostic indicators and laboratory test results. It usually takes several years of

---

[*] Corresponding author.

Y. Zhang et al. (Eds.): HIS 2014, LNCS 8423, pp. 261–273, 2014.

working for a full-time physician to accumulate a certain diagnosis experience. It is significance to abstract the experience and knowledge. We can provide them for the doctors to make decisions in a convenient form, it will reduce the subjective blindness in medical activities, make the diagnosis more scientific, and thereby improve the level of disease diagnosis and treatment [19]. Thus, clinical guidelines came into being.

Clinical Decision Support System can effectively address the limitations of clinician knowledge[11], reduce human negligence, and reduce medical costs relatively [1], [3], so as to provide a guarantee for the quality of care. Despite the CDSS has many advantages, but just a few of them are really accepted by a doctor and put them into use, the main causes are listed below: 1) different doctors' needs are different. Very experienced doctors only need few critical pieces of advice from computers; while unexperienced doctors may need detailed advice. (2) System cannot adapt to the rapid changes of the clinical guidelines [2]. We are in a era of knowledge explosion, emerging evidence-based medicine, clinical guidelines are constantly being updated. A perfect decision support system should support and adapt to the rapid changes in clinical guidelines. But most of the existing systems failed to do so. (3) During the diagnosis of complex diseases, it often needs a medical team made up of some experts to discuss the problem, but in real life these doctors work in different environment, collaborations has become an important obstacle to solve the problem[15],[18].

This paper propose that a MAS based on the Execution Engine can effectively address the above deficiencies.

First, in the MAS, the conclusions deduced by the system shows in a user friendly interface that also displays the ranking of advice, the doctors can choose and pick the most valuable advice for their situations or make their own decision.

Second, in the MAS, clinical guidelines is described by XML format, we designed a multi-agent Execution Engine to parse this type of XML file, and the system can have timely access to these updated content at runtime and do not interrupt the operation of the system.

Third, the paper presents the idea of Multi-Agent Systems, which can divide a problem into many small parts in order to achieve the goal that agents complete tasks through discussing in the way of communication in the distributed environment.

2   Approach Overview

2.1   Agent Technology Proposing

Object-oriented software development is mainstream, although it has a lot of advantages, also some shortcomings are exposed, the most important deficiencies can be summarized as: object-oriented technology is not the most appropriate for the real world simulation. Agent software development is designed to solve this problem, which is closer to the reality of the human society and the general problem-solving methods and habits of human beings [13].

The basic idea of object-orientation is starting from the existing things of the real world, stressed that understanding and thinking of problem should be centered in things of the problem itself. According to the essential characteristics of these things we abstract things as objects of the system and the object works as a basic unit in the system. Through the basic concepts of object, class, inheritance, encapsulation, messages, etc. to program.

The basic idea is of agent-orientation is starting from the people and the surrounds in the real world. It thinks that the properties of things, especially the dynamic ones, are heavily influenced by the related people and environment.It emphasizes the interaction among understanding, thinking and objective things. It combines the subjective and objective characteristics of things and abstracts them into agent of system. The agent works as a basic unit in the system, through the team work of the agents to release the goal the system is aimed at [8].

With the development of computer science and technology, agent provides the possibility for cooperating among people to solve complex problem.

2.2   Agent Concepts

Agent originates in a conceptual model of distributed artificial intelligence. It is a new method of computation to solve complex, dynamic, distributed intelligent applications. It usually refers to a target, behavior and knowledge, solving problem by planning, deducing and decision-making according to their capacity, resources, status, and related knowledge in an uncertain environment. It is a kind of entity can complete specific tasks and achieve a certain goal independently [12].

Agent generally has the following major features [5]:

1) Autonomy (autonomy): After initialized, without user intervention, the Agent can make some decisions independently.

2) Reactivity: Agent can react in time to the changes of environment.

3) Collaboration: Agent has the ability to resolve conflicts through negotiation, which is the key of MAS (Multi-Agent System) systems working successfully.

4) Adaptability: With the interaction between the user and the environment, Agent can actively adapt to the environment and expand their knowledge.

5) Communication: This feature is extremely important in MAS, Information between the different Agents can be exchanged each other by communication and does not affect the independence of the Agents. In the MAS system, The ability of communication is the foundation of their ability to learn, and also is the basis for coordination, exchange and competition between different Agents [10]. We select FIPA as the communication language. It draws up a series of technical specifications which contain the architecture, communication language, content language and interaction protocols [20].

Currently, the vast majority of Agent-based systems are single agent, but with the proposing of increasingly complex application problems and the maturation of technology, the single agent systems cannot solve these problems because of the individual Agent's limitation of knowledge and computing resources. Typically, the most powerful tool to deal with complex problems is abstracting and modular that the multi-Agent system just provides. If a problem is very complicated, the only way to solve this problem is to develop a large number of modular components with special functions (i.e., Agent) designed to solve a specific aspect of the problem. This decomposition allows each Agent to resolve corresponding special problem using appropriate examples. When interrelated problems appear, each Agent in the system must be coordinated to ensure proper handling of this correlation.

Multi-Agent System has the following characteristics: Each member of the Agents only has the incomplete information and problem-solving ability, lack of a global perspective to coordination; Knowledge and Data are dispersed or distributed; the process of calculation is asynchronous and concurrent.

Meeting the needs of Multi-Agent Systems theory and practical application, a new MAS development platform –JADE arises at the historic moment.   JADE (Java Agent Development Framework) is a multi-Agent Development Framework fully coded by Java [5], which follows the FIPA rules. It provides the basic naming services, yellow pages services, communication mechanisms, etc. can be effectively integrated with other Java development platforms and technology, which greatly simplifies the development of Multi-Agent systems in all aspects. JADE mainly includes the following sections: 1) A runtime environment on which agent to survive;2) a runtime library on which programmers to develop;3) a series of graphical tools, which can help users manage and monitor Agent status in runtime.

3   Case Study

Assuming that the patients have been enrolled in the scope of Urgent referral in the stage of breast cancer referral, this case study is about Triple assessment of the patients. Triple assessment is a common procedure in the UK National Health Service to determine whether or not a patient with suspected breast cancer does or does not have malignant or benign breast disease [4]. The process involves taking a comprehensive clinical history followed by decisions about imaging (typically mammography and ultrasound); biopsy (needle sampling) and the management of confirmed cancer. Genetic risk assessment is also included in this application.

The application includes decision support for four areas crucial to the evaluation of a patient attending a triple assessment clinic (updated from the original workflow). Triple assessment workflow is shown in Fig. 1.

1)   Genetic risk assessment
    The application helps assess familial and genetic risk of breast cancer. The RAGs applet is used here to construct a pedigree and calculate genetic risk for the individual patient, expressed as high, medium or low. Support for this task is based on NHS NICE Familial Breast Cancer guidelines.

2） Selection of correct mode of imaging (mammography, ultrasound or neither). The medical knowledge for this task is derived mainly from ACR guidelines.

3） Selection of the right mode of biopsy (if any). The knowledge for this task is derived from NHSBSP guidelines.

4） Selection of the optimum way to manage the patient based on examination, imaging and cytology results (it is assumed that core biopsy results if any would not be available on same day). The knowledge for this task is derived mainly from BASO guidelines [6, 7], [9].

'triple_assessment'defines the main tasks:examination, imaging_decision, ultrasound_enquire, biopsy_decision,and so on. These may need to be tagged with roles,for example Examination (Surgeon), Imaging_Decision/Ultrasound_Enquiry/ Mammography_Enquiry(Radiologist), Biopsy_Decision(Pathologist). Management Decision (Management).

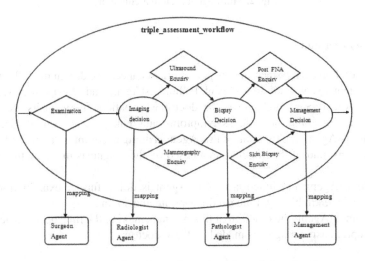

Fig. 1. Triple_assessment_workflow shows the main tasks and the role of necessary agents

4   Design and Implementation

4.1   The Architecture of the System

Multi-agent system architecture is shown in Fig. 2, In the MAS, when an event occurs (for example, a patient reports a symptom), it will trigger the first agent's behavior and process the message by performing the Execution Engine. The results produced by the Execution Engine will be sent to the next agent which is needed for cooperation(the collaborative agent is defined in the Behavioral Rule), the next agent processes received messages in the same way, until the completion of the task.

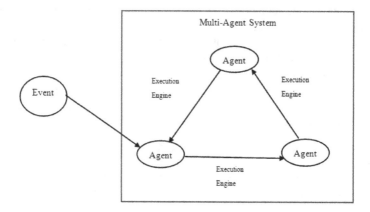

Fig. 2. Multi-agent system architecture

4.2   Agent Design

In the case of Triple assessment for suspected breast cancer, we design the following four agents: SurgeonAgent, RadiologistAgent, PathologistAgent, and ManagementAgent.

SurgeonAgent: SurgeonAgent is the doctor who patient firstly visits; he inquires basic information about the patient's symptoms, and makes the appropriate decisions.

RadiologistAgent: the function of this Agent is doing a mammogram of both breasts, or Do an ultrasound of the affected area based on the diagnosis made by the previous doctors.

PathologistAgent: the function of this Agent is doing further examination of the patient, such as Skin biopsy, Fine needle aspirate and so on.

ManagementAgent: the function of this Agent is making the final decision according to the comprehensive diagnosis made by all the doctors.

4.3   Execution Engine

Execution Engine is designed to get the latest XML content at runtime, without affecting the operation of the system. The structure of Execution Engine is shown in Fig. 3. It is made of Rule Repository, Rule Matching and Rule Interpretation Engine. When event occurs, the trigger agent first performs Behavioural Rule matching, and find the rules belonging to its own and can handle the current event from Rule Repository by Rule Matching component, and then return the rules to Rule Interpretation Engine component, which can parse the rules.When parsing <Processing> tag, it will do a derivation of the event according to Production Rule and get a result, and then select a branch which the condition equals the above result in Decision Tree. In accordance with the condition, the corresponding action will be performed and send the details to the defined receiver agent of the decision-making branch.

This design method not only can be used for diagnosis and treatment of breast cancer but also can apply to other diseases with the modification of the content in the BR and PR. We will introduce the Execution Engine in the following three parts and state the principle of the three components respectively.

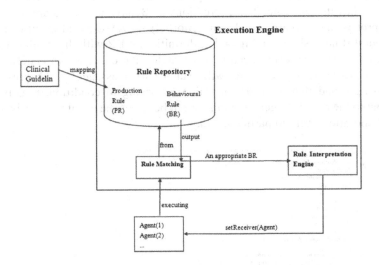

Fig. 3. Execution Engine Architecture, the key of the MAS

Rule Matching

When an event occurs, the agent will select a BR which can handle the current event according to the following conditions in Rule Repository: Sender, MessageContent and so on. It can be implemented in the following method:

```
//Get the current BR's Sender, MessageContent
for (int j=0;j<list.size();j++){
Element event=root.getChild ("event");
String Sender=event.getChildText ("sender");
Element message=event.getChild ("message");
String MessageContent =message.getChildText ("content");
// comparison
ACLMessage msg=receive ();
If(sender.equals(msg.getSender().getLocalName())&&Message
Type.equals(msg.getContent())){
    return list.get(j);
}
}
```

Rule Repository

Behavioural Rule is used to guide the behavior of the agent which is defined in the form of XML. All Behavioural Rules are placed in Rule Repository, each Behavioural Rule is defined for some agents to dealing with a certain events, and each agent has its own rule. The expressions of Behavioural Rule are as follows: {event, processing, decision (condition, action) n}.An XML-based specification of a Behavioural Rule is shown in Fig. 4.The definition of BR with the similar structure describes that when an event occurs, if it matches the event which is defined in a Behavioral Rule, then the agent will handle the message by the pre-defined <Processing>, and then perform an action according to condition. Finally, send the output to the receiver agent and this output becomes the event which triggers the next collaboration agent to participate in.

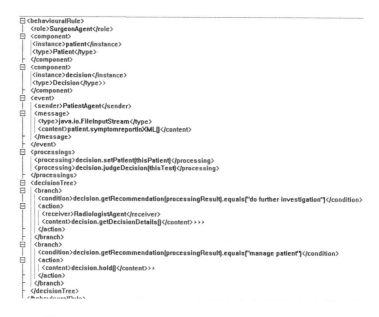

Fig. 4. Specifition of a Behavioral Rule for the SurgeonAgent

Rule Interpretation Engine

This component is responsible for parsing BR, and can be able to get the XML content dynamically at runtime. It can be implemented by the combination of parsing XML with JDOM and java reflection mechanism.

(1) DOM and SAX are two common ways to handle XML documents [16, 17]. JDOM is an open source project, which is based on a tree structure, using java technology to achieve the parsing, generation, serialization, and a variety of operations

of XML document. The API of JDOM integrates the advantages of DOM and SAX, which makes DOM and SAX cooperate more naturally and coordinate.

(2) Reflection is a very important characteristic that makes Java be considered as a dynamic language, which allows dynamically discovery and bind classes, methods, fields, and all other element generated by the language. In other words, by using a mechanism such applications can achieve a description of their behavior and monitoring, and adjust or modify the state and related semantics describes behavior according to the state and result of their own behavior. Java reflection mechanism mainly provides the following functions: judging which class any object belongs to at runtime; construct an object of any class at runtime; judging what member variables and methods any class has at runtime; invoking the method of any object at runtime.

For example we want to exceute the portion of <processing> in the BR by the Rule Interpretation Engine; the defined form of < processing > is as follows:

```
<Processing>decision.judgeDecision (thisTest)
</processing>
```

We can do a sample implementing:

```
/*Assume that there is only one processing, get the
processingcontent*/
String ProcessingContent=root.getChildText ("processing");
/*the processingcontent is the form of "object.method ()",
so we must use the java reflection mechanism.*/
/*before the first appeared point in the processingcontent
is the name of" object"*/
InstanceName=ProcessingContent.substring(0,processingCont
ent.indexOf ("."))
int firstCircle=ProcessingContent.indexOf("(");
/*between the first point and the left bracket is the name
of method*/
methodName=ProcessingContent.substring(firstPoint+1,
firstCircle);
Method
method[]=instanceName.getClass().getDeclaredMethods();
If method[i].equals(methodName){

Obj=method[i].invoke(instanceName.getClass(),parameters[]);
}
```

In the case of Triple assessment for suspected breast cancer, when a patient reports symptoms, PatientAgent will send the Patient as an object to the SurgeonAgent, after SurgeonAgent receives an event, it knows the Sender of Event is PatientAgent; the content of the event is patient. It will find the satisfying Behavioural Rule according to these conditions in Rule Repository. And the Behavioural Rule found will be sent to Rule Interpretation Engine for parsing. If the conclusion of the production is do further investigation, the content of first branch in BR's DecisionTree will be executed, and then the result will be sent to the receiver RadiologistAgent. RadiologistAgent processes the message by the same Execution Engine and communicates with the next one, until the completion.

4.4   Expected Results

In the case of Triple assessment for suspected breast cancer, four agents are distributed on three computers. They separately execute Execution Engine, and the results are sent to the appropriate agent. PatientAgent is deployed in the computer with IP address 192.168.0.5, SurgeonAgent is deployed in the computer with IP address 192.168.0.11, RadiologistAgent is deployed in the computer with IP address 192.168.0.17. When PatientAgent sends a message to SurgeonAgent, the results are shown as Fig. 5. SurgeonAgent (192.168.0.11) receives a message, and matched the corresponding rules which can process current event,The selected rule is "BehaviouralRule.xml", the results deduced is do further investigation. The corresponding receiver should be RadiologistAgent according to the content of the BR decision tree.

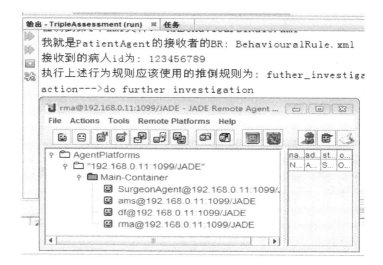

Fig. 5. SurgeonAgent receives messages sent by PatientAgent.and deduced a result by performing Execution Engine

As is shown in Fig. 6, the RadiologistAgent (192.168.0.17) receives the message sent by SurgeonAgent and it executes Execution Engine, with the corresponding decision made described as follows.

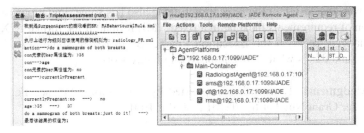

Fig. 6. RadiologistAgent receives messages sent by SurgeonAgent. and made a decision by performing Execution Engion

The results will be listed in a user friendly interface, and it is just a kind of suggest. Whether it is adopted or not is up to the doctors themselves. For example when SurgeonAgent do a decision, according to the production rules, there are three options that are listed below Fig. 7:

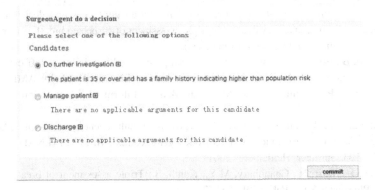

Fig. 7. SurgeonAgent do the option according to the decision made by system

5   Discussion and Conclusion and Future Work

Currently, lots of CDSSs have many disadvantages when used in the practical application.For example,It is difficult to update their knowledge and can't meet the new requirements so that it must be Re-development.This lead to increasing of the cost greatly.The last inconvenience is medical team often locate in different work environment but can't discuss each other.The system's design meets the aim to complete tasks and reach the final goals with cooperation and exchange in the way of communication between agents in the distributed environment. Each agent plays a different role and has a different function in the system. But in this MAS, any agent with its own role can complete their task by the same set of Execution Engine. It can also be used in diagnosis and treatment of many other diseases in addition to breast cancer. We can only modify the content of PR and BR. Therefore, the Execution Engine can be used commonly.

However, the design of the Execution Engine also has some limitations, such as the definition of requirements must be in a fixed XML format, if the format of XML need to be changed, so as to the Execution Engine. So there are some defection in the flexibility and this is what can be improved in future work.

Acknowledgments. This work is supported by the National Science Foundation of China under Grant Number 61202101 and 61151001.

References

1. Xiao, L., Cousins, G., Fahey, T., et al.: Developing a rule-driven clinical decision support system with an extensive and adaptative architecture. In: 2012 IEEE14th International Conference on e-Health Networking, Applications and Services (Healthcom), pp. 250–254. IEEE (2012)
2. Xiao, L., Greer, D.: Adaptive agent model: Software adaptivity using an agent-oriented model-driven architecture. Information and Software Technology 51(1), 109–137 (2009)
3. Patkar, V., Hurt, C., Steele, R., et al.: Evidence-based guidelines and decision support services: a discussion and evaluation in triple assessment of suspected breast cancer. British Journal of Cancer 95(11), 1490–1496 (2006)
4. Séroussi, B., Bouaud, J., Gligorov, J., et al.: Supporting multidisciplinary staff meetings for guideline-based breast cancer management: a study with OncoDoc2. In: AMIA Annual Symposium Proceedings of the American Medical Informatics Association, vol. 2007, p. 656 (2007)
5. Bellifemine, F., Poggi, A., Rimassa, G.: Developing multi-agent systems with JADE. In: Castelfranchi, C., Lespérance, Y. (eds.) Intelligent Agents VII. LNCS (LNAI), vol. 1986, pp. 89–103. Springer, Heidelberg (2001)
6. Ahmed, I., Nazir, R., Chaudhary, M.Y., Kundi, S.: Triple assessment of breast lumps. J. Coll. Physicians Surg. Pak. 17(9), 535 (2007)
7. Drew, P.J., Chatterjee, S., Turnbull, L.W., et al.: Dynamic contrast enhanced magnetic resonance imaging of the breast is superior to triple assessment for the pre-operative detection of multifocal breast cancer. Annals of surgical oncology 6(6), 599–603 (1999)
8. http://jade.tilab.com/
9. http://www.openclinical.net/demos/
   triple-assessment-guideline-for-secondary-care.html
10. Bellifemine, F., Poggi, A., Rimassa, G.: Developing multi-agent systems with a FIPA-compliant agent framework. Software-Practice and Experience 31(2), 103–128 (2001)
11. Xiao, L., Fox, J., Zhu, H.: Developing an Open and Adaptive Agent Architecture to Support Multidisciplinary Decision Making
12. Xiao, L., Greer, D.: Environment support for the configuration of adaptive agents. Multiagent and Grid Systems 5, 1–23 (2009)
13. Xiao, L., Fox, J., Zhu, H.: An Agent-oriented Approach to Support Multidisciplinary Care Decisions. In: 2013 3rd Eastern European Regional Conference on the Engineering of Computer Based Systems (ECBS-EERC), pp. 8–17. IEEE (2013)

14. Xiao, L., Hu, B., Croitoru, M., et al.: A knowledgeable security model for distributed health information systems. Computers & security 29(3), 331–349 (2010)
15. Musen, M.A., Shahar, Y., Shortliffe, E.H.: Clinical Decision-Support Systems Biomedical Informatics, pp. 698–736. Springer, New York (2006)
16. Harold, E.R.: Processing X M L. with Java: a Guide to SAX, DOM, JDOM, JAXP, and TrAX (2003)
17. Hunter, J.: JDOM makes XML easy. In: Java Developer Conference on Sun's 2002 Worldwide (2002)
18. Garg, A.X., Adhikari, N.K.J., McDonald, H., et al.: Effects of computerized clinical decision support systems on practitioner performance and patient outcomes. JAMA: The Journal of the American Medical Association 293(10), 1223–1238 (2005)
19. Pestotnik, S.L., Classen, D.C., Evans, R.S., et al.: Implementing antibiotic practice guidelines through computer-assisted decision support: clinical and financial outcomes. Annals of Internal Medicine 124(10), 884–890 (1996)
20. Bellifemine, F., Poggi, A., Rimassa, G.: JADE–A FIPA-compliant agent framework. In: Proceedings of PAAM 99(97-108): 33 (1999)

A Comfortable THz Source for Biological Effect

Huafeng Shi[1,2,*], Bin Yang[1,2], Wenlong Yu[1,2], and Lei Jin[1,2]

[1] Shenzhen Institutes of Advanced Technology Chinese Academy of Sciences,
1068 Academy Avenue, University Town, Shenzhen, China
[2] Shenzhen Key Laboratory of Medical Sleep and Health Research,
1068 Academy Avenue, University Town, Shenzhen, China
hf.shi@siat.ac.cn

Abstract. A terahertz (THz) pulse laser with a wavelength of 385 μm is optically pumped by a transverse excited atmospheric CO_2 laser based on molecular gas. The used CO_2 laser wavelength is 9.26 μm with an output peak power density of 3.0 MW/cm². The 385 μm THz pulse signal was observed at different D_2O vapor pressures. The energy of the THz pulse is performed as a function of the D_2O vapor pressure, and a maximum THz pulse signal energy was obtained. And this can be used for researching for biological effects comfortably.

1   Introduction

Terahertz (THz) is preliminary defined as the wavelength region of 1 mm ~ 30 μm (0.3 ~ 10 THz). Due to lack of THz source generation and detection methods, it is still a relatively unexplored gap in the electromagnetic radiation spectrum [1,2]. Since the THz spectrum plays an extremely important role in physical, chemical, biological, and medical applications, it's of great interest to pay much attention on THz research. Recent years, some THz source, transmission, and detection methods have been reported [3-5]. In some reported THz sources [6,7], optically-pumped molecular gas laser (OPMGL) technology will be a promising candidate in a wide variety of scientific and commercial applications, which decreases in cost, and increases in reliability. All OPMGL operate on molecular rotational transitions, including superradiance structure and stimulated Raman emission, which are very effective methods of pulse generation in the THz region. Therefore, in this letter, an optically pumped terahertz laser based on molecular gas is investigated.

2   Model

Heavy water (D_2O) molecule is a light asymmetric-top molecule as shown in Fig. 1(a). The structure consists of a tiny V-shaped and symmetric (point group C_{2v}) with two mirror planes of symmetry (the blue and red planes) and a 2-fold axis of rotation (axis z). It has a singular distinction of being the most powerful emitter in the THz

---

* Corresponding author.

Y. Zhang et al. (Eds.): HIS 2014, LNCS 8423, pp. 274–280, 2014.

spectral region [8,9]. The molecular dipole moment, from the center of negative charge (Deuterium atoms, green) to the center of positive charge (Oxygen atom, red), is formed. This is equivalent to a unit negative charge separated from positive charge. As the molecular dipole is aligning with a pump field, the dipole moment will change and the population inversion between the rotational states will transit to lower level, as a result, the pumped THz laser can emit.

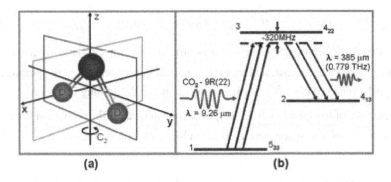

(a)   (b)

Fig. 1. (a) The heavy water molecule model, the deuterium atoms partially positively charged (green), while the oxygen atom partially negatively charged (red), and (b) a simple three-level system adopted for the D_2O molecules to laser THz signal.

Fig 1(b) shows a representative physical diagram of the THz lasing process, operating at a wavelength of 385 μm (0.779 THz). When the D_2O molecules were optically pumped by a CO_2-9R(22) line with a wavelength of 9.26 μm, an absorption occurred from the ground state [level 1 $(0, 5_{33})$] to the excited state [level 3 $(v_2, 4_{22})$]. The subsequent 385 μm THz laser emitted when the molecules transited from the level 3 $(v_2, 4_{22})$ to the level 2 $(v_2, 4_{13})$. Since the frequency of the pump field is lower by about 320 MHz than the resonance frequency of the absorption, implying the existence of the off-resonant pumped and stimulated Raman emission. This transition process in the three-level D_2O molecule system can be described by density matrix motional equation as follows:

$$\dot{\rho} = \Lambda - \frac{i}{\hbar}[H, \rho] - \frac{1}{2}\{\Gamma, \rho\} \tag{1}$$

where H is the system Hamiltonian, ρ is the density matrix symbol of ensemble formed by plenty of molecules, Λ is the pump excitation matrix, and Γ is the decay relaxation matrix. Under the condition of electronic-dipole approximation, slowly-varying-amplitude approximation, and rotating-wave approximation, the gains of the pump and the THz signals in per unit length can be obtained by solving the Eq. (1) and expressed as:

$$G_p = -\frac{2N_v \, |\mu_p|^2 \, \omega_p \tau}{\varepsilon_0 nc\hbar B_p} \mathrm{Im}(\rho_{31}) - \alpha_p$$

$$G_{THz} = -\frac{2N_v \, |\mu_{THz}|^2 \, \omega_{THz} \tau}{\varepsilon_0 nc\hbar B_{THz}} \mathrm{Im}(\rho_{32}) - \alpha_{THz}$$

$$(2)$$

Where G_p, μ_p, ω_p, B_p, α_p, $\mathrm{Im}(\rho_{31})$ and G_{THz}, μ_{THz}, ω_{THz}, B_{THz}, α_{THz}, $\mathrm{Im}(\rho_{32})$ are the gain, transition electric dipole moment, laser frequency, Rabi frequency, coefficient of loss, and imaginary part of density matrix of the pump and the THz signals, respectively, N_v is the density of molecules joining in the process, n is the refractivity of the medium, $\hbar$ is the plank constant, τ is the relaxation time, ε_0 is the permittivity of free-space, and c is the velocity of light in free-space.

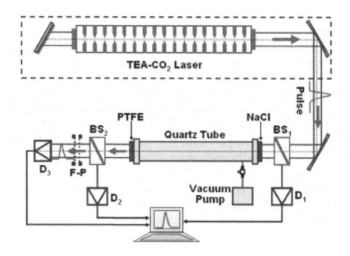

Fig. 2. Schematic experimental setup of the THz emission optically pumped by TEA CO$_2$ pulse laser. F-P is a Fabry-Perot interferometer and D3 is a pyroelectric detector.

3   Setup and Experiment

Fig 2 shows a sketch of our experimental setup. A grating-tunable transverse excited atmospheric (TEA) CO$_2$ laser is used as the pump source, dashed square showing the metal shielded room to avoid the THz emission from EMI (electro magnetic interference). The maximum output energy of the CO$_2$ laser is about 0.3 J/pulse for TEM$_{00}$ mode measured with a model EJ-10 laser energy meter. The measure pulse width is about 100 ns with a photonic drag detector. Thereby the maximum output peak power density can be up to 3.0 MW/cm^2. A high voltage power supply (27 kV) is used to operate the CO_2 laser. One block holds a grating (150 grooves/mm) used to select the emission line. By grating tuning, a desired laser line from more than 60 lines with wavelength from 9~11 μm can be selected. The main component of the experimental setup is a superradiation structure, i.e., an amplified spontaneous emission (ASE). It consists of a sample tube, input and output windows. The sample tube is made of 1 m in length and 5 cm in diameter quartz tube. The input window is a piece of NaCl crystal (6 mm thickness) which is good for 9~10 μm signal transmission. The output window is a polytetrafluoroethylene (PTFE) plate (4 mm thickness), which can be effectively opaque to 9~10 μm signal and allow the THz signals (including 385 μm) to pass efficiently. The D_2O vapor (specified isotopic purity: 99.8% D) filled at a controllable pressure observed by a pressure meter. The CO_2 source laser was focused by two concave mirrors into the filled quartz tube through the NaCl window. The THz laser produced, as the CO_2 source laser via the full filled quartz tube, then outputted by the PTFE window. For broadband detection, direct detectors based on thermal absorption are commonly used [10]. A pyroelectric detector (D3 in Fig. 2) with a rise time of ~25 ns is used to detect the THz signal. A Fabry-Perot interferometer (F-P in Fig. 2) is made by metallic mesh grids to measure the THz signal wavelength and the spectral characteristics. To decrease the error caused by the instability of pump laser, a power divider is placed between the output window of the sample tube and the F-P interferometer, as shown in Fig. 2. Most of the THz signals were transmitted through the divider and then coupled into the F-P interferometer. The rest of the THz signals were reflected by the divider and detected by D2. The stability of the THz laser was monitored in real time. By using the signals detected by D2 as the criteria and making a difference with those detected by D3, the measuring accuracy of the THz spectral characteristics can be improved. To study the transient behavior of the THz laser, both the pulse shapes of the CO_2 pump pulse and the THz signal were simultaneously recorded by a digital storage oscilloscope (DPO4104, quadruple channel, sampling rate 5GS/s, input bandwidth 1 GHz).

In experiment, there are several operating parameters will inflect the output THz signal power, but the D_2O vapor pressure is the most easily controlled and changed one. With other operating parameters keeping constant, the output THz signal power can reach a maximum by properly turning the D_2O vapor pressure and the corresponding D_2O vapor pressure (called the optimum vapor pressure). So here the D_2O vapor pressure is discussed. Fig 3 shows the temporal behavior shape of the 385 μm THz pulse signals (red curve 2) together with the pump CO_2 pulses (blue curve 1). In the experiment, the D_2O vapor pressures are changed from 0.55 to 1.25 kPa. Because of the threshold intensity for stimulated Raman emission and nonlinear amplification in the experiment, only the most intense peak of the pump CO_2 pulse generates THz emission. It can be seen from Fig. 3 that the behaviors are rather similar but the highest THz signal energy output appeared at the D_2O vapor pressures of 0.75 kPa in Fig. 3(b).

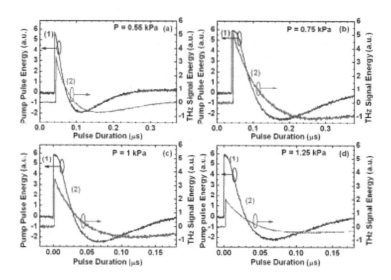

Fig. 3. The temporal behavior of THz pulse signals (red curve 2) together with the pump CO_2 pulses (blue curve 1) at different D_2O vapor pressures

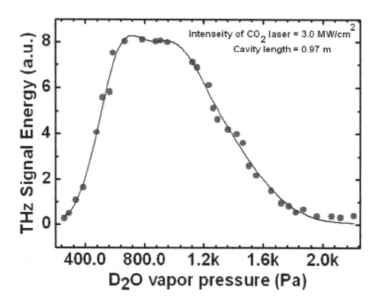

Fig. 4. The output THz energy as a function of the D_2O vapor pressure at room temperature. The red dots are the sampling datum from measurements and the blue line is the corresponding Gaussian fitting curve.

4   Results and Conclusion

Fig 4 shows the profile of the THz signal energy as a function of the D_2O vapor pressure at room temperature. The THz laser emission occurred over a wide pressure range from 0.2 up to 2.3 kPa, and the CO_2 pump pulse energy and other operating parameters were kept constant while the D_2O vapor pressure was varied. From Fig. 4, we can see that adequate adjustment of the D_2O vapor pressure (it is about 0.8 kPa) can lead to a maximum output THz signal power. The dynamics of this phenomenon is very complicated. At low pressure, the THz signal gain is proportional to the operating D_2O vapor pressure. When the D_2O vapor pressure is relatively low, the energy exchanged between the pump source and medium molecules is insufficient. The Raman interaction between independent energetic systems is very small, and two crests of Alternating Current (AC) Stark splitting are separated into Raman line and center line. With the THz signal gains at different D_2O vapor pressures obtained by Eq. (2), the spectra are shown in Fig. 5. Heighten the D_2O vapor pressure by filling more D_2O, more molecules will take part in the process. More molecules on the ground state absorbed the pump laser and contributed to the emission transition to excited state, resulting in the larger gain of the THz intensity, and the THz signal power increases. Meanwhile, the AC Stark splitting and broaden effect are notable. Two crests of the AC Stark splitting become overlapped gradually, as shown in Fig. 5. The overlapped part is taken as background signal and then amplified by the Raman process. As this process goes on, two peaks of the AC Stark splitting connected entirely into a relatively wide spectrum and they can also increase the THz signal power. When the D_2O vapor pressure is higher than a certain value (the optimum vapor pressure of about 0.8 kPa), the number of the molecules which stayed on the excited level become less due to the quickened energy exchange process (relaxation time shortened). Since the vibrational relaxation of the D_2O molecule is very fast compared with the CO_2 laser pump duration, a sufficiently large vibrational population can be excited and the overall ground state population will be depleted or simply bleached. Only a finite amount of power and energy density can be extracted on a per pulse basis, i.e. an equivalent vibrational saturation or bottleneck occurs, which had the effect of terminating the interaction. Furthermore, continuously heighten the D_2O vapor pressure, self-absorption coefficient of medium increased [11,12], the output power decreased in the contrary, leading to the curve fall down. So it's difficult to increase output power merely dependent on change of the D_2O vapor pressure, other parameters are necessary to take into account in further investigation.

In summary, a superradiant THz emission is investigated from D_2O vapor. It has a wavelength of 385 μm, pumped by the TEA CO_2 laser pulse with a wavelength of 9.26 μm. There exists an optimum D_2O vapor pressure value at round 0.8 kPa under which the output THz signal power reaches the maximum. Attempt explanations are presented, including the population, relaxation time, energy exchange, AC Stark splitting, and broaden effect. The preliminary results indicate that the OPMGL technique is a successful approach for the generation of THz laser. More detailed comparisons of theoretical and experimental evidence will be further investigated.

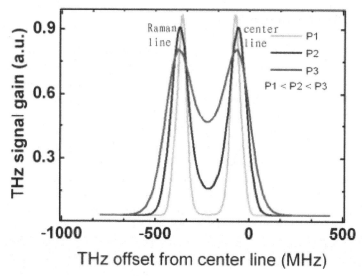

Fig. 5. The spectra of the THz signal gains at different D_2O vapor pressures. The curves broaden and separate into Raman line (left peak) and center line (right peak).

References

1. Sirtori, C.: Applied Physics: Bridge for the Terahertz Gap. Nature 417, 132–133 (2002)
2. Köhler, R., Tredicucci, A., Beltram, F., Beere, H.E., Linfield, E.H., Davies, A.G., Ritchie, D.A., Iotti, R.C., Rossi, F.: Terahertz Semiconductor-Heterostructure Laser. Nature 417, 156–157 (2002)
3. Carr, G.L., Martin, M.C., McKinney, W.R., Jordan, K., Neil, G.R., Williams, G.P.: High-Power Terahertz Radiation from Relativistic Electrons. Nature 420, 153–156 (2002)
4. Borak, A.: Toward Bridging the Terahertz Gap with Silicon-Based Lasers. Science 308, 638–639 (2005)
5. Watanabe, S.: Infrared Investigation of Deuterated Si(111) Surface Formed in Hot Heaby Water. Appl. Phys. Lett. 67, 3620–3622 (1995)
6. Siegel, P.H.: Terahertz Technology. IEEE Trans. Microwave Theory Tech. 50, 910–928 (2002)
7. Lee, Y., Hurlbut, W.C., Vodopyanov, K.L., Fejer, M.M., Kozlov, V.G.: Generation of Multicycle Terahertz Pulses via Optical Rectification in Periodically Inverted GaAs Structures. Appl. Phys. Lett. 89, 181104–181106 (2006)
8. Rønne, C., Thrane, L., Åstrand, P., Wallqvist, A., Mikkelsen, K.V., Keiding, S.R.: Investigation of The Temperature Dependence of dielectric Relaxation in Liquid Water by THz Reflection Spectroscopy and Molecular Dynamics Simulation. J. Chem. Phys. 107, 5319–5331 (1997)
9. Yuan, D.C., Siegrist, M.R.: Single-mode Operation of a Hybrid Optically pumped D_2O Pulsed Far-infrared Laser. J. Appl. Phys. 68, 1445–1449 (1990)
10. Ferguson, B., Zhang, X.C.: Materials for Terahertz Science and Technology. Nature Materials 1, 26–33 (2002)
11. Yu, B.L., Yang, Y., Zeng, F., Xin, X., Alfano, R.R.: Terahertz Absorption Spectrum of D_2O Vapor. Opt. Commun. 258, 256–263 (2006)
12. Rønne, C., Åstrand, P., Kerding, S.R.: THz Spectroscopy of Liquid H_2O and D_2O. Phys. Rev. Lett. 82, 2888–2891 (1999)

Author Index